Books by Mark Hyman, MD

The Young Forever Cookbook

Young Forever

The Pegan Diet

Food Fix

Food: What the Heck Should I Cook?

Food: What the Heck Should I Eat?

The Eat Fat, Get Thin Cookbook

Eat Fat, Get Thin

The Blood Sugar Solution 10-Day Detox Diet Cookbook

The Blood Sugar Solution 10-Day Detox Diet

The Blood Sugar Solution Cookbook

The Blood Sugar Solution

The Daniel Plan

The Daniel Plan Cookbook

UltraPrevention

UltraMetabolism

The Five Forces of Wellness (CD)

The UltraMetabolism Cookbook

The UltraThyroid Solution

The UltraSimple Diet

The UltraMind Solution

Six Weeks to an UltraMind (CD)

FOOD FIX
UNCENSORED

INSIDE THE ▬▬▬ FOOD INDUSTRY'S BIGGEST ▬▬▬ COVER-UPS

MARK HYMAN, MD

WITH BRIANNA BELLA-HYMAN
FOREWORD BY CASEY MEANS, MD

Little, Brown Spark
New York Boston London

This book is intended to supplement, not replace, the advice of a trained health professional. If you know or suspect that you have a health problem, you should consult a health professional. The author and publisher specifically disclaim any liability, loss, or risk, personal or otherwise, that is incurred as a consequence, directly or indirectly, of the use and application of any of the contents of this book.

Little, Brown Spark
Hachette Book Group
1290 Avenue of the Americas, New York, NY 10104
littlebrownspark.com

First Edition: February 2026

Little, Brown Spark is an imprint of Little, Brown and Company, a division of Hachette Book Group, Inc. The Little, Brown Spark name and logo are trademarks of Hachette Book Group, Inc.

The publisher is not responsible for websites (or their content) that are not owned by the publisher.

The Hachette Speakers Bureau provides a wide range of authors for speaking events. To find out more, go to hachettespeakersbureau.com or email hachettespeakers@hbgusa.com.

Little, Brown and Company books may be purchased in bulk for business, educational, or promotional use. For information, please contact your local bookseller or the Hachette Book Group Special Markets Department at special.markets@hbgusa.com.

ISBN 9780316598637
LCCN 2025941555

10 9 8 7 6 5 4 3 2

CCR

Printed in the United States of America

To the farmers, eaters, communities, advocates, activists, scientists, businesses, and policymakers who are working to fix our food system

Contents

PART III

INFORMATION WARFARE

PART IV

FOOD AND SOCIETY: THE DESTRUCTION OF OUR HUMAN AND INTELLECTUAL CAPITAL

PART V

THE ENVIRONMENTAL IMPACT OF OUR FOOD SYSTEM

Foreword

We are in a crucible moment for humanity. Lifespan in the United States is consistently declining, preventable chronic diseases are rising globally, obesity now affects 2.5 billion people, and infertility rates continue to climb. Meanwhile, our oceans are choking with plastic, our topsoil is vanishing, and biodiversity is collapsing worldwide. It's a rough moment for Planet Earth and its inhabitants!

Oddly enough, there's good news. There *are* answers—and they *all* lead back to our forks. Each of these crises can be meaningfully addressed by fixing food. The solutions are in this book.

As I write this foreword, we're witnessing a tug-of-war between progress and regression in the fight to improve the American food system. On the one hand, the Make America Healthy Again (MAHA) movement has swept the country, culminating in the appointment of Robert F. Kennedy Jr.—a staunch food-as-medicine and regenerative-agriculture advocate—as secretary of health and human services. In this role, he oversees roughly 25 percent of the budget of the largest government agency on Earth. Since his swearing in on February 13, 2025, we've witnessed unprecedented momentum on food: movement to ban artificial dyes in school lunches, eliminate soda purchases on the federal Supplemental Nutrition Assistance Program (SNAP), improve infant formula quality, and close the loophole that enables Big Food to self-affirm harmful additives as "generally recognized as safe."

At the same time, progress is being actively dismantled by industry-funded interests. A Bayer-funded industry group, Modern Ag Alliance, is pushing nationwide legislation to grant legal immunity to pesticide and herbicide manufacturers—blocking harmed individuals from suing for illness if labels comply with the standards of the Environmental Protection Agency. How do they aim to pressure the US government into providing them with immunity? In the spring of 2025, they threatened to stop producing agrochemicals. And who will suffer? American farmers, because China is the primary other major producer of agrochemicals. As a result of this legal maneuvering, combined with the instability around tariffs, our homegrown farmers and food supply are increasingly threatened. These bills are advancing in multiple state legislatures, protecting the agriculture cartel that this book courageously exposes. Simultaneously, the American Heart Association testified *against* a bill that would prohibit the purchase of junk food and sweetened beverages through the country's largest nutrition assistance program, SNAP. In response to public outcry, they reversed this stance on May 8, 2025.

In this moment, no book is more urgent than *Food Fix Uncensored*. If we fix food, we can begin to solve the most existential threats facing humanity and the Earth.

When I first read the original edition of *Food Fix* in 2020, I was at a personal inflection point. I had spent my life pursuing the pinnacle of conventional medicine—research training at the National Institutes of Health, earning dual degrees at Stanford, and dedicating myself to the high-stakes world of ear, nose, and throat surgery. I believed, deeply, in the promise of modern medicine, confident that if I worked hard enough, studied long enough, and sacrificed deeply enough, I would become a true healer.

But as I moved deeper into clinical medicine, that belief began to fracture. I was operating, prescribing, diagnosing—yet the patients kept returning. Sicker. More exhausted. More inflamed. Endless pills and procedures. I wasn't healing anyone. The system wasn't working. Within the sterile, gleaming efficiency of the hospital, I kept thinking, *Why are so many people getting sick? Why are chronic diseases all going up all at once? And why is the powerful, expensive, revered American health care system so ineffective at fixing the burden of chronic disease and its costs?*

Dr. Hyman has espoused for decades the simultaneously simple and hugely complex answer to these questions: Our health care system is fundamentally broken because it profits from long-term sick patients and loses money from healthy ones. Therefore, the root causes of chronic disease—like food—are insidiously ignored. Having witnessed this reality firsthand, I put down my scalpel in September 2018, committed to finding a path to become a true healer and address the real roots of chronic disease, including poor nutrition, metabolic dysfunction, environmental toxins, and bought-off science. In 2019, I cofounded the health and wellness company Levels to empower individuals to understand the impact of food on their health using continuous glucose monitoring.

Though I'd been a Mark Hyman superfan for years—devouring his books in stolen moments during residency—when I read *Food Fix* in 2020, it struck me as one of the most important texts I'd ever encountered. It was a lens into the industrial-scale corruption profiting from American illness—and it was a beacon for change. It confirmed everything I had witnessed in the operating room, in my family's health, and in the rising tide of chronic disease across the country. It didn't just explain—it revealed.

This book doesn't simply present data. It delivers clarity. It lays bare the machinery behind our nation's dysfunction: a food system that is actively manufacturing disease for profit. Page by page, it exposes how chronic disease is not just an unfortunate by-product of modern living—it's the logical outcome of a system engineered for earnings over life.

Food Fix Uncensored makes it unmistakably clear: Our health crisis is not accidental. It's by design. And it's costing us *everything*.

What this book reveals is a national emergency. The American food system has been hijacked by powerful commercial interests that control our governments, our choices, and our health. In just a few decades, we've seen an explosion in chronic disease: type 2 diabetes, heart disease, autoimmune conditions, cancer, Alzheimer's, infertility, mental illness, and obesity. More than 93 percent of American adults have some degree of metabolic dysfunction. And it's getting worse. Life expectancy in the United States is falling—even as we spend more on health care than any nation on Earth. The expected lifespan for American men is now just 77 years—averaging 7 years less than our peers in Japan and Switzerland and forty-ninth in the world.

We're told the science is settled. It is not. The science has been buried. In all my medical training, I never learned that each serving of ultraprocessed food consumed daily increases early mortality by 14 percent, and that 67 percent of children's calories come from ultraprocessed foods. No one taught me about the endocrine-disrupting chemicals in our pesticides, the microplastics accumulating in our brains, or the fact that 95 percent of the USDA's Dietary Guidelines Advisory Committee for 2020 had financial ties to Big Food. I wasn't taught that our health care system itself is the third leading cause of death in the United States.

You would think our health care institutions would be clamoring to reverse metabolic dysfunction and alleviate American suffering through the most important lever: food. But they are not. They not only remain silent but continue accepting millions from the industries causing the problems.

That's why *Food Fix Uncensored* is more than a book. It's a road map to reclaiming our vitality. By exposing the forces behind our broken food system, it offers not just insight—but hope. By shining light on the web of corruption keeping us sick, it enables us to begin pushing back.

This isn't just a health crisis. It's a spiritual one. We've collectively lost our reverence for life, for nature. We've fallen for the illusion that we can chronically poison ourselves under the guise of efficiency and advancement—and then fix it all with drugs. But there is another path— one rooted in common sense, transparency in science, and deep respect for the miracle of the human body and the Earth that sustains it.

I'm honored to write this foreword. The bravery of *Food Fix* didn't just widen my aperture of understanding—it helped crystallize my purpose and make me far bolder in my work. I believe it can do the same for many others. Share this book with your family, friends, schools, and children. Discuss it at your dinner table and in your book clubs.

We can restore health to America in just a few years. But it will take all of us. We need you—each of you reading this—to heed the call and muster courage. Make different choices for yourself and your families. Call out corruption. Inspire *and* demand the change we so urgently need.

Food Fix Uncensored is a rallying cry—for doctors, parents, policy-makers, business leaders, and anyone who believes we deserve better. Health is our natural state. Fixing food is how we heal not just our bodies but our nation.

—Casey Means, MD

FOOD FIX
UNCENSORED

Introduction

If you've read any of my previous books, you might be wondering, *Why is a doctor so obsessed with food? Shouldn't he be focused on medicine, hospitals, and treatments?* Well, I'm obsessed with food because our Standard American Diet (ironically, known by its acronym, SAD) is arguably the single biggest threat to our future as a society.

Every major crisis we face—skyrocketing disease rates, economic collapse, environmental destruction—traces back to one thing: our food.

This system isn't just broken—it's designed for profit, not nourishment. The way we grow, process, market, and consume food is fueling chronic disease, burdening our economy, widening inequality, polluting our land and water, and driving climate disaster. It's siphoning our human, social, economic, and natural capital faster than a busted dam releases water in a flood.

Sound extreme? The reality is far worse than you can imagine.

We have unwittingly become the lab rats of a radically altered food supply—one that has been hijacked by Big Food, Big Ag, Big Pharma, and enabled by regulatory capture. In just the past century—and even more drastically over the last 40 years—we've shifted from real, recognizable food to ultraprocessed, chemically engineered products that don't even meet the definition of "food." How is food defined in the dictionary? "Any nutritious substance that people or animals eat or drink or that plants absorb in order to maintain life and growth." What most Americans (and more and more of the global population) eat is not even food. It does not maintain life and growth. It does the opposite. It promotes death, disease, and decay.

Poor diet is now the single biggest killer on the planet, which forced me to ask a terrifying question: What the hell happened to our food—and who is responsible for the system that produces it?

As a doctor, my oath is to relieve suffering and illness and to do no harm. But as a functional medicine physician, my training goes beyond just treating symptoms—it's about finding and fixing the root causes of disease. And time after time, with every patient who walked through my door, I saw the same disturbing pattern: Their illnesses started with their forks.

The more I treated patients, the more I realized I was playing a losing game. I started to piece together an awareness that my tools of healing were futile when up against the reality of our modern lifestyles: that our diet is the number one cause of death, disability, and suffering in the world. It's fueling an explosion of chronic disease, robbing people of their health, and devastating entire generations. No matter how many medications I prescribed or how many treatment plans I designed, I was up against a force far greater than anything I could fix in my office—our modern food system.

So, I started following the trail—from seed to soil, from field to fork, from food to landfill. And what I uncovered was so shocking, so deliberately engineered, so systemically corrupt, that I knew I couldn't stay silent.

What I discovered is that there is a powerful web of forces working mercilessly to keep us sick, suffering, and trapped in a system engineered for profit, not health. Big Food, Big Ag, Big Pharma, and even our own government policies have created an industry designed not to nourish us but to exploit us. Every aisle in the grocery store, every school lunch tray, every hospital meal, has been hijacked—loaded with ultraprocessed junk, sugar, starch, chemicals, and additives that are literally killing us.

I realized that if I stayed silent, I would be violating my Hippocratic oath—the sacred duty of a doctor to protect and heal. I couldn't turn a blind eye while millions of people in America (and billions globally)—children included—were being set up for a lifetime of chronic disease. I had to speak up.

When I wrote *Food Fix,* it was a call to wake up to a crisis that most people hadn't yet begun to see clearly: that our food system is not just broken—it's been weaponized. In the mere five years since then, something remarkable has happened: The zeitgeist has shifted.

We're living through a moment when more and more people—citizen journalists, health advocates, doctors, parents, farmers, even teenagers on TikTok—are pulling back the curtain themselves. They're translating the science, connecting the dots, and exposing the corruption that's been hiding in plain sight.

And yet, the crisis has only deepened. Chronic disease continues to skyrocket. Mental health is deteriorating. Our kids are sicker, our soil is more depleted, and our food—what we still call food—is more ultraprocessed, more toxic, and more detached from nourishment than ever before.

That's why this updated edition is so important. The urgency is greater. The public is more awake. And the stakes couldn't be higher.

In this updated edition, I'm exposing how our food system has been captured by corporate power and regulatory failure—and what we can actually do about it. You'll see how food lies at the root of our most pressing issues—chronic disease, mental illness, environmental collapse, economic instability—and meet the villains profiting from this mess, as well as the heroes leading the fight to fix it.

This is more than just a book. It's a road map to reclaiming our food, our health, and our future. Are you ready to see the truth?

Spoiler alert: Fixing our food system *might* just save the world.

THE HIGH COST OF CHRONIC DISEASE

Imagine a world where we could reverse the chronic disease epidemic, heal the environment, slow climate change, end poverty and social injustice, reform politics, and revive economies worldwide—all by changing what we eat. It sounds radical, but the truth is, our food system is at the root of nearly every crisis we face.

The way we grow food, the way we process it, and what we end up eating (or not eating) doesn't just impact our waistlines—it's shaping the future of our health, our communities, our planet, and the global economy. And right now, we are headed in the wrong direction.

Chronic disease, including heart disease, diabetes, and cancer—largely driven by our modern diet—kills more than 43 million people every year,[1] accounting for close to 75 percent of all deaths worldwide.[2] That's more than twice the number of deaths caused by infectious diseases.

And the numbers keep getting worse. When I published the original version of this book in 2020, roughly 2 billion people were overweight, while 800 million went to bed hungry. Fast-forward just five years, and the problem has only intensified—today, more than 2.5 billion people are overweight or obese, while roughly 800 million are undernourished (due to either abject starvation or malnourishment resulting from inadequate dietary nutrition).[3]

And here in the United States? One in two Americans and one in four teenagers now have pre-diabetes or type 2 diabetes by conventional criteria—a condition that doesn't just shorten life expectancy but serves as a catalyst for nearly every other debilitating disease we're facing. Worse, 93.2 percent of Americans are metabolically unhealthy, suffering from high blood pressure, high blood sugar, or abnormal cholesterol, are overweight, or have had a heart attack or stroke. What does "metabolically unhealthy" mean? It is the equivalent of pre-pre-diabetes but still has all the risks of pre-diabetes or type 2 diabetes, including heart disease, cancer, dementia, infertility, and mental illness.

The imperative to transform our food system is not just medical, moral, or environmental, but economic as well. Chronic disease is now the single biggest threat to global economic development, estimated to siphon $129 *trillion* from the American economy alone in the next 35 years ($3.7 trillion per year today,[4] multiplied by 35 years). And the worst part is that 40 percent of our current direct health care costs in America, almost $5 trillion, is paid for by the government, funded by you, the taxpayer (through direct and indirect costs like Medicare, Medicaid, Veterans Affairs, Department of Defense, the Children's Health Insurance Program [CHIP], Indian Health Service, etc.). It accounts for one in three dollars of the federal budget and rising fast.

These high costs of chronic disease threaten our national security as well. As of 2024, at least 71 percent of young Americans aged seventeen to twenty-four were ineligible for military service without a waiver[5] because of poor health, and even those who do qualify are often battling obesity (defined as a body mass index above 30). Obesity-related health issues also lead to significant financial costs for the military, with the Department of Defense spending approximately $1.5 billion annually on obesity-related health care expenses.[6] In fact, allegedly in 2021, 72 percent of military evacuations were for chronic health issues caused by obesity, not combat injuries. Our country's strength, future, and, quite literally, safety are being undermined by what's on our plates. It's time to face the truth: Our food system isn't just broken — it's betraying us.

COMMERCIAL DETERMINANTS OF HEALTH

In 2005, the World Health Organization (WHO) convened a landmark summit in Thailand, producing *The Bangkok Charter for Health Promotion in a Globalized World*[7] — a bold acknowledgment that globalization, corporate interests, and aggressive commercial practices aren't just shaping economies, they're shaping public health.

From that summit emerged a chilling term: commercial determinants of health (CDoH) — a polite way of codifying how private industries are profiting from making us sick.[8] The WHO now defines CDoH as "private sector activities that affect people's health, directly or indirectly" — and surprise, surprise, it's Big Tobacco, Big Alcohol, Big Food, and Big Ag leading the charge. Their products subvert public health and privatize profits while socializing the costs, which are paid by governments and their citizens globally.

These industries don't just sell products — they manufacture demand for addiction and disease. Here are some examples of how they distort truth and create desire:

- Aggressive marketing — especially targeting children, low-income communities, minorities, and even hospitals
- Deep-pocketed lobbying — ensuring policies protect profits, not people
- Predatory product design — engineering foods, drinks, and substances that keep consumers hooked (biologically addicted) and unwell

- Using front groups that promulgate false "scientific" propaganda such as the American Council on Science and Health
- Co-opting professional associations that are designed to represent public health interests, like the American Heart Association and the American Diabetes Association
- Funding most of the "science" at academic centers, especially on nutrition
- Donating to social groups like the NAACP and the Hispanic Federation, enabling them to control their public actions

Why do they do all this? To circle the wagons, close off attack vectors, control the scientific and public narrative, and publicize their disease-promoting, addictive products while undermining both the truth and public health.

The WHO is finally taking action, advocating for higher taxes ("vice taxes"), stricter advertising laws, and corporate accountability.[9] But the reality is that all of this isn't just about policy; it's about power. For these industries, this is all existential. They will not roll over without a fight.

So, whatever you think of the WHO, one thing is clear: When a transnational institution starts calling out corporate interests, the problem is real. The WHO is now working to monitor and regulate the commercial forces driving the global health crisis—because public health shouldn't be dictated by the industries that profit from disease.

Here's how this game works: When money rules, public health loses. Our food system isn't broken—it's rigged. Decades of lobbying, political payoffs, and unchecked corporate influence have created a system where Big Food, Big Ag, and Big Pharma call the shots, while the rest of us pay the price in chronic disease, environmental destruction, and skyrocketing health care costs.

When industry lobbyists have free rein, we end up with a mess of conflicting, uncoordinated food policies that subsidize, protect, and enrich the food industry at the expense of public health, small farmers, and the environment. Corporations—not citizens—are placed at the center of decision-making, turning our food system into a race to the bottom. Science, public health, grassroots advocacy, and even school nutrition programs have all been hijacked—polluted by corporate-funded junk research and multimillion-dollar misinformation campaigns designed to keep us confused and compliant.

And today just a handful of CEOs control nearly everything we eat. Over the last 40 years, what was once a diverse and competitive food

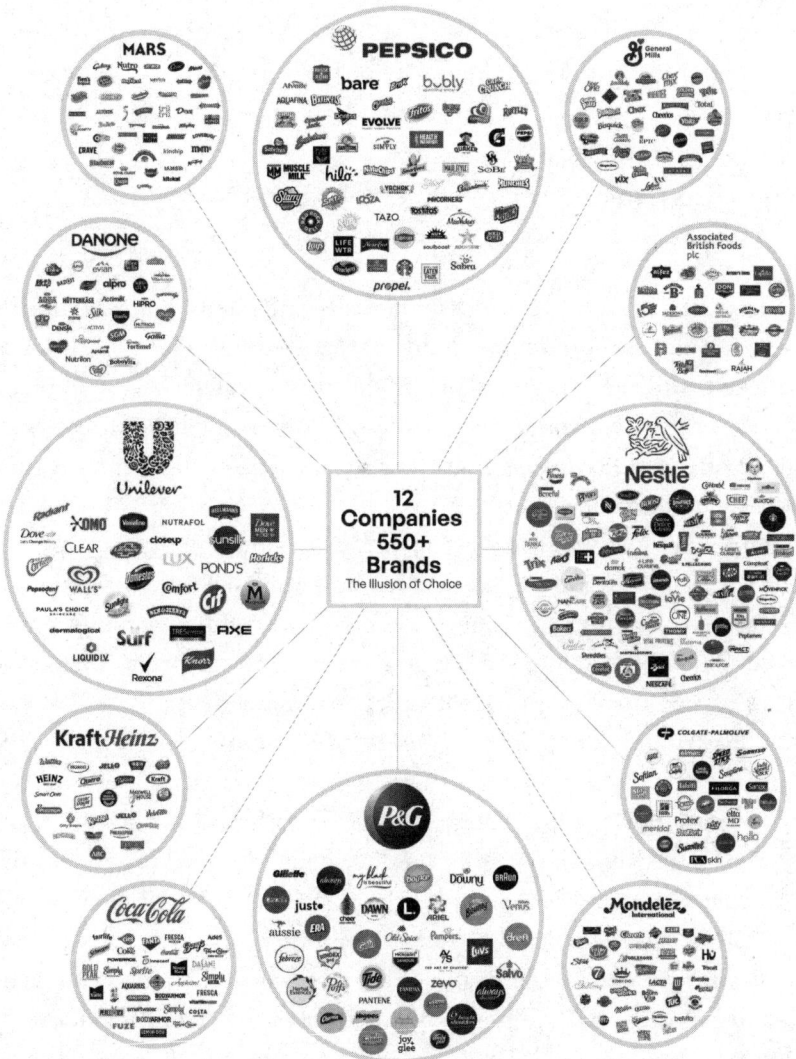

industry has been consolidated into a handful of megacorporations. The result? A $15.7 trillion global food empire[10] (agriculture, food processing and manufacturing, distribution, and retail)—accounting for 14.5 percent of the world's entire economy—where a very few executives dictate what food is grown and how it's processed, distributed, and sold.[11] In fact, most of the "healthy" brands are also now owned by Big Food.

This isn't just bad policy—it's a corporate takeover of our food, our health, and our future. The question is: How long are we going to let them get away with it?

THE COMPROMISE: OUR CHILDREN'S FUTURE

Our children's future is being sabotaged—one school lunch at a time. Instead of nourishing young minds, we're feeding them a cocktail of processed junk and sugar, right in their own cafeterias. Half of all schools serve brand-name fast food, and 80 percent have direct contracts with soda companies, pushing sugary drinks on kids as if they were essential to education.[12]

And it gets worse—food companies are spending billions targeting children and minorities with the worst junk imaginable. They're hooking them young, priming them for a lifetime of addiction to ultraprocessed, nutrient-dead "food" that fuels obesity, diabetes, metabolic disorders, cognitive dysfunction, and mental illness.

How can we expect kids to thrive academically, focus in class, or regulate their emotions when their brains are inflamed, running on toxic fuel? This sets entire generations up for failure—impacting learning, mood stability, and even brain development. Need proof? Studies show that violent crime in prisons drops dramatically with something as simple as better nutrition or a daily multivitamin.[13]

But this isn't just about health—it's about justice. Poverty, inequality, and even violence are fueled by the devastation of our nutritionally bankrupt food system. We are setting kids up for failure before they even get a chance to succeed.

There is a solution though, a *Food Fix*. Across the globe there are governments, businesses, grassroots efforts, and individuals who are reimaging food from field to fork, creating solutions that address the challenges we face across the landscape of our food system.

Dariush Mozaffarian, MD, the former dean of the Friedman School of Nutrition Science and Policy at Tufts, and director of the Tufts Food Is Medicine Institute, shared his hope for what may seem like an overwhelming problem, highlighting that "waves of innovation and capital are now sweeping food and allied disciplines, from agriculture to processing to restaurants and retail, and in health care, personalization, mobile tech, and employee wellness. Catalyzing this multibillion-dollar revolution, and ensuring its rapid trajectory is evidence-based and mission-oriented," he writes, "is an essential opportunity and challenge."

As a doctor, it is increasingly clear to me that the health of our citizens, our society, and our planet depends on disruptive innovations that decentralize and democratize food production and consumption—innovations that produce real food at scale and that restore the health of the soil, water, air, and biodiversity of our planet. I cannot cure obesity and diabetes in my office; it is cured on the farm, in the grocery store, in the restaurant, in our kitchens, schools, workplaces, and faith-based communities.

This recognition has reinforced my excitement about the Make America Healthy Again (MAHA) movement. Its progress over the past twelve months, along with action by the moms of MAHA, has been one of the most encouraging revolutions I've seen in my lifetime. For the first time in my 40 years' practicing medicine, I have seen the political zeitgeist shift to address the chronic health crisis and our food system head-on. I'm blown away.

MAKE AMERICA HEALTHY AGAIN:
A MOVEMENT BEYOND POLITICS

Let's get one thing out of the way—the MAHA movement has been politically co-opted. It's been branded and wrapped in rhetoric that understandably does not sit well with everyone. Sometimes the radical grandstanding even irks me a bit. But illness is not red, blue, or purple. Your cells don't have an ideology. Everyone is affected by this chronic disease epidemic and by our food system. It is a human problem, a shared suffering common to humanity.

The MAHA movement is the single most significant public health movement we've ever seen in this country. And if we're serious about fixing our broken food system, we can't afford to dismiss its merits based on political tribalism.

At its core, MAHA is about confronting the toxic grip that Big Food, Big Ag, and Big Pharma have on our health—and no matter which side of the aisle you're on, the facts remain the same: Ultraprocessed foods filled with sugar, starch, and harmful additives are driving the nation's chronic disease epidemic.[14] Despite spending significantly more than any other country on health care expenditures,[15] the United States leads the world in obesity, diabetes, metabolic dysfunction, and diet-related illnesses among developed nations.[16] We are now ranked forty-ninth[17] in life expectancy, coming in last among wealthy developed nations. Americans comprise 4 percent of the world's population yet accounted for nearly 17 percent of COVID-19 deaths worldwide.[18] Why? Americans are chronically ill and are pre-inflamed from eating our industrial diet, creating a perfect storm for the ravages of COVID-19. This is a crime given our advances in science, know-how, and an extraordinarily advanced health care system. And it's all because we have a food system engineered for profit, not health.

MAHA is focused on dismantling the broken food system by tackling it from multiple angles. It pushes for regulatory reform, demanding stricter oversight on harmful food additives and deceptive marketing tactics that mislead consumers and that flood our food supply with empty starch and sugar calories—the very foods driving everything from obesity and type 2 diabetes to heart disease, cancer, dementia, and, to a large extent, our mental health crisis. It emphasizes public education and transparency, shining a light on how ultraprocessed foods (mostly because they are vehicles for massive amounts of starch and sugar) are fueling the country's chronic disease epidemic. And it fights for policy changes that matter—from improving the nutritional quality of school meals and restricting junk food advertising aimed at children to getting sugar and ultraprocessed food full of harmful additives out of our food and reforming our biggest food program, the Supplemental Nutrition Assistance Program (SNAP, commonly known as food stamps). SNAP peaked at a $125 billion a year program,[19] of which 75 percent is spent on junk food, including 10 percent on soda.[20] The goal is clear: to reclaim our health from corporate interests and build a food system that nourishes rather than harms.

And for the first time, health leaders and influencers across the spectrum are rallying behind this movement. Experts like my friends and peers Drs. Casey Means, Marty Makary, Chris van Tulleken, David Ludwig, Don Layman, Dariush Mozaffarian, and Mehmet Oz, among many others—all of whom have sounded the alarm on the dangers of ultraprocessed foods—are stepping up to support real policy change. Entrepreneurs and activists like Calley Means, Jillian Michaels, Vani Hari, Gary Brecka, and Jason Karp are acknowledging that the war on chronic disease starts with reclaiming our food system from corporate control. This isn't just a policy push—it's a cultural shift, and the momentum is undeniable.

As triggering as politics can be, I hope you can give me the benefit of the doubt when I say that this isn't about Left vs. Right—it's about life vs. disease, health vs. corporate greed. If we can't set aside ideological differences to address the single biggest driver of our nation's health crisis, then we've already lost. MAHA isn't perfect, but it's a start—and it's the best shot we've ever had at reclaiming our food, our health, and our future.

For years, I have felt like I have been standing on a beach watching a tsunami approaching while everyone around me is sunbathing and playing in the water, oblivious to the implications of what is about to happen. And now, *finally*, after I and a few others have been sounding the alarm bell for decades, America is waking up to the disaster that is our food, agriculture, and health care system. More than 30 states are passing laws to ban harmful chemicals in food, stop the purchase of soda through SNAP, mandate nutrition education for physicians, and more. A presidential commission was tasked with reporting on the root causes of our chronic disease epidemic,[21] especially how it affects our nation's children, and created a historic analysis and road map to address the complex causes underlying our current health crisis and to provide a strategy to fix the root causes of our chronic disease epidemic through policy.

Our broken food system is the most urgent catastrophe of our times.

But here's the good news: It's also one with clear solutions. One that we have the power to fix.

Note to Reader: To access more resources, at the end of each chapter, look for a QR code. Simply scan the code with your smartphone camera or QR code reader app to instantly access additional resources curated for that chapter. These may include extended reading, key research studies, video content, action guides, tool kits, and ways to get involved. We created these digital supplements to help you go deeper, stay informed, and take meaningful action beyond the page.

PART I

IS OUR FOOD SYSTEM BANKRUPTING OUR HEALTH AND ECONOMY?

People are fed by the food industry, which pays no attention to health, and are healed by the health industry, which pays no attention to food.
—WENDELL BERRY

Before I assault your limbic system with shocking statistics, I want to read you in on the thesis of this book: There are solutions that can solve all the problems I describe here. I am calling it the Food Fix Action Guide, a complex set of related strategies for citizens, businesses, philanthropists, and governments to fix our food system that can occur on a global level. It will not be easy, but it is necessary for our survival as a species, for the economic and political stability of world governments, and for the health of the planet.

The Food Fix Action Guide has the potential to be an enormous driver of economic growth and innovation. Billions of dollars of investment are flooding into the food and agriculture sectors, creating new businesses, jobs, and national and global economic growth for innovations in farming, food manufacturing, retail, restaurants, health care, and wellness that improve the health of people and the planet. The side effects will be significant economic growth, jobs from entire new industries, and trillions in cost savings from addressing chronic disease, restoring ecosystems including soil, water, and biodiversity, and reversing climate change. The countries that get this right will not only help humans and the Earth but leap ahead in the twenty-first century in jobs and economic growth.

In the pages ahead, we will unpack how all these factors contribute to suffering and lack in the world. We will learn how we as citizens, businesses, philanthropists, and governments can begin to restore the health of our people, our communities, our economies, and the environment. There is a Jewish concept called tikkun olam, which roughly translates to "repair of the world." That is what our work must be; it is the hope of this book.

CHAPTER 1

THE HIDDEN PRICE TAG
OF OUR FOOD

One hundred twenty-nine trillion dollars—$129,000,000,000,000—is an almost unimaginable number. Yet, by extrapolating the current costs, this is an estimate by the Milken Institute of the burden to the American economy of chronic disease over the next 35 years in both direct health care costs and lost productivity and disability.[1] To put it in perspective, that is more than four times the US gross domestic product of $29.18 trillion a year. According to the World Bank, in 2023, the *entire world's* GDP was just $106 trillion.[2]

For that amount of money, here's what we could do:

- Erase the federal deficit
- Provide free education
- Provide free health care
- Eradicate poverty
- End food insecurity and hunger
- Solve social injustice, income, and health disparities
- End unemployment
- Ensure our national security
- Enhance our global economic competitiveness
- Rebuild our infrastructure and transportation systems
- Shift to renewable energy
- Draw down carbon emissions and reverse climate change

■ Transform our industrial agricultural system, which is destructive to humans, animals, and the environment, into a sustainable, regenerative system that reverses climate change, preserves our freshwater resources, increases biodiversity, protects pollinators, and produces health-promoting whole foods

That $129 trillion is referring to the total cost of chronic illness in the United States over the next 35 years based on both direct health care costs and the loss of productivity due to heart disease, diabetes, cancer, mental illness, and other chronic conditions.[3] Most of those diseases are caused by our industrial diet,[4] which means they are overwhelmingly avoidable if we transform the food we grow, the food we produce, and the food we eat.

Clearly not all chronic disease will disappear, nor will all those who are chronically ill be able to go back to work. But if even a conservative fraction of that money, an estimated $15 trillion (about three years of our total federal tax collections),[5] became available, it would provide crucial resources to solve our most critical problems.

These chronic diseases are not just the problem of the government or the individuals who suffer from them—*your* tax dollars are directly funding and causing disease. One hundred percent of Medicare and Medicaid spending comes from federal and state taxes, which means every taxpayer contributes to managing the escalating costs of chronic illnesses. Is this really how you want to be spending your hard-earned dollars?

In 2024, Medicare and Medicaid spending exceeded $2 trillion,[6] with chronic diseases accounting for roughly 90 percent of these costs,[7] translating to a *massive* (and growing!) taxpayer burden. In fact, of our almost $5 trillion in annual health care spending in the United States, the government foots nearly 40 percent of the bill.[8] One out of every three dollars of the federal budget pays for health care, dollars that come directly from you, the American taxpayer.[9]

This strain is compounded by a soaring national debt, which breached $35 trillion in 2024—a historic level that poses risks to both economic stability and national security. If we can effectively reduce the chronic disease burden through prevention and lifestyle interventions, the savings could significantly alleviate pressure on taxpayers, free up funds for other critical investments, and help stabilize our nation's fiscal health (which matters a lot in this new multipolar world, in which many superpowers are vying for advantage). Addressing these diseases is not just a health care imperative — it's a matter of national security and economic survival.

But I get it — the complexity of the problem prevents people from connecting the dots and taking action. Most of the true costs are not even recognized, limiting the motivation to change the system, but know this: Our food system is quite literally stealing from our children's futures. We may have no choice but to pay attention.

THE COSTS OF CHRONIC DISEASE

You may not be aware that at least 11 million people die every year from a bad diet,[10] making our diet the *number one killer* globally. More than 2.5 billion adults and 390 million children and adolescents around the world are overweight and sick[11] from eating our processed, industrialized diet, entirely devoid of the nutrition necessary to develop healthy bodies and brains.

In July 2024, the Centers for Disease Control and Prevention shared a report on the health and economic costs of chronic conditions in America that details the staggering impact of chronic illness created by our current food system.[12] It's overwhelming, but between that report and the Centers for Medicare and Medicaid Services data, here are just a few key facts:

- As of 2023, chronic diseases and mental health conditions accounted for 90 percent of the nation's $4.9 trillion in annual health care expenditures,[13] or 17.6 percent of the US gross domestic product.
- This means that approximately $4.41 trillion was spent on managing chronic and mental health conditions in 2024, which is about 15.2 percent of the GDP, about $29 trillion for that year.
- This reflects a significant increase from just over two decades ago, in 2002, when direct health care costs were $1.6 trillion.[14]

- Notably, the 2023 spending of $4.9 trillion marks a 7.5 percent increase from 2022.
- The indirect costs, including just lost income, reduced productivity, and impact on caregivers, but not including the impact of our food system on the environment and the climate, totaled another $2.6 trillion.[15]
- Most of the diseases driving the costs are related to obesity and poor diet: heart disease, abnormal cholesterol, osteoarthritis, type 2 diabetes, high blood pressure, stroke, cancer, Alzheimer's, and kidney failure. It's important to note that these costs do not include prediabetes (which affects somewhere between one in two and one and three Americans and causes heart attacks, strokes, and dementia even if it never leads to full-blown type 2 diabetes).
- The number of individuals aged fifty and older with at least one chronic disease is expected to rise from approximately 71.5 million in 2020 to 142.7 million by 2050, nearly doubling over three decades.[16] Those aged fifty and older with multiple chronic conditions are projected to increase from about 7.8 million in 2020 to 15 million by 2050, a 91 percent increase. And that's just for those over fifty. Population-wide, seven in ten Americans have a chronic disease — that's nearly 200 million people.[17]
- Seventy-three percent of US adults are either overweight or obese — that's about 250 million Americans! Forty-ish percent are obese,[18] tripling from 13.4 percent in 1962.[19]

Yes, I realize these are confronting stats.

If the burden of chronic disease will cost just the American economy $129 trillion over the next 35 years, and we extrapolate those costs globally, this becomes a truly existential threat.

Global (non-US) per capita health care costs are a mere *one-tenth* of that of the United States, yet the global obesity rates are lower. The United States has about 4 percent of the global population, so if we extrapolated the 70 percent overweight statistics to the world stage, it would affect roughly 5.7 billion people, costing the global economy *quadrillions* of dollars. That's a lot of zeros.

Where Obesity Places The Biggest Burden On Healthcare

Average annual health expenditure per capita due to obesity from 2020-2050*

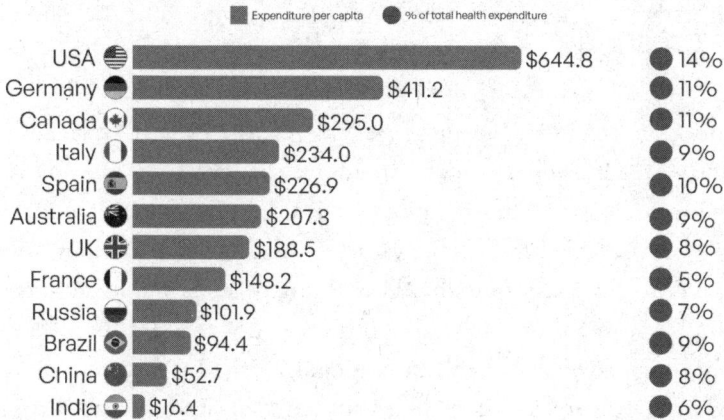

■ Expenditure per capita   ● % of total health expenditure

	Expenditure per capita	% of total health expenditure
USA	$644.8	14%
Germany	$411.2	11%
Canada	$295.0	11%
Italy	$234.0	9%
Spain	$226.9	10%
Australia	$207.3	9%
UK	$188.5	8%
France	$148.2	5%
Russia	$101.9	7%
Brazil	$94.4	9%
China	$52.7	8%
India	$16.4	6%

*U.S. dollars - purchasing power parity.

And while locally we see the Right and Left bickering over the costs of benefits, with Democrats arguing to create Medicare for All and Republicans insisting on reducing entitlements to bring down our more than $36 trillion national debt, as of mid-2025, both are missing the plot: Fix the reason why we have those costs in the first place. Stop the flow of sick people into the system and the harm to our environment by fixing the cause: our food system. Not addressing the root causes of these downstream chronic health issues and expecting the government to foot the bill is like mopping up the water from an overflowing tub while continuing to run the tap. Doesn't it make more sense to just turn off the faucet?

Yet most of our government's policies promote the growing, production, marketing, sale, and consumption of the worst diet on the planet, including billions in subsidies (known as crop insurance or other supports) for commodity crops turned into processed food and food for factory-farmed animals. Fifty-nine percent of our farmland is used to grow commodity crops (corn, wheat, soy) that get turned into ultraprocessed foods, which we know are deadly, and which make up about 60 percent of our diet and 67 percent of children's diets!

In America, only 3 percent of our farmland is used to grow fruits and vegetables, despite the recommendation of the US Food and Drug Administration (FDA) that more than 50 percent of our diet should be fruits and vegetables.[20] The calculus just doesn't add up. The government appears to be talking out of both sides of its mouth.

The Congressional Research Service estimates that as of 2025, 40 percent[21] of our *entire* mandatory federal spending will be for health programs such as Medicare and Medicaid, much of this addressing entirely preventable lifestyle and chronic disease.[22] Bill Haslam, the former governor of Tennessee, shared with me that *one in three* dollars of its state budget is spent on Medicaid. This does not account for all the federal programs covering health care, including the Department of Veterans Affairs, Department of Defense, Children's Health Insurance Program, and Indian Health Service, among others.

All in all, our states and federal government combined cover roughly 48 percent of health care costs in America.[23] The Government Accountability Office (GAO) has reported that federal spending for Medicare and Medicaid has grown by approximately 80 percent over the past decade,[24] with projections indicating continued growth, possibly as high as $3.5 trillion in federal spending in the next decade. To put that in perspective, our entire federal individual income tax collections in 2024 were only $2.4 trillion; the total tax collections from all sources were $4.9 trillion.[25] There will be almost nothing left for the government as a whole—for defense, education, transportation, or anything else. Neither cutting Medicare nor creating Medicare for All will solve this problem.

In the fall of 2024, in an attempt to explore solutions, Congressman Vern Buchanan, vice chair of the House Ways and Means Committee and chairman of the Health Subcommittee, organized a pivotal hearing titled *Investing in a Healthier America*. The session focused on the role of lifestyle and preventive medicine in combating chronic diseases and the escalating obesity epidemic that had, until then, been uncannily absent from public discourse. In it, I testified, along with four other industry experts, advocating for the recognition of the national emergency that is our current state of health.

I sat before Congress to tell the hard truth: America is sick because of what we eat—yet instead of reform our food system, we continue to spend $4.8 trillion a year on a broken health care system that treats symptoms instead of root causes. The American diet—60 percent (67 percent for children) of which is comprised of ultraprocessed junk loaded with sugar, refined starch, additives, and chemicals and stripped of real nutrients—is the canary in the coal mine.[26] These foods aren't just bad for us; they are directly fueling obesity, type 2 diabetes, heart disease, and cancer. And this ultraprocessed junk is everywhere— nearly 80 percent of the food in grocery stores is ultraprocessed. This isn't by accident. It's a system designed for profit, not for health.

In my testimony, I made it clear: We need a radical shift. Our health care system is failing because it treats chronic disease with pills instead of prevention or lifestyle treatment interventions. Food is medicine, and it should be the foundation of our health care system. But right now, medical schools barely teach doctors anything about nutrition, so even our doctors don't know how to address these problems.

I called on Congress to invest in nutrition education for doctors, integrate dietary counseling into standard medical practice, and push for policy changes that put real food back at the center of health care. My testimony was limited to the areas that the Ways and Means Committee oversees, namely, the government health care programs that are left to treat all the illness caused by food.

But my message was clear: This isn't just a health issue. It's an economic and national security crisis. If we don't fix the way we eat, no amount of money, drugs, or medical interventions will stop the chronic disease epidemic.

We must take proactive steps to improve the health and well-being of our citizens, which includes promoting better nutrition and healthy lifestyles.

HOW TO FIX HEALTH CARE: BEYOND CUTTING ENTITLEMENTS OR MEDICARE FOR ALL

During the 2013 World Economic Forum, I spoke at a prestigious gathering of the world's health care leaders from government, the pharmaceutical industry, insurers, and health care systems. My talk followed a distinguished panel focused on fixing health care by better health information technology, improved care coordination, reduction of medical errors, improved efficiencies, and improved payment models—all necessary but not sufficient. The discussion was revealing to me in the way traditional health care and policymakers think about "improving" health administration. Akin to rearranging the deck chairs on the *Titanic,* their ideas were no more than window dressing on a house whose foundation is crumbling.

I just couldn't wrap my head around the logic behind their proposals: "Wouldn't it make more sense to address the *root causes* of chronic disease that are driving the costs, rather than trying to clean up after the fact?," I asked. The room of 300 people went silent. It was as if I had just revealed the meaning of life. Afterward, the panel moderator, the dean of Columbia University's School of Public Health, told me how profound this insight was and how all the health leaders were talking about it after. Really? I was shocked. This is so obvious, yet apparently none of these esteemed experts had thought of it.

That year, the World Economic Forum declared chronic disease to be the single biggest threat to global economic development,[27] a trend reflected in the fact that General Motors spends more on health care than on steel,[28] and Starbucks spends more on health care than on coffee beans.[29]

According to the World Obesity Federation 2023 report,[30] by 2035, the global economic impact of overweight and obesity is projected to hit a staggering $4.32 trillion per year (not including all the chronic diseases it causes, including heart disease, cancer, type 2 diabetes, dementia, depression, and more), which is roughly equivalent to the global impact from smoking, armed violence, war, and terrorism *combined*. That's about 4 percent of global GDP, almost on par with the economic toll of COVID-19 in 2020. Additionally, that same report estimated that close to $370 billion a year of this burden will be shouldered by low- and middle-income countries alone.

If we don't take serious action to improve prevention, treatment, and support, more than half the global population could be struggling with excess weight in just a decade. In addition to the direct costs of treating obesity and its related chronic diseases, the McKinsey Global Institute reports that obesity accounts for $2 trillion in lost annual economic productivity.[31] Any way you slice it, the costs of obesity and chronic disease are literally weighing down the world.

Further complicating the implication of these illnesses on the global stage, lifestyle diseases like obesity and type 2 diabetes, once considered diseases of affluence, have now been exported to the lowest-income nations worldwide. Indeed, roughly 80 percent of obesity and chronic disease now exists in the developing world, in low- and middle-income countries.[32] They face what the WHO classifies as the "double burden of malnutrition"[33]—the simultaneous presence of undernutrition and overnutrition in the same population—and are completely unprepared for this epidemic. You might be surprised to know that obesity, food insecurity, and malnutrition occur at the same time, in the *same people*. We are overfed, but undernourished. There is little health care infrastructure, few doctors and nurses to treat these problems, and even less money.

What kicked off this trend? It was the hope and promise of the then well-intentioned Green Revolution—a 1960s movement originally intended to combat hunger by transforming global agriculture through the introduction of high-yield crop varieties, chemical fertilizers, pesticides, mechanization, and advanced irrigation techniques. While successful in achieving calorie security, it saw some dramatic unexpected consequences. It certainly did succeed in its use of agricultural technology to create abundant cheap food to feed the world. But the emphasis on staple crops like wheat, rice, and corn reduced the cultivation of nutrient-rich traditional crops, contributing to hidden hunger and micronutrient deficiencies. The reliance on chemical inputs like fertilizers and pesticides has resulted in polluted ecosystems and exposed farmers to health risks, while intensive farming practices have simultaneously degraded soil and water resources. Illustratively, India is projected to have only twenty-five harvests left because of soil depletion caused by ideas like the Green Revolution. Mechanization and monocultures widened social inequalities, displaced small farmers, and reduced agricultural biodiversity. Poignantly, suicides are not only the leading cause of death for farmers in the developing world, but also the leading cause of death for farmers in the United States. Over time, this shift not only contributed to chronic diseases linked to poor diets but also created long-term sustainability challenges, from climate impacts and pollinator depletion to water scarcity.

This allegedly "cheap" food has ironically turned out to be very, very expensive.

And while chronic disease is costly (and kills millions), it is only a small part of the total cost driven by our food system. Below, we explore some of the costs.

THE INVISIBLE COSTS OF OUR FOOD SYSTEM

All of us pay the invisible costs. We pay for them indirectly through the loss of our social capital (human happiness, health, productivity, etc.), our natural capital (health of our soil, air, water, climate, oceans, biodiversity, etc.), our economic capital (our ability to address economic disparities and social, environmental, educational, and health care problems), threats to national security, and more. According to the 2021 Rockefeller Foundation report *True Cost of Food,* for every one dollar we spend on food directly, there are three dollars in costs for collateral damage to our social, natural, and economic capital.[34]

You know who the true costs are *not* paid by? The food system that generates said costs. This is why the companies profiting from them are so hell-bent on maintaining the status quo. If they had to compensate the public for their "externalities"—a euphemism for the entirely predictable second- and third-order consequences—we would be seeing a drastically different economic and health landscape. As concerned citizens, we must demand a true accounting for this cascade of unintended (and in some cases intended) consequences of our food system, including environmental degradation through the depletion of fresh water, forests, and soil, damage to our oceans, loss of biodiversity, pollution, and chronic disease and its economic burden.

Shifting our thinking from seeing health care, disease, social justice, poverty, environment, climate, education, economics, and national security as separate problems, to reflecting on the interdependencies and the systems nature of this problem—in other words, connecting the dots—is critical to solving it. It will require collaboration and action by governments, businesses, nonprofits, and citizens to solve. But the first step is to understand these connections.

ACCOUNTING FOR SUSTAINABILITY AND CONSEQUENCES OF OUR FOOD SYSTEM

The true cost of food is not on the price tag. If the true cost of food were built into the price we pay, or if Big Ag and Big Food had to pay for the harm caused by the food they produce—the pollution, the loss of biodiversity, the loss of soil and cropland, the depletion of our water resources, chronic disease, the loss of intellectual capital from harm to our children's brains from ultraprocessed food, environmental toxins, farmworker and food worker injustices, the threat to national security and other damaging outcomes—then your grass-fed steak and organic, regeneratively grown produce would be *much* cheaper than the industrial food we've become accustomed to.

Sometimes it takes litigation to hold these companies accountable for the true costs.

For example, over a 30-year period General Electric dumped 1.3 million pounds of polychlorinated biphenyls (PCBs) into the Hudson

River.[35] Eventually the company was held to account. Robert F. Kennedy Jr., then the chief prosecuting attorney for Riverkeeper[36] (an environmental nonprofit organization dedicated to protecting the Hudson River), and his colleagues forced General Electric to undertake a historic cleanup costing more than $1.7 billion.[37] More recently, in June 2023, industrial manufacturer 3M (which makes everyday household staples like Scotch tape) agreed to a $10.3 *billion* settlement to resolve claims that it contaminated public drinking water systems across the United States with per- and polyfluoroalkyl substances (PFAS), known as the infamous "forever chemicals," which have been linked to a smorgasbord of health issues, including many forms of cancer.[38]

Also in June 2023,[39] DuPont, along with its spinoff companies Chemours and Corteva, agreed to establish a $1.185 billion[40] fund to address allegations of PFAS contamination in numerous US drinking water systems. This settlement aims to compensate affected public water systems and support efforts to remediate PFAS pollution, coming on the heels of the major wins in 2004[41] and 2017[42] against the same company for its known use of perfluorooctanoic acid (PFOA), colloquially known as Teflon. These class action suits won $343 million and $671 million, respectively, after confirming a "probable link" between PFOA exposure and several life-threatening diseases, all of which were known by the company's leadership and concealed from the American public for more than 50 years.[43]

My point: All of the costs of the food industry need to be quantified. To quote the phrase often attributed to legendary management expert Peter Drucker, "What gets measured gets managed."

A movement is now under way to truly account for the real costs—to humans, to the environment, and to economies—of our current industrial food system. It is called *true cost accounting*. Some costs are easy to measure, like direct health care costs. Some are harder to measure, due to the amorphous and complex nature of large systems. But many groups are working hard to assess all these factors and map out an honest view of the consequences of how we grow food, what we grow, and how it affects those who grow it and eat it, as well as the impact on governments and economies. Changes in our food policy to account for this cost, leveraging both taxes and incentives, can have a profound impact on improving the overall health of humanity and the planet. If we think about it from this perspective, why should junk-food companies get a tax deduction for marketing food known to cause obesity and chronic disease?

THE TRUE COST OF YOUR FOOD: MORE UNINTENDED CONSEQUENCES

By now you might be getting the picture, recognizing all the additional costs of our food system—the ones you don't pay at the grocery store or restaurant. But what if the real cost of food and our food system was actually built into the price? What if farmers who provide ecosystem services (building soil, improving water use and biodiversity) were paid for those services, while Big Ag companies—seed, chemical, and fertilizer companies that destroy ecosystems (depleting organic matter in the soil, overusing and polluting freshwater resources, destroying biodiversity such as pollinator species, and contributing to climate change)— were charged for their impact on ecosystem destruction? Maybe the factory-farmed burger *should* cost $1,000 a pound. Maybe the can of soda *should* be $100. And maybe the cost of grass-fed steak should be only $3 a pound.

Here are some of the other costs hidden in your feedlot steak or burger (or pretty much any food grown our industrial agricultural system):[44]

- Pesticide poisoning and related illnesses cost $1 billion a year.[45]
- Other pesticide costs including death of birds and insect pollinators (bees and butterflies), loss of biodiversity, crop loss, and groundwater contamination are about $7 billion a year.[46]
- Cleanup of manure from CAFOs (confined animal feeding operations) costs about $4 billion a year. There are millions of those animals, and they produce more than 300 million tons of manure a

year, which is held in open pits or manure lagoons and contaminates land, water, and air.[47] This cost doesn't account for all the illnesses, like asthma, in nearby communities from aerosolized toxins caused by this pollution.

- Declining property values around CAFOs are $26 billion a year,[48] costing farmers their asset security. Who wants to live near a stinky, polluted hog, chicken, or beef operation?

- Taxpayer subsidies from the US Farm Bill, which include these factory farms among their recipients, have averaged about $16 billion a year over the past decade.[49] In December 2024, the American Relief Act of 2025 was enacted, including an additional $31 billion in economic and disaster aid for farmers and ranchers.[50]

- Fast-food employees—roughly 6 percent of SNAP recipients— make so little money to serve up your burger (and fries and soda) that they need food stamps to buy their own food. That costs the US government (and taxpayers) about $7 billion a year in aid through SNAP—the Supplemental Nutrition Assistance Program.

- Increasing CO_2 in the atmosphere acidifies the oceans, killing phytoplankton, which produce 50 percent of the oxygen we breathe.[51] How do we even calculate the price of losing 50 percent of our oxygen?

- Antibiotic use in animal feed to promote growth and prevent infection from overcrowding is the primary contributor to antibiotic resistance in humans and the related gut and immune issues, which kill more than a million people a year and cost at least a trillion dollars globally every year.[52] The antibiotics also end up in manure and slurries that are spread on fields (including organic crops) and destroy the soil microbiology.

This is not an exhaustive list, but you get the point. The global cost is not in the billions or even trillions but in the *quadrillions*. Much of it is hard to measure. How do you measure the loss of biodiversity or the destruction of coral reefs, or the decimation of phytoplankton, which produces so much of the oxygen we breathe? Who is paying that cost?

You are. I am. We are. The planet is. Natural habitats and oceans are. Even the historical diversity of seeds used to grow our food is suffering.

Agriculture's Impact on Climate Refugees

Climate refugees are real, displaced by natural disasters and extreme weather events. A leading international think tank projects that by 2050 there will be 200 million to 1.2 billion climate refugees.[53] That was the entire population of the world in 1820, just two centuries ago. To put it in perspective, the Syrian refugee crisis, which was in part due to climate change–induced drought, amounted to just 7.4 million refugees (about 0.6 percent of that UN projection).

Vulnerable populations around the world are exposed to increasingly catastrophic weather, increased infectious disease, and threats to their food security. In 2024, extreme weather events led to significant economic losses worldwide, causing an estimated $310 billion in damage,[54] marking a 6 percent increase from the previous year. In just the first week of 2025, the Los Angeles wildfires alone caused estimated damages and economic losses between $250 billion and $275 billion, landing it the distinction of being one of the costliest natural disasters in US history.[55]

In 2023, global heat exposure led to an estimated 512 billion potential work hours lost, a record high, representing approximately 1.5 times the average from 1990 to 1999.[56] Higher temperatures also fuel infectious disease—cholera, malaria, and dengue fever, among others. The heat also worsens health and increases the demand for limited health care services for those with heart disease, type 2 diabetes, and lung diseases.

Agriculture is affected by climate change and increasing temperatures, too, with downward trends in yields in thirty countries threatening food security. This is clearly not all about our food system, as many other factors drive climate change, but since the full value chain of our food system is the single biggest contributor, if we fix it, it would also be the single biggest solution. The *Climate Change 2023 Synthesis Report* by the Intergovernmental Panel on Climate Change, their sixth assessment report (AR6) of this kind, emphasizes transforming agricultural systems as a key solution to climate change and food and political security.[57]

A Complicit Government

We also have a co-opted government. When I asked Ann Veneman, the former secretary of agriculture under George W. Bush, why we couldn't have science guide our policies for food and agriculture, or why we don't stop the marketing of junk food to kids, or have more transparent food labels, or stop subsidies for commodities turned into processed food, or create subsidies for fruit and vegetables, she told me point-blank that it was the food and agriculture industry's influence on Congress and the administration. Her hands were tied.

The Farm Bill—a massive piece of legislation in the United States that determines how the government spends money on farming, food production, and nutrition programs—covers things like subsidies for farmers, SNAP, and conservation efforts. Because it has such a big impact on who gets money and support in the food and agriculture industry, companies and organizations with a stake in farming—like seed producers, agro-chemical companies, fertilizer companies, and food corporations—want to influence what's included in the bill.

To do this, they hire lobbyists, who are professionals paid to... persuade...lawmakers to include policies that benefit their clients. They're like the hired mercenaries of industry. Problems outsourced; blame deflected. In the case of the 2014 Farm Bill, more than 600 companies spent a staggering $500 million to ensure their interests were represented.[58] Companies like Monsanto, sold to Bayer in 2018[59] (which sells genetically modified, or GMO, seeds and the herbicides and pesticides applied to them), and Syngenta (a major agricultural chemical company) have continued to give money to politicians on the Senate and House Agricultural Committees because those lawmakers directly shape the bill. For example, it's been rumored that 73 percent of senators and 90 percent of representatives on these committees received donations from these companies, which, if true, raises concerns about whether the policies they support truly serve the public—or the corporations funding them.

THE AGRICULTURE CARTEL'S PREDATORY POWERS

The agriculture cartel's powers begin with the seeds. GMO seeds are sold to farmers by Big Ag seed monopolies. Five big companies, Bayer (Monsanto), ChemChina and its subsidiary Syngenta, Corteva, and BASF, formed by giant mergers over the last few years buying up dozens of seed companies, control most of the seeds in the world, including 60 percent of the vegetable seeds.[60] These companies benefit from the predatory oligopolistic powers that burden farmers with less choice and higher prices, making them dependent first on the seeds they breed and then on the chemicals they produce to inoculate seeds bred specifically to necessitate their chemicals. These companies produce the seeds but also the pesticides and herbicides that have become necessary for their crops. Convenient, right? The consolidation and centralization of seed production means that we have less food biodiversity and resiliency, which threatens our food security (more diversity in natural systems generally means more resiliency). It also means the loss of autonomy to save and collect seeds for farmers, especially for the 2.5 billion small farm holders across the globe.[61]

In the United States, many farmers are further constrained from investing in long-term regenerative practices because crop insurance policies often favor conventional farming methods and genetically modified seeds from major agribusiness conglomerates. In many cases, farmers cannot even get crop insurance unless they prove they're using industrial seeds. This system actively punishes diversification and innovation, leaving farmers beholden to a rigged structure that prioritizes industrial agriculture and depresses their margins. Tragically, farmers face significant financial and mental health pressures, contributing to one of the highest suicide rates[62] among all professions in the country.

Soda and Sugar-Sweetened Beverages

The soda and sugar-sweetened beverage story is pretty much the same as that for your burger or steak—damage to the environment, huge costs to society, and massive economic consequences from drinking the high-fructose corn syrup that sweetens your soda, energy drinks, teas, and coffees. But there is one big difference. Feedlot (factory-farmed) meat isn't great for you. The use of antibiotics to promote faster growth and weight gain and prevent disease or contamination due to the over-crowded and unsanitary living conditions the poor animals live in— aside from being an animal welfare catastrophe—also contributes to antibiotic-resistant bacteria in humans, which cause all kinds of down-stream health issues for us. Nonetheless, eating it doesn't kill people (at least, not directly). But sugar does. Especially high-fructose corn syrup, which is now pervasive in our sugar-sweetened beverages.

Sugar-sweetened beverages are associated with approximately 1.2 million new cases of heart disease and 340,000 deaths worldwide each year,[63] in addition to causing diabetes and increasing the risk of cancer. The risk goes up with every additional soda: Another study found that your risk of death from heart disease was 31 percent higher if you con-sumed two sugar-sweetened beverages a day, and every extra drink caused the risk to go up by another 10 percent.[64]

And the ubiquity of soft drinks certainly doesn't help. On Amazon .com, Smartwater (made by Coca-Cola) is 9 cents an ounce. Coca-Cola is 4 cents an ounce (in a 2-liter bottle). When water is more than double the cost of soda, we have a problem.

The other big problem with the soda industry is that as taxpayers we pay for 31 billion servings of soda to low-income households through SNAP. Sugar-sweetened beverages are the single biggest line item for SNAP,[65] accounting for nearly 10 percent of the "food" purchased by SNAP recipients. That means taxpayers are spending $12 billion a year to enrich Coca-Cola and, quite literally, poison their fellow citi-zens.[66] Not only is there zero nutrition in soda, but it is one of the few things that has been proven causal to obesity, a disease that is a force multiplier for most other chronic illnesses that burden our health care system, the bills for which are covered by taxpayers.[67]

But there is a happy aside now, five years since publication of the first edition of *Food Fix:* As of March 28, 2025, there is a significant push at both federal and state levels to restrict the purchase of sugary sodas and other junk foods using SNAP benefits. Health and Human Services Secretary Robert F. Kennedy Jr. has announced that states will be granted waivers to prohibit the use of SNAP funds for purchasing sugary beverages. West Virginia has become the first state to seek such a waiver, with Governor Patrick Morrisey expressing intentions to implement this restriction! West Virginia is also the first state to ban food additives. I actually helped advise the governor when the food industry tried to manipulate him by telling him that grandmothers who used red dye in their cupcakes for school bake sales would go to prison if he passed the law. Sadly the industry resorts to this and worse to protect their profits.

ANOTHER CULPRIT: THE UNDERBELLY OF CORN

As a nation, we pay four times for our corn. We privatize the profits and socialize the costs.

First, through the taxpayer-funded Farm Bill mentioned earlier, corn subsidies have totaled more than $116 billion from 1995 to 2021, averaging roughly $4.1 billion per year—the highest subsidies of any crop.[68] About 3 percent[69] of that corn is used to make high-fructose corn syrup.[70] The rest is used for feed for factory-farmed animals, ethanol, cooking oil, alcohol, industrial products, and processed-food additives.

Second, we pay for the environmental consequences of modern corn production. Modern chemical-intensive till farming causes loss of topsoil. This causes an increase in greenhouse gases because industrial monocrop chemical agriculture depletes carbon-containing organic matter in soils (the soil is the planet's biggest carbon sink). Then we pay for all the damage from the nitrogen runoff to waterways and oceans, the harm from the pesticides and herbicides, and the depletion of our water resources.

Third, through our food stamp program, SNAP, we pay for much of the junk food and sugar-sweetened beverages made from corn syrup. In 2024, Matthew Dickerson, director of budget policy at the Economic Policy Innovation Center, released a report titled *Food Stamps: A Culture of Dependency* that detailed where SNAP dollars are going.[71] Between 2001 and 2023, SNAP enrollment grew by 150 percent.[72] During that time, taxpayer spending on the program surged from $31 billion (inflation-adjusted) to $135 billion.[73] Despite this massive increase, SNAP has no nutritional standards, meaning a significant portion of these funds are spent on ultraprocessed foods. There is a big difference between *food security,* or having enough calories, and *nutrition security,* which is having enough nutrients. Paradoxically, the most obese also suffer from the most nutritional deficiencies. Among the most purchased items are soft drinks, candy, frozen pizza, ice cream, and cookies—raising concerns about the program's role in fueling diet-related diseases. And that doesn't include noncarbonated sugar drinks that masquerade as health drinks like Powerade or Vitaminwater.

If you aren't convinced yet, consider that 39 percent of Coca-Cola's annual revenue of $45 billion in 2023 (or roughly 17 percent of their global annual revenue) comes from the United States.[74] Much of that comes from SNAP, likely making Coca-Cola a multibillion-dollar welfare recipient!

Rank	Item Purchased	Rank	Item Purchased
1	Soft Drinks	11	Candy
2	Fluid Milk	12	Infant Formula
3	Ground Beef	13	Frozen Pizza
4	Bag Snacks	14	Refrigerated Juices/Drinks
5	Cheese	15	Ice Cream
6	Baked Breads	16	Coffee and Creamers
7	Cold Cereal	17	Cookies
8	Fresh Chicken	18	Water
9	Frozen Handhelds and Snacks	19	Shelf Stable Juice
10	Lunchmeat	20	Eggs/Muffins/Potatoes

And fourth, we pay for all the health care costs of obesity and chronic diseases (caused mostly by diet), or about $4.9 trillion a year (up by more than $1 trillion since the first edition of *Food Fix* was published in 2020!). As a direct consequence of our nutritionally bankrupt diet in the United States, the growth of roughly 4 percent of our children is stunted,[75] causing permanent developmental, neurological, and long-term economic impacts for them and for our nation writ large.

And we pay for it all through our government support for industrial agriculture, which includes the euphemistically named "crop insurance"—the profits from which primarily benefit the oligopolistic racket of industrial firms that produce the chemicals, seeds, and fertilizer that supply those farms. Remember that taxpayers fund SNAP. Weirdly, the USDA won't disclose where those dollars are used, alleging that it is protecting the privacy of big retailers like Walmart and Kroger. Shouldn't taxpayers know exactly how much of and where their tax dollars are being spent?

A South Dakota newspaper decided this data should be public under the Freedom of Information Act (FOIA) and has filed a lawsuit to make the data public. In 2019,[76] the case went to the Supreme Court, which ruled in favor of the Food Marketing Institute, determining that such data is exempt from disclosure under FOIA's Exemption 4, which protects "confidential" commercial information.[77] Why isn't the government protecting its citizens, and not corporations? What are they hiding?

Even more egregious, we indirectly support the food industry's marketing of junk food to unwitting children, low-income individuals, and disproportionately minorities, by allowing them to deduct $7.5 billion a year, with restaurants accounting for $9 billion and canned and specialty foods accounting for another billion in advertising costs, all the while absolving them of the responsibility to pay for the chronic disease *directly* caused by that food.[78] Through Medicare, Medicaid, and other government-funded health programs that cover more than half the US population, taxpayers end up paying multiple times for chronic disease, while large corporations continue to profit from the system. As Dr. Casey Means says, "The primary place that we're getting our information is deeply influenced by a force that wants us to be chronically ill so that we can be customers of the pharmaceutical industry." And I would add the food and agriculture industries.

This simply isn't just. It must be fixed. We need to demand full transparency and honesty about the costs of our current food system for each one of us and for our communities, society, economy, and environment.

FOOD FIX: THE TRUE COST OF FOOD

There is not one simple solution to the challenges of the threats to farming, diet, public health, the economy, the environment, the climate, workers' rights, education, national security, social justice, income inequities, health disparities, and more. But they are all connected in one way or another by one thing: food.

In 2018 I met with then Representative Tim Ryan of Ohio and suggested that all our government's various policies on health, nutrition, agriculture, and food were not integrated, often working at odds with one another, and were overseen by eight different agencies, without any awareness of their effectiveness, influence on public health, or economic impact. That led to a request by Congress for the Government Accountability Office (GAO), the government's independent assessors of the effectiveness and cost of government policies, to examine these issues in detail and report on recommended actions to fix them. It discovered that there were more than *200* agencies in twenty-one departments working at cross-purposes, and in many cases directly contradicting one another.[79] The GAO recommended the creation of a federal strategy to reduce the burden of chronic disease, and to get it established in the Department of Health and Human Services (HHS). The establishment of the Administration for a Healthy America (AHA)[80] within HHS can hopefully fulfill this promise.

We need to think about these issues like systems thinkers, recognizing them as an interconnected, intersecting set of challenges that we can and must address collectively. Not to sound alarmist, but we are seriously running out of time to reverse the anthropogenic meta-crises we have created: the burdens of obesity, chronic disease, and infectious disease; loss of all our topsoil, causing nutrition insecurity; depletion of our freshwater resources, poisoning our marine life; loss of the Earth's biodiversity, increasing desertification; hunger; malnutrition; and the instability of governments and economies, to mention just a few.

I am not going through this to overwhelm you—but to help you connect the dots so we can solve this problem as a whole. The Big Food propaganda narrative that espouses the belief that Americans should eat less and exercise more only blames the victim. It is the very nature of the food industry to produce that addictive burger and soda that over-rides willpower, hacks your biology, and hijacks your metabolism.

Many of our greatest challenges today are, paradoxically, the unin-tended consequences of solutions to other problems. These "externalities" are a common feature of complex global systems—where addressing one issue often triggers a cascade of new ones. What began as well-meaning decisions and policies, guided by the best of intentions, has, over time, given rise to unforeseen and far-reaching complications.

The food system we have is not an accident but is mostly the result of good intentions and conscious goals that were mostly met. Though 750 million people around the world still suffer from hunger and many more from food insecurity, the efforts of the mid-twentieth-century food system were very successful (in their original purpose of increasing calorie abundance). But the unintended consequences were the focus on a few staple commodities, the hyper-processing of foods, which led to the erosion of land, soil, water resources, and climate, and the failure to increase protective minimally processed foods, all leading to the chronic disease and sustainability crises we see today.

That is why I wrote this book: to present practical and achievable solutions to this seemingly intractable problem. Some are well-formed programs that already exist. Some are proposed solutions by experts. Some are easy to implement, others more difficult. They are meant to highlight what is needed and what is possible, rather than a comprehen-sive set of solutions. Citizens, farmers, businesses, investors, nonprofits, and governments all must play their part. This is a starting point for a deeper exploration as a society, a road map for the change that is needed to address these challenges together. These ideas are meant to inspire, educate, and motivate individuals, businesses, and government policy-makers to innovate and think differently about these issues—to see the linkages, the need for systems thinking, the need for thoughtful inte-grated solutions.

We need new ideas, strategies, policies, and business innovations to fix these problems and bring diverse groups together to solve them. It is possible. Solutions exist. They are achievable, and we need the push from the grass roots and from the top down to shift public opinion, to create a movement that forces legislatures and policymakers to take notice and take action. We can use the power of our forks and our collective behaviors to move in the right direction. Throughout *Food Fix Uncensored* we will explore the specific ways in which citizens, businesses, and policymakers can solve the biggest problem we face today — our broken food system and all its consequences.

I hope you will join my efforts to find a Food Fix, by taking personal action and by urging our policymakers to fix our food system so we can improve the health of millions of Americans, our economy, and our environment. To learn more and join the movement, go to www.foodfixuncensored.com.

CHAPTER 2

THE ROLE OF OUR FOOD SYSTEM IN THE EPIDEMIC OF CHRONIC DISEASE

The food you eat can be either the safest and most powerful form of medicine or the slowest form of poison.

—ANN WIGMORE

On January 21, 2025, Larry Ellison, CEO of tech behemoth Oracle, went on record announcing a major investment in artificial intelligence.[1] His claim[2] was that the advancement in large language model artificial intelligence technology was ready to tackle the problem of treating chronic diseases like cancer. They would do so by developing personalized vaccines targeted for each individual cancer and genetic profile.

On the surface, this sounds like a momentous achievement. Why wouldn't I, as a medical doctor, be thrilled that we might see a breakthrough in cancer treatment? Well, of course, this may prove to be a lifesaving innovation. And I certainly hope that it does. But the subtext of Larry's announcement is that cancer is a given and we must mobilize our economic, intellectual, and engineering firepower toward finding treatments. This rhetoric is common among technologists, and sadly, even most of the mainstream medical establishment. But what they are missing is that chronic diseases like cancer are actually *preventable* and in many cases *reversable!* Degenerative diseases like many cancers don't just develop randomly; their development is based on a set of fairly predictable conditions, many of which are lifestyle related. And of those causes, many of them relate to our food system, in one way or another.

My radical assertion is this: The chronic diseases that are ravaging our population and burdening global economies *cannot* be cured by better medication or medical care. While these are important, they often come too late. What we need is *prevention,* or early intervention; we need to look upstream and fix the *source* of the problem: food.

A DECLINE IN LIFE EXPECTANCY

The data is clear: Those who consume the greatest amount of those ultraprocessed "foodstuffs," the staple building blocks of industrial food (aka synthetic, lab-grown chemicals), are the sickest.[3] They have higher body weight, putting stress on the body, more visceral (belly) fat, which compromises organs and systemic health, and worse cholesterol and blood sugar — all of which cause many other downstream chronic diseases.[4] Thus, they are in decline for longer and are more likely to die sooner.

And for the first time in our history, life expectancy in the United States is falling. As of 2024, our average life expectancy was just 77 years, ranking us forty-ninth globally, just behind Cuba(!).[5] Any American around in the 1960s should shriek at the irony of that.

Over the 4 million years of human evolution, life expectancy increased. At the turn of the twentieth century, the global average was about 31 years. And from 1900 to 2000, life expectancy increased about 37 years, from 31 to 68 years.[6] In America we have more than doubled life expectancy through public health measures including sanitation, a dependable food supply, and vaccines.

But today, our current toxic food system is eroding these advances.

Children born today are expected to live shorter, sicker lives than

Average Life Expectancy

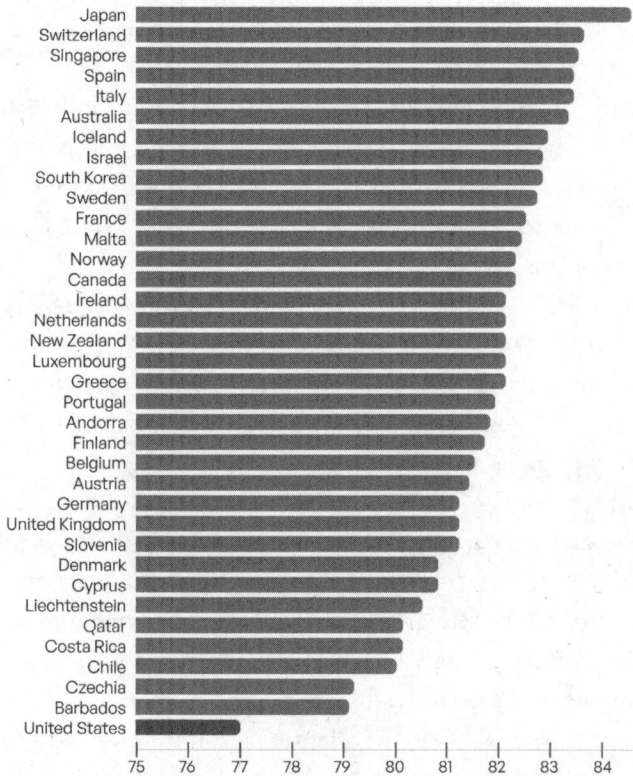

their parents.[7] The average child born today will live five fewer years than their parents, and if they are from a low-income background or are socially disadvantaged, they will live 10 to 20 fewer years.[8] One in three children born today will have type 2 diabetes in their lifetime.

For the past three consecutive years, we have seen life expectancy go down. Certainly, some of this decline may be a result of the tragic opioid epidemic, drug overdoses, suicide, mental health disorders, and COVID-19. But to put these in perspective, while opioid deaths have risen to approximately 80,000 a year in America,[9] this number pales in comparison to the almost 700,000 deaths a year in the United States from lifestyle-related cardiovascular disease alone (70 to 80 percent of this from diet).[10] There has been talk of declaring a national emergency to stem the deaths from opioid overdose. Why aren't we talking about a similar initiative to address deaths from poor diet?

And while technologists and transhumanists might claim otherwise, no amount of vaccines, medical therapeutics, or technological advancements can save us from our diet. Our bodies evolved to require nutrients found in nature, not in labs. We are simply not going to innovate our way out of this problem.

The geographic maps of life expectancy within the US present an irrefutable conclusion: When overlaid on the maps of obesity and type 2 diabetes (most prevalent in the southern American states), there is almost a complete correlation between the states with the highest obesity and diabetes rates and those with the lowest life expectancy. Death rates from heart disease, diabetes, chronic liver disease (which we now know to be at least partially caused by sugar and starch), stroke, and Alzheimer's are on the rise.[11] The disparities in life expectancy in this country are driven by disparities in education, income, and socioeconomic status affecting people with low income and minorities, which result in obesity and metabolic disease caused by poor diet.[12]

There has also been a rise in allergic, autoimmune, and inflammatory conditions linked to poor diet.[13] Mental health has declined precipitously, with increasing rates of depression, suicide, behavior problems, and neurodevelopmental disorders, much of which has been linked to poor nutrition.[14] We keep seeking beneficent solutions to the mental health crisis, but the harsh reality is that a brain devoid of essential nutrients—the literal building blocks of its structure and function—simply cannot produce the happy hormones and neurotransmitters we need to thrive.[15] The easiest and cheapest solution to resolve this crisis is to start with diet, but unfortunately this is not a cash cow for Big Pharma, so this cold hard truth is oft ignored.

In 2019 *The Lancet* published an analysis of dietary risk factors in 195 countries based on the Global Burden of Disease Study, the most comprehensive study of the effects of diet on health ever conducted, covering a 27-year period.[16] Despite its limitations, the study's takeaway was this: Diets absent a sufficient amount of nutrition (from fruits and vegetables, nuts and seeds, whole grains, etc.) and saturated with too many bad foods (processed foods, refined grains, sugar-sweetened beverages, trans fats, etc.) accounted for *11 million deaths* and 255 million years of disability and life years lost. Most striking was the finding that the lack of "protective foods" (foods rich in essential vitamins, minerals, and other nutrients that are strictly necessary to maintain the immune system, protect the body from diseases and deficiencies, and facilitate vital physiological functions) was as important in determining risk of death as the overconsumption of processed foods, if not more so. What does that mean in English? That you will decline rapidly and die prematurely if you do not consume sufficient quantities of essential nutrients. That is a big deal, because that means that we have *choice*.

Imagine if an infectious disease like Ebola or Zika or AIDS killed 11 million people a year. Look what happened during COVID-19—a worldwide lockdown for months, and in some countries years, for a virus that caused roughly half that many deaths over a five-year period.[17] If we were honestly facing the reality that our food system kills twice as many *each year* as COVID has in total, wouldn't we be forcing a worldwide reckoning? If we treated this crisis with the same degree of urgency that we gave to COVID-19, we would have mobilized governments, scientists, philanthropists, and businesses to fight this threat.

Yet the silence is deafening when it comes to our global response to these most common kinds of preventable deaths.

Illustratively, a few years ago, I was at the Milken Global Conference listening to a panel of the leading thinkers and actors in health care—the head of the National Institutes of Health, the CEO of the Bill and Melinda Gates Foundation, the head of the Centers for Medicare & Medicaid Services, and the CEO of Kaiser health systems. They spoke of important things—eradicating polio, malaria, and AIDS, gene editing to cure rare genetic disorders, improving the interoperability of medical records, data sharing, and improving medical payments systems to pay for value. All great advances.

But not one person mentioned the elephant in the room: the tsunami of disease, death, and costs driven by our poor diet, not to mention the effects of our food system on the environment, the climate, and even social justice. This dwarfs every other problem. Why are we neglecting this?

Generously, I could entertain the idea that our systems have simply been blindsided by the onslaught of our chronic disease epidemic. Too much, too fast, and too big a problem.

To me, this problem seems simply too obvious and too dramatic to dismiss. It is ubiquitous. It's at the checkout line at the supermarket. It's on the billboards on the freeway. It's in your neighborhood church. So the skeptic in me might suggest that there's a darker force inhibiting our response. Something more akin to, at best, willful ignorance, and at worst, deliberate collusion.

The reality is that the food we eat (or possibly more importantly, the food we don't eat) is the single biggest cause of death worldwide, exceeding tobacco and every other known risk factor, *ever*. Historically, infections, poor sanitation, or what we call "communicable disease" caused most deaths. Now more than 70 percent of deaths worldwide[18] are from what we call "noncommunicable disease," predominantly lifestyle-related conditions like heart disease, obesity, type 2 diabetes, cancer, and dementia. However, as we'll see in later in the book, there is a problem with the term *noncommunicable*. It implies that these conditions—such as heart disease, cancer, diabetes, dementia, and depression, among others—appear randomly, or worse, that they are the result of poor judgment. But in reality, these diseases are highly contagious and driven by the structural environment—government policies, poverty, and a pervasive and increasingly toxic global food system and environment that create conditions ripe for disease to flourish.

We have become culturally accustomed to blaming the victim for these diseases. But no one blames someone for getting malaria or tuberculosis. It seems as if the social conventions are rewritten when it comes to chronic disease. We blame individuals, accusing them of lacking personal responsibility, disparagingly labeling them as "lazy" or "undisciplined."

I don't believe that. Here's my (fairly educated) theory: The narrative that blames individuals for being sick or overweight—insisting it's their fault—is a carefully crafted deflection by Big Food. Their goal? To divert attention away from the real culprit: the very products they create. It's reminiscent of Big Oil's PR strategy of introducing "greenwashing" to mislead environmentalists and sow division. Similarly, I would not be surprised if the fat-shaming culture and even the subsequent body-positivity movement were proven to be products of Big Food's propaganda machine. In both cases—deliberate or not—they've masterfully redirected blame, exonerating themselves while leading innocent people down predictable, preventable paths of health decline—all while profiting from the chaos they've caused.

Let me take off my tinfoil hat for a moment to say it is certainly true that our social environment drives disease. If we live in a world where our food system produces mainly disease-causing foods, where a food carnival makes it almost impossible to make the right choice, where our government supports the production and sale of these harmful foods, and where these foods are consciously designed to be biologically addictive, and available everywhere—then personal agency certainly is...a fiction.

The science is clear: Noncommunicable diseases, it turns out, are actually *highly* communicable. You are statistically more likely to be overweight if your friends are overweight than if your family is overweight.[19] Depending on your neighborhood, your life expectancy may be 20 to 30 years shorter than that of folks from another county, city, or state. Simply moving an overweight person with diabetes from a low socioeconomic neighborhood to a slightly richer one leads to weight loss and improvement in diabetes, without any other intervention.[20]

This is far more than an issue of personal choice and motivated behavioral change. The food we have available to eat (predominantly "ultraprocessed" food, which bears little resemblance to its natural constituents) and the food we don't eat (fruits and vegetables and whole foods) are determined by the food system itself—what we grow and produce and how we market and distribute it, and what we don't. Most of these decisions are made for us by our government and corporations.

They choose what we eat and where it is available. We have historically had little to no influence in this.

But all of that is about to change.

According to the lead author of the *Lancet* study, "There is an urgent and compelling need for changes in the various sectors of the food production cycle, such as growing, processing, packaging, and marketing. Our research finds the need for a comprehensive food system intervention to promote the production, distribution, and consumption of healthy foods across nations." Much of our food production system from the field to the fork has devolved into the production of foods that make us sick and fat and cause us to degenerate prematurely, rather than of foods that make us healthy, prevent disease, and help us live a long, productive life. Sadly, both the intended and unintended consequences of our global food system provide too much of the bad stuff and not enough good stuff...and this is quite literally killing us.

THE PERILS AND PROMISE OF FOOD

Not to be crass, but in the late nineteenth and early twentieth centuries, obesity was so rare that it was considered a spectacle in circus sideshows. "Fat Ladies" and "Fat Men" were marketed as curiosities or marvels of human anatomy. When I was a young boy, I remember we went to the circus to see the "Fat Lady." You couldn't find them anywhere else.

And if you spend any time in the social mediaverse, I am sure you've seen the viral photos of beaches from the 1960s. You can scan them thoroughly and not find a single image of anyone overweight, never mind obese, among a sea of humans. Juxtaposed to the present day, the same snapshots would be overwhelmingly the inverse.

I often reflect that when I graduated medical school in 1987, there was not a single state with an obesity rate over 20 percent.[21] Now there is not a single state with an obesity rate under 20 percent, and within the last few years we have seen many states surpass an adult obesity rate of 40 percent, with most others landing over 30 percent.[22] Obesity, now officially considered a disease, and its downstream conditions (heart disease, cancer, type 2 diabetes, dementia, arthritis, and others) are literally weighing down our species, our communities, our environment, and our economy, depleting human, social, economic, and natural capital in ways both visible and invisible.

Not long ago, type 2 diabetes was known as adult-onset diabetes, as it was virtually unheard-of in children. Just a few decades ago, a pediatrician could go an entire career without encountering a single case. Today, it's alarmingly common, with physicians increasingly turning to weight-loss drugs like Ozempic and Wegovy to treat children and adults alike. These drugs have even been recommended as the first line of defense by the American Academy of Pediatrics for kids as young as twelve, who will be destined to be on these drugs for life![23] A lifetime customer is definitely a good business model, but it's not exactly what I'd call a healthcare success.

GLP-1 receptor agonists like Wegovy are being heralded as a quick fix for diabetes and obesity, but at a staggering cost—$16,000 per patient annually.[24] If prescribed to the roughly 73 percent of US adults age twenty and over who are classified as overweight or have obesity, this would burden American taxpayers with an estimated $3 trillion each year.[25] To put this in perspective, in 2023, the combined spending on Medicare and Medicaid was only $1.9 trillion![26] Why should the public foot the bill for the failures of our food system, which prioritizes profit over nourishment? The solution isn't to subsidize more drugs—it's to overhaul the food system itself.

But let's rewind. How did this happen?

Over the last 40 years, since the government's first dietary guidelines encouraged us to cut the fat and increase the carbs (a deadly idea), and since the expansion of the extractive, industrial agriculture that has produced hundreds of thousands of food-like substances from very few raw materials (predominantly wheat, soy, and corn), we are now a nation where being an optimal weight is an anomaly.

Today, approximately 60 percent of our calories in the United States come from ultraprocessed foods, with low-income, minority, and less-educated people consuming the most.[27] Even worse, we're setting up our children to fail: They're currently averaging about 70 to 75 percent of their daily calories from these Frankenfoods, which are concurrently devoid of any nutritional benefit, and, due to their toxic load through synthetic dyes and untested chemicals, cause rampant inflammation, insulin resistance, and obesity. We're drowning in calories, yet 90 percent of Americans are deficient in one or more nutrients at the level that creates known deficiency diseases such as scurvy, rickets, and others.[28] The paradox is that we provide our population with too many calories and not enough nutrients. As I alluded to above, the most obese adults and children are counterintuitively the most malnourished.[29]

Globally this problem is even worse. We have created the worst diet in the world and exported it to every country on the planet.

What is the root cause of this tsunami of chronic disease that affects more than one in two Americans (and increasingly our global population)? Think of it as some combination of physical inactivity, smoking, excess alcohol consumption, and junk-food diet, with diet being the overwhelming driver for most.

Our food system is by far the biggest contributor to the structural factors that have led to this epidemic of chronic disease. The shift in our food quality, our food and health policies, our agricultural practices, and business "innovations" in product development and marketing in the more than $9.5 trillion food industry[30] (food and agriculture) have unleashed a disease-inducing Medusa.[31] Indeed, the deeper down the rabbit hole I have gone on this investigative inquiry, seeking to understand the root cause of our health epidemic, the more obvious it has become that this is not an accidental outcome but a set of deliberate practices and policies driven by an amoral food system hungry for profit and market (or stomach) share.

We can, however, change this trajectory—first in our own homes, then in our country, and finally globally. Stay tuned and I'll show you how.

THE PROBLEM OF ULTRAPROCESSED FOODS

Despite the fact that we produce more than enough food for our global population, more than 800 million people go to bed hungry and 2.5 billion go to bed every night overweight. All of these more than 3 trillion people—more than one-third of the entire world—are suffering from harmful nutrient deficiencies that result in stunting, impaired cognitive development, mental health conditions, increased risk for infectious disease, and chronic diseases, among many others.

As we will discuss later, the current world food system produces an average of 2,750 calories per day for the 8.2 billion humans on the planet. The average calorie need is arguably about 2,000 calories for women and 2,500 calories for men per day, for an average of 2,250 calories per person. Just doing the math, globally we produce 500 calories more than we need per person per day, or about enough food to feed 10.2 billion people.[32] But even in the United States, food insecurity affects about 13 percent of the population, or about 18 million people, 6.5 million of whom are children.[33] The 41 million Americans on the Supplemental Nutrition Assistance Program (SNAP; formerly known as food stamps),[34] half of whom are children, are at risk for hunger and food insecurity.[35] The calories, while abundant, are nutritionally deficient, technically leaving much of the planet nutrient-poor because of lack of access to whole, fresh, nutrient-dense foods.

The most food-insecure populations are often the most obese, have two-to-seven times the risk of type 2 diabetes,[36] and are malnourished—all at once. How? Because much of what we produce isn't food in the true sense of the word. It's calorie-dense, nutrient-poor, ultra-processed "food-like substances." By definition, food is a substance consumed to provide essential nutrients for growth, energy, and the maintenance of the body. Most ultraprocessed products found in supermarkets fail this definition. Stripped of real nutrition, they're little more than "food-stuffs" engineered for shelf life and profit—not health. They are technically not even food.

The cost dynamic only compounds the problem. With $1 in hand, you can buy either 1,200 calories of potato chips or cookies—or 250 calories of carrots. For low-income families in food deserts, even finding a carrot is a challenge, let alone affording it. Ultraprocessed foods are cheap per calorie but shockingly expensive when you consider nutrients—or the lack thereof—and the downstream costs to humans, the environment, and society.

We have created a system that is efficient at producing calories but disastrous at nourishing people. And as long as we cling to outdated definitions and profit-driven food paradigms, we'll continue paying the ultimate price: widespread malnutrition, preventable chronic disease, and a population fed but not truly nourished.

But don't take my word for it. A recent study of more than 44,000 people published in *JAMA Internal Medicine* found that for every 10 percent increase in the intake of ultraprocessed food, the risk of death increases by 14 percent.[37] If 60 percent of our calories come from processed foods, the math adds up to a lot of unnecessary, food-caused, preventable deaths.

Just as the wrong foods can cause disease and death, the right foods can dramatically reduce disease and death. Mounting research proves that food is medicine and demonstrates how whole foods, especially an increase in vegetables and fruit, can prevent or reverse chronic disease.[38] At Geisinger Health System, providing food-insecure type 2 diabetics with a year's worth of whole foods reduced health care costs by 80 percent and dramatically improved their health outcomes.[39] At Virta Health, a type 2 diabetes reversal program using a ketogenic diet, achieved a full reversal for 53 percent of participants without the use of diabetes-specific medications![40]

Many of our problems can be traced back to how we define them and the lens through which we choose to view the world. Take food security, for example—commonly defined as "access to affordable, nutritious food." But on the back of the Green Revolution, "nutritious" seemed to have been re-interpreted as "vitamin-fortified, starchy calories." Rooted in an outdated medical and agricultural paradigm, this definition is painfully medically inadequate. Yet powerful vested interests, profiting handsomely from this antiquated system, ensure that resistance to change remains formidable. Even recently, FDA officials have told me that nutrient-fortified refined grains are a major source of vitamins and minerals and that advising Americans to avoid refined grains (which are directly linked to nearly every chronic disease) could cause unintended nutrient deficiencies. While I understand this logic, wouldn't it be better to create a food system that provides naturally nutrient-dense food for Americans that doesn't come with the consequences of type 2 diabetes, cancer, dementia, heart disease, infertility, and depression? You may not become deficient in folic acid if you eat enriched white flour, but you sure will increase your risk of type 2 diabetes. We have to "enrich" the food because it starts out so "impoverished."

Sadly, the decisions made around our produce cultivation decades ago created an agricultural system that doesn't produce enough fruits and vegetables for everyone to eat even the minimum requirement. We have all heard the adages that we should eat five to nine servings of fruits and vegetables, but in practice, our system is not designed to facilitate that choice. Just follow the money: The government's dietary guidelines advise us to eat 50 percent of our plate as fruits and vegetables, but government agricultural subsidies for fresh produce only amount to 4 percent of the total budget. Fruits and vegetables, often referred to as "specialty crops," receive minuscule direct subsidy support compared to commodity crops.[41] This disparity in subsidy allocation has significant implications for both agricultural production and the resultant dietary patterns in the United States. The emphasis on commodity crops contributes to an abundant supply of ingredients for processed foods, while the limited support for fruits and vegetables directly affects both their availability and their affordability. In other words: If we don't fund the growth of healthy produce, the population cannot choose to eat it. This misalignment between subsidy distribution and nutritional guidelines underscores the need for policy reforms that promote a more balanced and health-oriented agricultural framework.

We're telling people to eat more fruits and vegetables, but we don't prioritize growing them. How does this make any sense?

FOOD FIX: WHAT THE HECK SHOULD I EAT?

If you read literally anything about nutrition online, you're probably confounded about what qualifies as "nutritious." One of the most contentious topics out there, nutrition science, is muddled with conflicting opinions, pseudoscience, and corrupt research.

Sadly, the public is at the mercy of these constantly changing debates. Eggs were bad, then they were good. Fat was bad, now it's good, but controversy exists about whether to cut saturated fat or decrease refined plant-based oils. Some science shows that meat is bad and increases the risk of heart disease, cancer, and death; other science reports that meat is strictly necessary for optimal function. (Chapter 11 will help clear up some of the confusion.) The diet wars are bigger than ever in history. Vegan, Paleo, keto, low-fat, high-fat, low-carb, high-carb, raw. *What the heck should I eat?*

It would seem we should have a simple answer to this question, but there is vast disagreement from a variety of experts. I have spent the last 40 years studying nutrition, grappling with the changes in recommendations and diets, and treating tens of thousands of patients with food as medicine.

I'll read you in on a big little secret.

While the specifics *are* complex—and unique genetics and environment definitely play a role—there are some fundamental truths we can all live by. Any earnest physician or academic not bought by corporate greed will tell you that the basics are actually quite straightforward: Eat food as close to its natural state as possible, prioritizing clean protein (wild or regeneratively raised animals are the best), healthy fats, and a boatload of fresh produce (fruits and veg). If you do just that, skipping 100 percent of the processed Frankenfoods and packaged treats, and limit alcohol and sugar, you're more or less living in accordance with your evolutionary nature. Which is what your body is *desperately* craving.

I have reviewed the research on nutrition and what makes up a diet that is good for you, good for the planet, and good for society. I have laid this all out in my book *Food: What the Heck Should I Eat?* And I provided a way to do it in my cookbook *Food: What the Heck Should I Cook?* To get a nuanced view of the research, an honest and nondogmatic, non-philosophical view based on 40 years of studying nutrition and 30 years of applying it to thousands of patients, you can read the book, or check out the QR code on the next page for a quick guide on what to eat.

Scan the QR code below for a summary on what you should eat for you and for the planet.

FOOD FIX: FOOD AS MEDICINE

Not too long ago, a group of medical doctors and public health experts at Massachusetts General Hospital noticed something striking: Many of the patients who routinely showed up in the emergency room requiring the most medical services were also the patients who seemed to be the most nutritionally vulnerable. They were frequently patients with heart disease, type 2 diabetes, cancer, and other largely-food-related chronic diseases. For hospitals and health insurers, these are among the highest-cost, highest-need patients. While this may seem like common sense now, this correlation was not widely accepted in conventional medical wisdom at the time.

Motivated by this discovery, the doctors decided to launch a study with a local nonprofit group called Community Servings to see whether providing these patients with nutritious meals would have an impact on their health outcomes. The researchers recruited Medicaid and Medicare patients and split them into groups that either received nutritious healthy meals or did *not* receive nutritious meals. The study found that the patients who had nutritious meals had fewer hospital visits, ultimately resulting in a 16 percent reduction in their health care costs. And that was *after* deducting meal expenses. The average monthly medical costs for a patient in the nutrition group shrank to about $843—nearly half the roughly $1,413 in medical costs per patient in the control group.[42]

Another group of public health experts in Philadelphia studied what happened when a nonprofit health group called the Metropolitan Area

Neighborhood Nutrition Alliance delivered healthy meals to people with diabetes, heart disease, cancer, and other chronic diseases. Over twelve months, the patients in the nutritious meal group visited hospitals half as often as a control group and stayed for 37 percent less time. Ultimately, their health care costs plummeted more than 50 percent, or $12,000 a month per patient.[43] Considering that the sickest 5 percent of patients account for 50 percent of overall health care costs in the United States, according to the Agency for Healthcare Research and Quality,[44] providing meals to the sickest provides a major return on investment.

A similar effort is under way in California, where researchers are studying the health care impact of providing nutritious meals to 1,000 chronically sick patients insured by California's Medicaid program, known as Medi-Cal.[45] Studies have shown a 32 percent reduction in health care costs and a 63 percent reduction in hospitalizations.[46] Many of these programs are funded through private donations and coordinated by the national Food Is Medicine Coalition, which is a group of nonprofits that want to use nutrition to solve the health care and chronic disease crisis. The Food Is Medicine group hopes to get these medically tailored meals included in health care coverage.

These groups recognize what our federal government sadly does not: To tackle the crisis, our national food policies must be aligned with our health care policies. Instead of just treating rampant chronic diseases with medication and surgery, we have to start preventing and treating with food.

You might be thinking, if this is so simple, why isn't this already the medical status quo? The problem comes down to the incentives. The insurance (payer) model in the United States in particular is the barrier to entry for many of these types of not-so-radical but highly practical medical interventions. More on this later.

FOOD FIX: SPREAD THE WORD

Change your eating habits for your health's sake and then take this way of eating into your world. Instead of being influenced by your family, your neighborhood, or your workplace, be the influencer.

1. **Try my 10-Day Detox Program.** This program is an elimination-diet program done in community that helps you to reset your body and start to feel unburdened by your chronic symptoms, in just ten days! It will show you how you, too, can start living your best — and just how much food is contributing to chronic symptoms and how quickly they can resolve by a simple change in diet. You can learn more on my website at www.10daydetox.com and bring it to your community center, workplace, neighborhood, or family.

2. **Join a Diabetes-Reversal Program.** Virta Health's online program helps patients reverse diabetes using a ketogenic diet. Within one year, they see a diabetes reversal rate in 60 percent of the participants, with 94 percent reducing or eliminating[47] their primary diabetes medication, insulin, and with an average weight loss of 12 percent, or 30 pounds. These results are rarely seen in medical research, where a 5 percent change (in any variable) is considered success.[48]

What you choose to eat every day is the single most important thing you can do to create health, spread social justice, repair the environment, and reverse climate change. It is not all-or-nothing. Do your best. One bite at a time.

Scan the QR code to learn how to participate in the 10-Day Detox or the Virta Health program.

CHAPTER 3

THE GLOBAL REACH AND DUPLICITY OF BIG FOOD

In the 21st century, the real wealth is in controlling the food supply.
When you control the food, you control the people.

—ATTRIBUTED TO HENRY KISSINGER

The origins of our industrial food system—rooted in mass agriculture and processing—were (I suspect) not born of malice. In the early twentieth century, hunger, starvation, and vitamin deficiencies were rampant, and while food insecurity persists in parts of the world, we've made remarkable strides in combating these crises through the production of abundant, calorie-dense (albeit starchy and processed) foods, fortified with essential nutrients. However, like much of our industrialized world, over the past 50 years, the very food systems that once propelled humanity forward now imperil it. The entrenched methods and products of this agricultural-industrial complex have become a juggernaut, stubbornly resistant to change and clinging to outdated practices out of fear of disrupting profits. What once nourished the world now risks becoming its undoing.

Thus, the modern world faces a paradoxical crisis: overconsumption and undernutrition *coexist*, fueling an epidemic of obesity, chronic disease, and environmental degradation. The destructive agricultural practices that drive environmental destruction now demand a fundamental shift in perspective and application. While consumer demands—especially from millennials valuing sustainability, health, and brand integrity—are spurring rapid innovation in the food and agriculture sectors, vested interests have deployed aggressive and sophisticated misinformation campaigns to undermine these movements. A clear-eyed examination of the food system and the corporations shaping it is critical to identifying both the obstacles and the opportunities for transformative change.

What's worse is that what was once a first-world problem—obesity and chronic disease—has now become a global pandemic. The industrialized diet, arguably the worst on the planet, has migrated worldwide, creating a fast-food footprint that spans six continents. As processed-food sales decline in the United States and Europe,[1] they are skyrocketing in Asia, Africa, and Latin America[2]—by design, not by accident. The globalization of ultraprocessed, industrial food has allowed Big Food and Big Ag to infiltrate local diets, uprooting traditional, nutrient-rich staples that have sustained communities for centuries and replacing them with disease-driving Frankenfoods. From Mexico to Nigeria, India to China, this dietary imperialism is reshaping the world—for the worse.

"Growth is stagnant for global food companies in places like Western Europe and the United States and Japan because they've saturated the market," says Barry Popkin, an expert on global obesity and professor of nutrition at the University of North Carolina at Chapel Hill. "All the profit gain that every global food company sees is in low- and middle-income countries."

Not only are multinational companies pushing aggressively into developing markets, but they are also emphatically presenting their strategy to investors. "Half the world's population has not had a Coke in the last 30 days," Ahmet Bozer, the former president of Coca-Cola International, told a group of investors in 2014. "There's 600 million teenagers who have not had a Coke in the last week. So, the opportunity for that is huge."[3] With a wealth of data showing that soda kills and that sugar is addictive, this type of thinking (in my opinion) is profoundly immoral.

Chains like McDonald's, Burger King, and KFC now have more locations in other countries than they have in the United States. Only a couple of decades ago, Yum! Brands, the parent company of KFC, Pizza Hut, and Taco Bell, derived less than a third of its profits from outside the United States. Today, more than 60 percent of its profits[4] come from outside America. As of 2019, the company had more than 1,000 Pizza Hut and KFC locations in Indonesia, 600 locations in Mexico, and more than 800 fast-food outlets in India.[5] In Ghana, where KFC has a growing presence, obesity rates have increased by 650 percent[6] since 1980.[7] Like the chronic diseases their foods fuel, the American-born fast food complex is spreading across the globe like wildfire and shows no signs of slowing down.

A top company executive told investors at a conference in December 2018 that the company was operating at an unprecedented scale: "We've got 46,000 restaurants. We're opening seven new restaurants a day. In the last 12 months alone, we've got 10,000 more restaurants doing delivery."[8]

This phenomenon has had a dramatic effect: According to the World Health Organization (WHO), the worldwide prevalence of obesity among adults more than doubled between 1990 and 2022, rising from 7 percent to 16 percent.[9] In the same period, the prevalence among children and adolescents aged five to nineteen years quadrupled, increasing from 2 percent to 8 percent.[10] A study[11] published by Imperial College London in 2024 found that the total number of children and adolescents affected by obesity reached nearly 160 million in 2022, compared to 31 million in 1990, a fivefold increase in just 30 years.

In countries such as Vietnam, China, Indonesia, and Brazil, up to two-thirds of households suffer from this dual burden of malnutrition, creating what one report in the *International Journal of Obesity* called "a significant public health concern."[12] The Population Reference Bureau, a nonprofit that works to protect public health and the environment, studied the double burden of disease and found that it was a direct result of steering people in developing nations away from their traditional diets and physically active lifestyles.[13]

Traveling to countries where political barriers have kept Big Food at bay offers a striking contrast. During a recent visit to Cuba, where trade embargoes have long prevented the influx of American corporations, I found a country untouched by fast-food chains and largely free of the ubiquitous influence of major food brands. Obesity is virtually nonexistent. Remarkably, despite spending less than 10 percent per capita of what the United States allocates to health care, Cuba boasts a higher life expectancy. Who could have predicted that decades of international isolation would inadvertently position Cuba as an example of resilience in health outcomes?

BIG FOOD GOES GLOBAL

Food industry marketing in these emerging markets is annoyingly clever and profoundly insidious.

In the Western world, fast food is associated with low socioeconomic status. McDonald's, Burger King, and KFC are not exactly fancy food choices in the bustling metropolises of New York and London. But in lower-income countries, fast-food companies market their brands as "aspirational"—symbols of wealth and status. In China, KFC ads use cosmopolitan young professionals to create the impression that their fried chicken and biscuits can provide a taste of high society.

In addition to slick and manipulative marketing, fast-food chains establish a foothold by catering to local tastes. In Ghana and Nigeria, for example, Domino's Pizza franchises have offered pizza topped with jollof rice—a popular West African staple made with spices, peppers, and onions. Fast-food companies use these local favorites that would otherwise be nutritious and satisfying on their own as a Trojan horse to addict the unsuspecting youth. Travel to China and you could get a dried pork and seaweed doughnut full of sugar and oxidized vegetable oils at Dunkin'.[14] In Japan at one point you could get a giant pizza topped with tuna at Domino's Pizza. Take a trip over to India and you can pick up a veggie burger dripping with melted paneer served alongside a mango lassi (shake) at one of the more than one hundred Burger King locations across the country.

The effects of Big Food's incursions into these countries are clear. India is now known as the diabetes capital of the world, with more than 212 million people suffering from the disease,[15] a near threefold increase[16] since I published the first edition of this book in 2020. One public health watchdog[17] in India described the country as sitting on a volcano of diabetes. This is a country where obesity was unheard of only a couple of decades back. Not long ago, infectious diseases like malaria, pneumonia, and tuberculosis were the leading causes of death in India, but today those infections have been radically eclipsed by the epidemic of heart disease — caused primarily by insulin resistance[18] and obesity[19] — which is now India's number one killer.[20] What is worse is that those infectious diseases haven't gone away.[21] They still kill hundreds of thousands of Indians every year.[22] It's just that now the country's health care system is taxed with grappling with the double burden of infectious and chronic diseases simultaneously.

China is not far behind. Diabetes is spreading so quickly there that some experts say the country cannot build enough hospitals to keep up. When I published the first edition of this book just five years ago, the International Diabetes Federation projected that by 2030 roughly 130 million people in China would have diabetes. The country has now already surpassed that figure, with a current estimate of 148 million[23] suffering from *diagnosed* diabetes. That's more than 1 in 10 people, whereas 30 years ago it was 1 in 150, and that doesn't account for those with pre-diabetes who are trending toward the diagnosis, which is estimated at roughly one-third of the entire population.[24]

The Arab world has also been flooded with soft drinks and processed food. The Middle East and North Africa have the highest increase in diabetes globally;[25] the number of people with the disease is projected to soar more than 95 percent (!) by 2035.[26] In some Arab countries, one in three or four people have type 2 diabetes.[27] In just a couple of decades these populations transformed from a nomadic people with nearly no chronic disease[28] to a people with the fastest increase of obesity and type 2 diabetes in the world.

The unintended consequences of free trade in Mexico (NAFTA)

allowed the American food industry to quickly expand there as purvey-
ors of soda and fast food.[29] Now water costs three times as much as
Coke in Mexico. In the United States one in ten American adults have
type 2 diabetes; in Mexico one in ten *children* have it.

The fast-food pandemic has spread to some surprising places too.
Thailand is well-known for its large population of Buddhist monks,
many of whom follow an age-old tradition of daily intermittent fasting
to protect their health and aid their meditation sessions. But in 2018,
public health experts reported[30] that nearly half of all Buddhist monks
in Thailand are obese and at least 10 percent are diabetic. When
researchers studied the monks' dietary habits, they were initially baf-
fled. The monks generally consume fewer calories than the average
man in Bangkok, and they fast daily. What could be making them so fat
and sick? Then they discovered the problem: The monks tend to sip
soda throughout the day to keep up their energy levels. "When we
really do research about this, we are surprised," the Thai nutritionist
who conducted the study told the Australian Broadcasting Corporation. "It is the drink."[31]

Not long after Thai health experts raised the alarm about the outbreak of obesity among Buddhist monks, the WHO declared that the
home of the world's so-called healthiest diet, the Mediterranean, was
also being ravaged by the spread of ultraprocessed food.[32] Mediterranean countries now have some of the highest rates of obesity in Europe.
In Italy, Spain, Greece, and Cyprus, childhood overweight and obesity
rates have surged past 40 percent.[33] If the birthplace of the world's
healthiest diet is not safe, then no place is—and the food industry is
making sure of that.

ARE OUR BABIES AT RISK?

In the 1980s and 1990s, the infant formula industry came under intense
scrutiny over both the composition and the marketing of their products, particularly concerning the health risks and the aggressive promotion in developing countries.

Infant formulas during this period often contained high levels of processed ingredients, including excessive protein content—sometimes double that of natural breast milk.[34] This imbalance was linked to health issues such as insulin resistance and increased adiposity (body fat accumulation) in infants. Additionally, there were more than twenty recalls of infant formula since 1980 due to contamination with pathogens,[35] adulteration with foreign substances like glass,[36] harmful levels of toxic metals like arsenic (as recently as 2025),[37] and deficiencies in essential nutrients.[38]

Yet companies like Nestlé actively marketed infant formula in low- and middle-income countries, often portraying it as superior to breast milk.[39] Companies continue to promote formula as a superior alternative to breast milk,[40] leading to decreased breastfeeding rates and associated health risks for infants. The promotion of formula in areas lacking clean water and proper sanitation exacerbated health risks, because formula prepared under such conditions heightens the likelihood of infections among infants.

Recent studies have also raised concerns about the nutritional content of infant formulas. A study[41] by the George Institute for Global Health found that none of the infant or toddler food products in Australian supermarkets met the WHO's standards, with more than three-quarters failing to satisfy nutritional requirements due to high sugar and calorie content.

In response to these practices, international boycotts and advocacy campaigns emerged, targeting companies like Nestlé for their predatory marketing strategies. These efforts, in part, facilitated the adoption of the International Code of Marketing of Breast-milk Substitutes by the World Health Assembly in 1981,[42] aiming to regulate the promotion of infant formula and encourage breastfeeding. Despite these measures, insidious marketing of infant formula persists, often exploiting digital media to reach new mothers, thereby continuing to influence infant feeding decisions adversely.

As recently as May 2025, a shocking new study from the University of Kansas revealed that most infant formulas in the United States are loaded with added sugars instead of natural lactose, potentially harming early development and setting infants up for lifelong health risks.[43] I highlighted this to Health and Human Services Secretary Robert F. Kennedy Jr., and he then launched Operation Stork Speed to update regulations on infant formula designed to protect our children. According to the study, infants who are exclusively formula-fed may consume up to 60 grams of added sugar per day—the equivalent of two soft drinks!

Researchers warn that these findings expose the staggering extent to which sugar-laden infant formulas violate federal dietary guidelines—and worse, parents have little to no way of avoiding them. "Most of the formulas that parents and caregivers rely on likely present a substantial risk to infant health and development," the study states. "Caregivers and infants in the U.S. deserve a formula market that promotes healthy development—not one that primes infants for obesity and metabolic disease before they can even walk."[44] This bombshell report raises urgent questions: Why is the United States allowing ultraprocessed, sugar-heavy formulas to flood the market while other countries enforce stricter standards? And why are we setting up our youngest, most vulnerable population for a lifetime of chronic disease?

The legacy of these controversies underscores the need for vigilant regulation and public education to ensure infant health is prioritized over corporate profits.

PLANET FAT: THE FOOD INDUSTRY'S TACTICS

In 2017, the *New York Times* published an investigative series called "Planet Fat" that exposed some of the more brazen and shocking tactics that Big Food is using to uproot traditional diets in its quest to squeeze profits out of developing countries. The series showcased how the world's largest food company, Nestlé (again), recruits thousands of women[45] in some of the lowest-income towns in Brazil to go door-to-door selling candy and processed foods as part of its plan to expand its reach to a quarter million Brazilian households. The series profiled one young woman named Celene da Silva, a twenty-nine-year-old mother of three who sells candy in Fortaleza, where many people do not have access to grocery stores.

From the *New York Times* article:

> As she dropped off variety packs of Chandelle pudding, Kit-Kats and Mucilon infant cereal, there was something striking about her customers: Many were visibly overweight, even small children. She gestured to a home along her route and shook her head, recalling how its patriarch, a morbidly obese man, died the previous week. "He ate a piece of cake and died in his sleep," she said. Mrs. da Silva, who herself weighs more than 200 pounds, recently discovered that she had high blood pressure, a condition she acknowledges is probably tied to her weakness for fried chicken and the Coca-Cola she drinks with every meal, breakfast included.[46]

In Colombia, where soft drinks are cheaper than water, public health advocates were threatened when they pushed for a 20 percent soda tax and produced television commercials warning the public that soft drinks could lead to diabetes. One outspoken anti-soda advocate raced through the streets of Bogotá as food industry strongmen on motorcycles chased her, warning her to keep her mouth shut. Other anti-soda advocates in Latin America accused the industry of tapping their phones and computers with spyware. News outlets that published stories and columns criticizing the soda industry in Colombia faced enormous pressure from the food industry and censorship by the government. Even health groups that tried to run ads warning about the health hazards of soda found themselves censored.[47] The food industry made the government an offer they couldn't refuse, "encouraging" them to pass a law making it illegal to talk about soda taxes in the media or advertising.

"They have threatened advocates in Colombia physically," Popkin told me. "Walking, driving by them and making threats. They have worked their power to ban marketing in a country like Colombia, where you had to take them to court to stop it. They are doing everything they can to stall."

FOOD FIX: TRANSFORMING FOOD LABELS AND REINING IN JUNK-FOOD ADS

Big Food finally met its match in Chile, where more than half of all six-year-olds and three-quarters of adults are overweight or obese.[48] Furious that the country's health care system spends roughly $800 million every year[49] on obesity-related conditions, a doctor from Santiago, Guido Girardi, vowed to take on the food industry by aggressively going after companies' predatory marketing practices. In 2006[50] he was elected to the country's senate and became president of the Chilean Senate's Health Commission, allowing him to spearhead an alliance of nutrition experts to study and gather evidence on the best ways to rein in Big Food. That alliance brought in advisers from around the world, such as Barry Popkin. What did they come up with? A groundbreaking and sweeping new law called Ley de Etiquetado Nutricional y Su Publicidad, which roughly translates to the Food Labeling and Advertising Law. The law combined front-of-package labeling, advertising restrictions, and school policies into a unified national strategy for a relatively comprehensive strategy to combat the Machiavellian goals of Big Food.

The first of its kind worldwide, it set a groundbreaking precedent in public health policy because of its strict and comprehensive approach to regulating food labeling and advertising, the success of which has inspired similar legislation in other countries such as Mexico, Peru, and Uruguay.[51] While there are admittedly some challenges in its approach, the overall effort is revolutionary. Here are some of its major wins:

1. Food companies must display big black warning logos[52] in the shape of a stop sign on processed foods that are high in sugar, salt, saturated fat, or calories. If a food is high in one of these, then it gets a single black warning logo. Packaged foods that are high in all four of these get four warning logos on their labels. While this unduly focuses on factors such as calories, saturated fat, salt, and sugar, which are easy for processed food companies to manipulate (remember "low-fat" SnackWell's cookies?), rather than on overall diet quality and protective food, it is a step in the right direction. But this type of oversimplification, known in the scientific community as *nutritionism,* though well-intentioned, may, in fact, lead to other unintended problems, as we saw with the low-fat revolution that resulted in our current obesity crisis.

2. Strict new limitations have been instituted on food advertisements, especially those aimed at children younger than fourteen.[53] The measure bans the use of cartoon characters to market junk food to kids. Tony the Tiger was removed from Frosted Flakes. Toucan Sam was pulled from boxes of Froot Loops. Candies that use trinkets to lure kids, like Kinder Surprise, were banned. This may be the most important and effective piece of the legislation.

3. There are restrictions on the sale and marketing of junk food to children.[54] No longer can ice cream, potato chips, and chocolate chip cookies be sold in schools or advertised during cartoons or on websites that target kids. Junk-food commercials are banned from television or radio between six a.m. and ten p.m.

4. Food companies must incorporate messages that promote physical activity and healthy eating in their advertisements.[55] Advertising for certain products—particularly those high in sugar, sodium, saturated fats, or calories—must include educational messages to promote balanced diets and physical activity.

All of this came on top of a whopping 18 percent tax on sugary drinks[56]—among the highest in the world. Girardi and his alliance tried to push the sweeping new measures into law but had to overcome ferocious resistance from the food industry, which packed the halls of congress with food lobbyists determined to block it.

For a while, the food industry's lobbying efforts worked. The former Chilean president, Sebastián Piñera, a conservative businessman, vetoed the measure in 2011,[57] offering a hollow alternative: a health initiative financed by Big Food companies that emphasized the importance of exercise and moderation—common talking points of the Big Food apparatchiks. But Girardi and his allies refused to give up. They spent weeks protesting outside Piñera's home, holding cardboard signs accusing him of turning his back on the Chilean people.

"When transnational companies put pressure on Piñera to veto the law, we mobilized," Girardi said in an interview. "I was president of the senate, and I went to the presidential palace with a big sign that said, 'President Piñera is selling out the health of the kids to McDonald's and Coca-Cola.' I was there many days with the sign, and Piñera came out and asked me to leave because it was embarrassing. I said I'm not going to leave until you discuss this law with me. So, he took away the threat of the veto and we began to have a discussion."

In 2014 Piñera was swept out of power and a new president came to power, Michelle Bachelet, a pediatrician and former health minister who was passionate about halting the chronic disease epidemic. Bachelet resisted the food industry's lobbying efforts and in June 2015 approved the new regulations. The government rolled out the changes over the next three years.[58]

Researchers are now studying exactly what impact the measures have had on consumers, but already there's been a sea change in behavior. "Kids are telling their parents, 'Don't buy these foods because the teacher says they're not healthy if they have the black logo,'" Popkin says. "That's norm changing." Popkin was crunching the numbers and in the process of publishing the data in a peer-reviewed journal when I spoke to him. He told me that the results of the regulations are "four-fold in impact of what we've seen on any tax or anything else in the world on sugar-sweetened beverages, let alone junk food and other things. The impact has been amazing."

No wonder the US food lobby works mightily, spending hundreds of millions, to prevent any restrictions on food marketing or labeling by the FDA or the Federal Trade Commission.[59]

Chile's pioneering Food Labeling and Advertising Law has inspired a wave of similar initiatives in Latin America and abroad, including both neighbors of the US—Canada and Mexico. Notably, eight nations in the Americas have adopted policies requiring black "stop sign" warning labels[60] on foods and beverages high in nutrients of health concern, mirroring Chile's approach. One of the most admirable new food-labeling systems is in Israel,[61] where health authorities have created new laws requiring negative warning labels for junk foods and positive logos for nutritious foods like fresh produce, whole grains, and legumes. That may be the best way to get people to purchase more whole foods. Girardi says that it's important to spread these policies because consumers need to be aware about the food choices they're making. How can we be expected to make sound health decisions without being adequately informed?

Even beyond food labeling, the radical new system in Chile that Girardi spearheaded proves that strict regulations and taxation are necessary levers that can force multinational food companies to change — because they will not do it voluntarily. In the United Kingdom, for example, food companies complied with new regulations[62] forcing them to reduce the amount of sodium in their products. But they did not make those same changes to their products in the United States until the New York City Department of Health under Michael Bloomberg required them. It was the same with trans fats: Even though they had the technology to replace these deadly fats with healthier ingredients, many food companies refused to make the change until laws in various countries required them to do so.

In January 2025, the FDA proposed[63] a new rule requiring front-of-package nutrition labels on most packaged foods, aimed at making key nutritional information (like sodium, added sugars, and saturated fats) more visible to consumers. While the initiative appears to be a step forward for public health, a closer examination reveals it could serve as yet another loophole for Big Food to maintain the status quo under the guise of transparency.

Here is why: The proposed labels, which would categorize nutrient levels as "low," "medium," or "high," fail to address the deeper systemic issues within the food industry. By simplifying complex nutritional data into ambiguous categories, the labels risk misleading consumers into thinking that marginally improved processed foods are "healthy" choices. Moreover, the thresholds for these categories—set by the FDA—are likely to be influenced by lobbying efforts from the food industry, enabling companies to market their products as nutritionally sound while still packing them with harmful levels of sugar, salt, and fat. This undermines the very intent of the labels and allows Big Food to perpetuate unhealthy eating habits without meaningful accountability.

Public health advocates also highlight the absence of more stringent labeling requirements for ultraprocessed foods, which are among the biggest drivers of obesity and chronic disease. The new rule focuses narrowly on individual nutrients, ignoring the broader context of highly engineered, addictive products that dominate the US food supply. In addition, by leaving room for voluntary compliance during the initial phases and extended timelines for full implementation, the FDA has handed the food industry ample opportunity to dilute or delay the impact of these regulations.

Ultimately, while the front-of-package labeling proposal is framed as a consumer empowerment tool, it risks becoming little more than a public relations win for the food industry. Without stricter regulations and enforcement mechanisms, the measure may create an illusion of progress while allowing Big Food to evade real reform and continue profiting at the expense of public health.

For a quick reference guide on the Food Fixes and resources on improving our food safety, go to www.foodfixuncensored.com.

CHAPTER 4

THE PRICE OF HEALTH: TACKLING OBESITY AND DISEASE WITH FISCAL POLICY

As we've explored in the first three chapters, the global pandemic of obesity and chronic disease is as much an economic crisis as it is a health one. Warren Buffett famously called rising health care costs the "tapeworm" of American business[1]—and he wasn't wrong.

In just 50 years, health care spending in the United States has ballooned from 5 percent of GDP to nearly 18 percent,[2] which is clearly not working given the health expenditure stats relative to life expectancy (see chart following). At the same time, the cheapest and most accessible foods in most countries are often the ones most likely to make people fat and sick. This economic dynamic is fueling an epidemic of heart disease, diabetes, obesity, dementia, and cancer—the "big five" killers—and fiscal policies will be key to reversing the trend.

Consider the success of tobacco taxes. Once the leading cause of preventable death, smoking has plummeted dramatically thanks to aggressive taxes and public health policies. Today, poor diets have taken tobacco's place as the top preventable killer. A similar approach—like taxing soda—has the power to reshape eating habits and drive down obesity rates, with potentially lifesaving results.

Life Expectancy Vs. Health Expenditure
FROM 1970 TO 2014

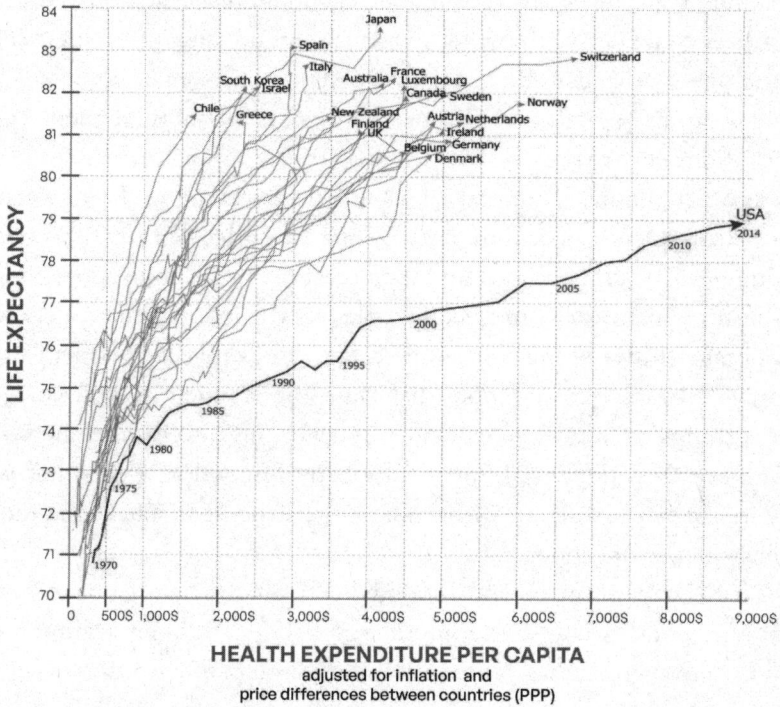

LIFE EXPECTANCY vs. **HEALTH EXPENDITURE PER CAPITA**
adjusted for inflation and
price differences between countries (PPP)

FORCING THEIR HAND

Some of the brightest minds in economics have endorsed the idea of taxes on unhealthy foods. In 2018, Larry Summers, the former treasury secretary and president of Harvard University, joined forces with former New York City mayor Michael Bloomberg and others to launch a global group called the Task Force on Fiscal Policy for Health.[3] Their goal: to advocate for taxes as a solution to rising health care costs and the obesity crisis.

"What I came to realize was that in terms of human betterment in the health care area, there was enormous potential," Summers told me.

"In terms of the impact you could have, even with a limited number of dollars, there was probably no sector more promising than health." Looking at global health through an economic lens, he realized that countries could derive tremendous returns by investing in health, making it one of the best financial investments. "In some contexts, the returns can be as high as 9:1 or even 20:1 in terms of the benefit-cost ratio," Summers says.

As an economist, Summers is a big believer in using the power of prices to influence behavior. First, people are price sensitive. Second, taxing products like tobacco and soda creates a lot of noise about those products, which itself can make people leery of buying them. "Taxes discourage things—and it's better to tax things that we want to discourage, like tobacco and foods that cause obesity and disease, than it is to tax things we want to encourage, like working and saving," he says. "We have evidence that humans rationally respond to prices and we buy less of things when they become more expensive. That's the most basic principle of economics."

That's why Summers and Bloomberg created their organization to advocate for taxes as a way to improve global health. Their argument is that the government has a responsibility to protect the health of its citizens. Taxing junk foods is a great way to do that because, well, it works. Singapore, for example, has long been a leader in using fiscal policy to shape public health and social behavior. Its taxation system on "vice" goods—products like tobacco and alcohol—is a prime example of how strategic economic levers can drive healthier choices. These taxes are designed not only to generate revenue but also to curb consumption of goods that harm public health. These tax policies are complemented by public awareness campaigns that educate citizens on the health risks associated with these products, reinforcing the behavioral shift.

Combined with incentives for healthy food, or innovations in market-based solutions and tax code incentives, it is a proven way to boost public health outcomes and reduce health care costs. How do we know? Well, if it didn't, then the soda industry wouldn't spend hundreds of millions of dollars fighting such taxes: Whenever a soda tax is proposed, the beverage industry mobilizes significant resources to oppose it.[4] Their significant financial opposition underscores their concern that soda taxes could substantially impact profits. "The fact that the food industry objects so strongly is confirmation that these taxes are effective and have significant and meaningful impacts—and if they didn't change the demand for their products, the food industry wouldn't care," Summers says.

One of the main criticisms against soda taxes is that they are regressive, causing a disproportionate impact on low- and middle-income families. This is a primary talking point for the soda industry. Some politicians have embraced it as well. The thing about junk-food taxes is that they are indeed regressive: People with low income pay a higher share of their income in taxes. But they also suffer a larger share of the adverse health consequences. "So, the benefits, in terms of reduced health care spending, in terms of longer life expectancy, and general well-being, will be disproportionately felt by the poor," Summers says. "So, I'm completely comfortable with the idea that we should put a universal tax on sugary foods, recognizing that it may indeed be socially regressive, but that it will be offset in other ways."

Admittedly, taxes on bad food need to be combined with incentives and price reductions on healthy foods for this taxing to benefit everyone. The revenue generated from these taxes must be paired with incentives that support cheaper prices for consumers, business incentives for research and development, and marketing and distribution of protective, healing foods. This is important to avoid unintentionally driving lower-income or price-sensitive individuals toward other forms of engineered Frankenfoods that bypass the limits on certain ingredients by replacing them with something worse (like we did when we replaced saturated fat with deadly trans fats, which are fortunately now banned).

All in all, when money is used to uplift underserved communities with social programs, support for education, and more, as was done with the Philadelphia soda and sweetened beverage tax[5]—which so far has provided $500 million[6] to fund universal pre-K, public schools, and recreation centers—soda taxes gain wide acceptance and give back to those most affected. Some soda lovers have crossed over to Delaware to buy non-taxed soda, but the net decrease in consumption, the community and health benefits, and the reduction in health care costs outweigh any downsides.

THE PARTNERSHIP OF TAXES AND SUBSIDIES IN SAN FRANCISCO

In 2010, Laura Schmidt, a professor of health policy at the University of California, San Francisco (UCSF) medical school, was working on a program to improve health in underserved Bay Area communities. Schmidt had previously worked on alcohol addiction but switched her focus to sugar when she discovered that one of the leading causes of liver transplants in America is not alcoholism but sugar and its consequences, obesity and diabetes: "Nonalcoholic fatty liver disease" (which, since I published the OG version of this book in 2020, has been renamed "metabolic dysfunction–associated steatotic liver disease" to better represent the cause, which didn't exist decades ago). Schmidt knew that the way to tackle the country's sugar addiction was to use some of the same tactics that worked on alcohol, such as taxes and warning labels.

With Schmidt's help, the city of San Francisco took aggressive action on sugary drinks. It introduced a penny-per-ounce soda tax,[7] passed an ordinance slapping health warnings on soft drink advertisements (which ultimately was defeated by a massive beverage industry lawsuit against the city of San Francisco claiming the warnings violated "free speech"), and banned the use of city funds to pay for sugary drinks. But the city did something else remarkable. It used the roughly $15 million in annual revenue[8] brought in by the soda tax to help pay for nutritious school meals made with locally grown produce and to install water hydration stations in schools and public buildings. An additional portion of the money was then used to subsidize healthy eating vouchers for low-income San Franciscans.[9] Thanks to Schmidt and her colleagues in the public health community, San Francisco installed one hundred brand-new water stations in parks and other public locations, mainly targeting low-income neighborhoods.[10]

The insights taught Schmidt and her colleagues a valuable lesson. Much like the reform of the Supplemental Nutrition Assistance Program (SNAP), it is not enough to ban or discourage bad foods. We also have to create incentives or subsidies that encourage people to consume the right foods (or drinks) too.

"We realized that if the city is going to tax soda, put warning labels on it and stop selling it themselves, then what are people without access to clean water going to do?" she said. "How can we help them? And do we really want people buying more bottled water? Wouldn't it be better to have them drinking safe, clean tap water?

"Taxes are regressive," she added. "And so, I think it's kind of ethical, if you're going to pass a tax, that you provide people with a healthy and free (or at least, affordable) substitute. Don't make people pay the jacked-up prices on bottled water (which itself faces health scrutiny due to the phthalates and 'forever chemicals' in the plastics). That to me is the ideal soda tax: You take some of the proceeds and you roll them into providing people with clean water."

Hospitals, Schools, and Public Institutions as Soda-Free Zones

Thankfully, Schmidt did not stop there. As she was leaving a lecture on sugar and disease at UCSF one day, she walked by a food court at the medical center and noticed one obese person after another guzzling soda. The imagery struck her. Here she was, a public health expert warning people about the dangers of sugar, and yet her own institution was profiting from the sale of sugary drinks to sick patients and their families. "I thought to myself, 'I feel like a total hypocrite, this is disgusting,'" she said.

Schmidt had spent years working on policies that governments could enact to promote healthy behaviors. But she realized that workplaces, private institutions, medical centers, and universities could do a lot. So, in 2015, Schmidt and her colleagues at UCSF pressed the school's chancellor to stop selling sugar-sweetened beverages on the campus. It was a seemingly herculean task since UCSF is one of the largest employers in San Francisco, with more than 24,000 workers on a sprawling campus that extends across the city.[11] But the university found the policy surprisingly simple to execute. The school's beverage supplier simply started stocking the university cafeterias, vending machines, gift shops, conference rooms, and stores with water and zero-calorie beverages instead of soda. Even fast-food chains on the campus, like Subway and Panda Express, agreed to swap out sugar-laden beverages with healthier options. The initiative led to a 48 percent reduction in soda consumption[12] and an improvement in weight, cholesterol, and metabolic markers of pre-diabetes.

BUT...ARE WE JUST CREATING A NANNY STATE?

Anytime a city or country tries to impose a soda tax, the beverage industry bombards the public with pamphlets, billboards, and commercials telling people to reject this so-called nanny state. It's an argument that my friend Dr. Aseem Malhotra, one of the most influential cardiologists in England and now a leading food industry watchdog, has thought long and hard about. I asked him to explain why the food industry's favorite talking point is fatally flawed.

"When you talk about nanny states, this is a term that's used [in my view] as propaganda," Dr. Malhotra says. "It's used by people that want to keep perpetuating the status quo where they're benefiting and profiting from regulations that are so weak that they can mislead the people into buying products that ultimately cause them harm."

But what, exactly, do nannies do? They protect children—who lack the information, experience, or autonomy to make decisions in their best interest. While we don't want to infantilize our citizens, treating them as incapable of discernment, we must confront a deeper truth: Government and corporate policies largely shape the choices people make. When pricing, availability, and marketing are designed to steer consumers toward unhealthy options, true agency is an illusion. In such a system, protecting public health is not overreach—it's responsibility.

We have mandatory seat belt laws, mandatory vaccinations, mandatory car seats for children, and other public health measures. How is this any different? When the government proposed mandatory seat belt laws decades ago, the car industry vehemently opposed the idea. Carmakers were also against mandatory airbags and fuel emissions standards. These were all "nanny state" ideas, they cried. But now that we've had these safety measures in place for a while, the public has grown accustomed to them and the car industry is doing just fine. We accept these as reasonable regulations because they are good for society. They save lives and protect the environment. It's the same with smoking. Many critics of public smoking bans have now come around to the idea that less smoking is a net positive for society.

"I think as awareness grows, then this nanny state argument will not stand up, and politicians will respond to the public," Dr. Malhotra says. "The way the public gets their information is also the media. Mass media has a huge impact on public opinion. We really need to engage journalists and editors so these discussions can be heard. We can't keep this information from the public."

Historically this has been challenging because mainstream media is mostly supported by Big Business ads, making it hard for them to do true muckraking journalism, but with the rise in citizen and independent journalism along with long-form, nuanced podcasting, we are finally able to unlock true, honest investigative journalism again. I have been personally told by anchors at CBS and CNN that they were prohibited from covering these issues because their advertisers were almost all junk food and pharmaceutical companies. Thanks to the courageous efforts of media warriors like Bari Weiss at the Free Press, heavy hitters like Joe Rogan, and other crusaders like them, we are finally able to hear the real motivations behind these types of Big Business propaganda campaigns.

Proposed Policy Solutions

In 2018, Dr. Malhotra proposed a bold new plan that could reverse the diabetes crisis in three years. He created it with two other highly respected public health experts: Dr. Robert Lustig, a pediatric endocrinologist at UCSF, and Professor Grant Schofield from the Auckland

University of Technology in New Zealand.[13] Here are some of the controversial but potentially extremely effective solutions they proposed:

- Education for the public should emphasize that there is no biological need for or nutritional value of added sugar. The food industry should be forced to label added or processed sugars in food products in teaspoons rather than grams, making it easier for the public to understand. If a can of soda says it contains 39 grams of sugar, do people really understand that it has almost 10 teaspoons of sugar? I certainly wasn't aware that roughly 4 grams of sugar is equal to 1 teaspoon until I started working in the space. Labels like these are *designed* to obfuscate the truth and confuse consumers.

- Companies that make sugary products should be banned from sponsoring sporting events, and we should encourage celebrities in the entertainment industry and professional athletes to publicly dissociate themselves from sugary product endorsements. Examples of star athletes who have already done this include Indian cricketer Virat Kohli,[14] basketball star Steph Curry,[15] football legend Tom Brady,[16] and singer Beyoncé.

- Sugary drink taxes should extend to sugary foods as well.

- There should be a complete ban on ads for sugary drinks (including fruit juice) on TV and internet on-demand services.

- Government food subsidies should be reduced for commodity crops such as corn turned into sugar, which contributes to health detriments, and the delta in subsidies should be reallocated to farmers growing "specialty crops" (healthy produce). This is because subsidies distort the market and increase the costs of nonsubsidized crops, making healthy food unaffordable for many.

- New policies should be implemented to prevent all professional dietetic organizations from accepting money or endorsing companies that market processed foods. Alternatively, if they do, they should not be allowed to claim that their dietary advice is independent.

- Healthy eating and physical activity should be split into separate and independent public health goals. Avoiding a sedentary lifestyle through the promotion of physical activity to prevent chronic diseases is necessary for all ages and sizes. But it is important to remember that "you can't outrun a bad diet." You have to walk roughly four miles to burn off one 20-ounce soda. Physical activity is often perceived as an alternative solution to obesity based on the idea of calories in, calories out. But the reality is that the quality of calories matters more than the quantity. Sugar and broccoli calories are not the same inside your body. A Big Gulp with 750 calories of sugar has profoundly different effects on your metabolism and your essential bodily functions than the same caloric value in broccoli. You may have heard of the concept of "energy balance," also known as the "calorie hypothesis of weight gain," which is effectively the idea that weight gain (or loss) is a simple mathematical equation of the ratio of calories consumed relative to those expended. Under this theory, weight gain = more calories consumed than expended, and weight loss = more calories expended than consumed. But this theory ignores the metabolic complexity of the dynamic human system, and it unnecessarily pits two independently healthy behaviors against each other. To relieve the burden of nutrition-related disease, we need to improve our diets, not just depend on physical activity. Big Food focuses on exercise, moderation, and energy balance as the solution. This essentially blames the victim, implying that you have obesity because you eat too much and don't exercise enough; in other words, obesity results from being a lazy glutton. In the face of the science that all calories are not the same, and that ultraprocessed foods hijack your brain chemistry and metabolism, this is utter and unproven nonsense.

FOOD FIX: TAX JUNK FOODS

As outlined above, one powerful way to influence food prices is through fiscal incentives—tax breaks, subsidies, or other financial rewards used to encourage or discourage certain behaviors. Right now, we dole out these incentives to companies that spend billions marketing junk food to children and low-income communities. Maybe it's time to stop handing out tax breaks to industry lobbyists and companies that spend billions advertising obesity- and disease-causing ultraprocessed food to children and low-income communities. We should eliminate those tax breaks and instead use that money to produce and increase the availability of healthy foods. A policy to end tax breaks for harmful practices has already been proposed in Congress, but it has stalled in committee. The Food Is Medicine Working Group needs to repackage it into a new bill that rebalances the price structure of junk and healthy foods. It wouldn't raise income taxes—rather, it would only apply to specific items like soda, chips, fast food, and candy.

Taxes on unhealthy foods could fund subsidies for nutritious options, making the policy cost-neutral. Right now, the devastating consequences of our food system—for chronic disease, children's health, and the climate—are completely absent from the price tags at the grocery store, restaurants, or fast-food chains. It's time to change that and ensure the real costs are reflected in what we pay.

In an ideal world, every government should institute a junk-food tax of some kind, and sugar-sweetened drinks are the logical place to start. Sugary drinks are clearly not the sole cause of obesity, but they represent the largest source of added sugars in the modern diet,[17] and they have a disproportionate impact on obesity, diabetes, and heart disease. The revenue that such taxes would bring could be mandated to fill budget shortfalls or to pay for important public services like pre-kindergarten and after-school programs and other community benefits. Soda taxes are the low-hanging fruit for policymakers who understand that we have to do something about our out-of-control health care costs.

The evidence is clear: Soda taxes work. Multiple studies[18] and nationwide experiments have proven their effectiveness in reducing consumption, making it imperative for governments worldwide to consider implementing them. Whether at the national level or through provinces, states, and municipalities, soda taxes can play a transformative role in public health. The most impactful approach is a tiered soda tax, which taxes beverages based on their sugar content. Under this model, drinks with lower sugar levels face lower taxes, while the most sugar-laden products are taxed at the highest rate.

This strategy is far superior to a flat tax, which unfairly applies the same rate to a kombucha with 4 grams of sugar as it does to a Pepsi with 41 grams. Studies[19] show that tiered taxes face less opposition because they incentivize innovation, they encourage companies to reformulate products to avoid the highest tax brackets, and of course, they benefit consumers by reducing unconscious sugar consumption. It's a rare win-win scenario: The public gets healthier choices, and the industry is nudged toward producing better products.

According to the World Bank's Global Sugar-Sweetened Beverage Tax Database, as of August 2023, there are 132 sugar-sweetened beverage taxes in effect (a fivefold increase from when I published the first edition of this book in 2020), including 119 national-level taxes across 117 countries and territories, covering approximately 57 percent of the world's population.[20]

The impact on reducing consumption and forcing Big Food to reduce sugar in its products has been significant. In 2017, Saudi Arabia enacted one of the strictest policies in the world, with a 50 percent tax on soft drinks and a 100 percent tax on energy drinks.[21] The United Arab Emirates did the same thing. To combat these taxes, the CEO of Red Bull called the UAE government, complaining that sales were down 70 percent. But since corporations have no ability to lobby these governments and these countries receive no tax revenue from those businesses, their protests are largely ignored. Following suit, India imposed a 40 percent tax on sugary drinks in 2017.[22] The Philippines passed a tax on drinks containing caloric and noncaloric sweeteners in 2017, but those made with high-fructose corn syrup are taxed at double the rate of other drinks.[23]

Mexico is perhaps the most powerful example of why we need more soda taxes. The country holds the dubious distinction of being one of the world's largest consumers of soft drinks (the former president, Vicente Fox, was previously the head of Coca-Cola for all Latin America), so it's no surprise that it has one of the highest obesity rates. Yet in

2014, the Mexican government enacted a 10 percent tax on sugary drinks, and a 5 percent tax on junk foods. Researchers found that after just one year, sales of soft drinks plunged 12 percent while sales of bottled water climbed 4 percent (the increase in water consumption was likely much greater because the study didn't look at tap water intake).[24] The findings provided the first hard evidence that such taxes do, in fact, nudge people in the right direction. Later studies also revealed some encouraging trends. The greatest reductions in soda intake occurred among low-income Mexicans and in households with children. One study in the *Journal of Nutrition* found a 16.2 percent jump in water purchases among low- and middle-income households.[25] If that data weren't impressive enough, a study in the journal *PLOS Medicine* estimated that over the course of a decade the tax could help save almost 19,000 lives, prevent close to 200,000 new cases of diabetes, and lower Mexico's health care costs by as much as $983 million![26]

The United States doesn't have a federal soda tax. But 117 countries do,[27] and more than a half dozen US cities and counties across the country have instituted soda taxes on their own—and more are expected. Upon the institution of the first city-wide soda tax, in 2015, researchers at the University of California, Berkeley, found that soda consumption in low-income Berkeley neighborhoods fell by more than 20 percent and water intake jumped significantly.[28] Philadelphia followed, imposing a soda tax in 2017 for both sugar-sweetened and artificially sweetened drinks, and saw that soft drink intake dropped significantly among low-income children.[29]

FOOD FIX: SUBSIDIZE HEALTHY ALTERNATIVES

The oft-ignored truth is that the price tag on most foods is a lie—it doesn't come close to reflecting their true cost to society. Crop subsidies, sugar tariffs, tax breaks, and dirt-cheap corn syrup make it possible for a can of Pepsi to sell for less than $1. But the real price? Trillions of dollars in taxpayer-funded health care costs for obesity, diabetes, and metabolic diseases. The fallout doesn't stop there: The industrial production of corn syrup and ultraprocessed foods is wrecking our soil, polluting our air and water, and driving climate change. So why do we accept this? Why don't we demand that the true costs of these foods — on our health and planet — be reflected in their price?

Imagine flipping the script on our food system: impose a 20 to 30 percent tax on packaged and processed junk, and funnel that money into subsidizing truly nutritious, minimally processed foods. Suddenly, instead of paying 99 cents for a 36-ounce soda, you'd pay 20 cents for an apple or orange. That $15 wild salmon at Whole Foods? It could be yours for $4 or $5. Organic, grass-fed beef, chicken, and eggs would finally be affordable.

The revenue from junk-food taxes should be used to make healthy food more affordable while supporting farmers, not driving them out of business. Price is an absolutely crucial tool in shaping behavior. Just look at tobacco taxes — they've shown us how effective pricing can be in driving healthier choices. The government has the power to use price as a lever to make nutritious food accessible and address the root causes of our public health crisis.

It's time to stop normalizing cheap junk and start building a food system that prioritizes health, affordability, and sustainability.

FOOD FIX: DEMAND SODA-FREE ZONES

Just as we did with smoking, we can create soda-free zones. Public and private institutions across the country — and the world for that matter — are now showing how this can be done. More than thirty medical centers[30] and universities in the United States alone have stopped selling sugary beverages. Many have also implemented policies to make clean drinking water and healthy foods more available.

In 2018 the Geisinger Medical Center in Pennsylvania, which provides health care to thousands of patients, eliminated sugar-sweetened beverages, removed deep fryers, and started limiting sodium and using locally grown fruits and vegetables in its meals. The Indiana University Health system removed sugary beverages[31] and deep fryers and made healthy food options less expensive. It also began marking foods with a color-coding system, showing red, yellow, and green to help people identify the healthiest options.

The Hospital Healthier Food Initiative, which the Partnership for a Healthier America launched, says that at least 700 hospitals nationwide have committed to serving more nutritious patient meals, implementing stricter cafeteria standards, and selling more fruits, vegetables, water, and other healthy foods on their campuses.[32] As one of the first back in 2010, the Cleveland Clinic removed sugar-laden drinks from its campus, prioritizing offering healthier food options.[33]

Many large companies are transforming their food environments to promote healthier workplaces. Services like SnackNation make it easy for businesses to swap out junk food for better options, offering snacks like fresh fruits, nuts, seeds, trail mix, and low-carb protein bars. Another great example is Farmer's Fridge, which provides fresh, wholesome meals like salads, grain bowls, and wraps through smart fridges placed in offices. These initiatives not only support employee health but also foster a culture of wellness that benefits both individuals and organizations.

For a quick reference guide on the Food Fixes and resources on how you can demand clean foods, go to www.foodfixuncensored.com.

PART II

THE DIRTY POLITICS OF BIG FOOD

If I had to sum up America's food policies in one word, it would be "chaos"—and if I could use two, they would be "unmitigated disaster."

Our food system is governed by eight different agencies with 200 departments, each operating in its own silo, rarely communicating, almost never collaborating on shared objectives, and mostly working at cross-purposes. The result? A tangled web of confused, conflicting, and often outright contradictory policies. One agency might be promoting healthier diets while another is subsidizing the very crops used to create ultraprocessed junk. It's not just inefficient—it's sabotaging our health, our economy, and our future. It's systemic failure on a national scale.

On top of that, most of our food and agriculture policies undermine public health and harm the environment, all to pander to corporations whose sole goal is to increase private profits. Through corporate lobbying efforts, the food industry hijacked some of our most important food programs, profiting from sickness and disease and environmental malfeasance—and it sticks you, the taxpayer, with the bill. It's borderline criminal.

Big Food companies claim to be good stewards of public health. They argue that obesity is a complex issue and that they have an important role to play in addressing it. Engaging government agencies and working on policy issues is a critical part of this effort, they say. But food companies have a much more insidious motive. The real reason they spend so much money in Washington is so they can block policies that hurt their bottom lines and promote policies that make them money. Food corporations have to answer to their shareholders; they have a fiduciary responsibility to maximize shareholder profits, and they pursue this mission zealously—regardless of whether the outcomes are harmful to society and the environment or not.

Our nation's disjointed food policies are driving a disease-creating economy (not to mention climate change, social inequities, and a host of other "externalities"), and most people have no idea.

CHAPTER 5

HOW BIG FOOD AND BIG AG CONTROL FOOD POLICY

In February 2017,[1] not long after Donald Trump was sworn into office, the members of the House Committee on Agriculture convened a hearing on Capitol Hill to address a controversial issue: Should the government stop people from using food stamps to pay for soft drinks and other junk foods? Two months prior to the congressional hearing, the federal government released a report showing that approximately $7 billion[2] worth of food stamps is spent on sugary beverages every year.[3] That's 20 to 30 billion servings of soda a year that we give to low-income households.[4] Seventy-five percent of the foods purchased with Supplemental Nutrition Assistance Program (SNAP) funds are ultra-processed junk food:[5] Oreo cookies, Lay's potato chips, ice cream, and more. It's no surprise that studies show that people who use SNAP have high rates of heart disease, diabetes, and, therefore, premature death compared to the rest of the population.[6]

While Uncle Sam can't force anyone to eat fruits and veggies, the government can at least make sure that taxpayer dollars aren't used to subsidize the Frankenfoods that are driving the belt-popping rates of obesity and chronic disease.

For many nutrition experts, the central question of the hearing was a no-brainer, but due to the influence of Big Food's money in politics, making positive change is never easy.

TIME TO PRIORITIZE NUTRITION QUALITY, NOT JUST *QUANTITY*

The government created SNAP in 1964 to help malnourished Americans. Today the program is a crucial safety net that helps low-income families put food on their tables and avoid hunger and food insecurity. It does a great job at doing exactly that.

But while the health of those on SNAP is better than the health of those who are eligible but have not signed on, the barometer for their health is dangerously low.

Today, SNAP is the country's largest food assistance program, providing benefits to more than 42 million low-income Americans each month (12.6 percent of the US population),[7] at a cost to taxpayers of more than a hundred billion dollars a year (in 2021, it peaked at $125 billion).[8] SNAP beneficiaries cut across all races and age-groups. Roughly 36 percent of them are white, 25 percent are Black American (though they make up only 12 percent of the population), 17 percent are Hispanic, and about 4 percent are Asian or Native American, while the rest are unknown.[9] Millions are veterans, seniors, or people with disabilities. Almost one in two SNAP recipients is a child.[10]

While SNAP is undeniably a vital anti-hunger and anti-poverty tool, it is also a system in desperate need of reform. It has inarguably succeeded in addressing calorie deficiencies for more than 40 million Americans, but it has utterly failed to solve the deeper problem of nutritional poverty. It provided *food security* (enough calories), but not *nutrition security* (enough nutrients). The reality is that America's lowest-income households aren't struggling with a lack of calories—they're drowning in cheap, empty, disease-causing ones.

Thanks to taxpayer-funded subsidies for corn, soy, and grains, junk food is more affordable than ever, flooding low-income communities with ultraprocessed, nutrient-devoid calories. SNAP has inadvertently become a conveyor belt for the very foods driving the obesity and chronic disease epidemics. One study[11] by Harvard found that SNAP participants consume 61 percent more sweetened drinks, 56 percent more potatoes, and 46 percent more processed red meat—while eating 39 percent fewer whole grains—compared to nonparticipants at the same income level. Children in SNAP households were found to consume staggering amounts of empty calories, sugary drinks, and processed meats.

The Farm Bill, which funds SNAP, spends billions subsidizing cheap calories but fails to invest in nutrient-rich foods that could actually protect public health. Despite being the largest and most expensive component[12] of the Farm Bill, SNAP hasn't protected its recipients from the ravages of obesity, type 2 diabetes, and other diet-related diseases. Instead, it perpetuates the cycle of poor nutrition among our most vulnerable populations.

This isn't just a policy failure—it's a public health crisis hiding in plain sight. If we truly want to help America's neediest, it's time to overhaul SNAP and ensure it delivers not just food—but real, life-sustaining nutrition.

BIG FOOD TARGETS THE VULNERABLE

Why do SNAP recipients eat so poorly? The answer lies in the ruthless precision of Big Food's marketing machine. Grocery stores and food companies know exactly when SNAP benefits are distributed, and they pounce. A 2018 study[13] in the *American Journal of Preventive Medicine* found that in low-income New York neighborhoods, shoppers were two to four times more likely to encounter soda displays and sugary drink ads during the first week of the month—the very week food stamps are issued. Ads for healthier, low-calorie drinks "coincidentally" didn't spike. Notably, wealthier neighborhoods, with fewer SNAP recipients, saw no such surge in junk-food promotions. The implication is glaringly obvious: Big Food targets low-income Americans with junk, and it's not by accident—it's by design.

Why target SNAP recipients with soda and chips instead of fresh produce? Simple: profit. Sugary beverages and ultraprocessed junk carry massive profit margins compared to fruits, vegetables, meats, and seafood. As David Ludwig, Harvard obesity expert, puts it, "Sugary beverages are incredibly profitable. They're heavily advertised, placed at the front of the store, and put on sale—specifically aimed at SNAP recipients." Big Food and retailers aren't just fueling (and feeding) a public health crisis—they're directly, and occasionally deliberately, profiting from it, exploiting our nation's poor for the sake of their bottom line. It's calculated, predatory, and shameful.

Almost every other government food program—from school lunches to military food programs to WIC (the Special Supplemental Nutrition Program for Women, Infants, and Children)—has at least *some* nutrition standards. But SNAP has none. And it's created a huge economic and public health catastrophe. A 2017 study[14] by researchers from Tufts examined almost half a million adults over the span of a decade and found that SNAP participants had substantially worse health than other Americans: twice the rate of heart disease, three times greater likelihood to die from diabetes, and higher rates of metabolic diseases.[15] SNAP beneficiaries account for at least 61 percent of the adults on Medicaid and 13 percent of people on Medicare.[16] The math is pretty simple: Providing healthy and nutritious foods to SNAP recipients would reduce chronic disease rates and sharply lower health care costs. It would benefit the millions of people who depend on SNAP and ultimately save taxpayers billions or potentially even trillions of dollars in downstream healthcare costs.

The federal government has a duty to set nutrition standards for the food stamps program, which it ignores. Increasing access to healthier foods and removing obvious junk foods from the program would reduce obesity and diabetes rates and dramatically lower health care costs. As David Ludwig puts it, "We've allowed SNAP, due to food industry lobbying and neglect, to become a conveyor belt of terribly unhealthful calories. With modest reforms, we can continue to address the important problem of hunger in the United States and at the same time help reduce diet-related chronic diseases that are devastating low-income communities."

POLITICAL SWAY

To give you an idea of how challenging it can be to introduce even modest reforms into public programs like SNAP, let's go back to the 2017 hearing of the House Agriculture Committee, which oversees the roughly $1.5 trillion Farm Bill over a decade, including SNAP. Some on the panel of food and poverty experts at the hearing argued that eliminating sugary drinks from the program was a badly needed measure that could improve the health of millions of Americans, sharply reducing health care costs in the process. Other experts who opposed them said the restrictions would stigmatize SNAP users and create too much red tape. "Confusion at the checkout aisle," they cried.[17] This is a specious argument because SNAP already limits certain purchases, such as certain energy drinks,[18] alcohol, and hot foods. Every checkout clerk knows what's covered and what's not...plus the government publishes a list.[19]

But the most striking comments came from the lawmakers themselves. One by one, dozens of congressmen and -women took turns dismissing the link between junk-food diets and obesity. Republican Congressman Roger Marshall, an obstetrician from Kansas, said a lack of exercise was the primary factor driving obesity rates. Then Democratic Congressman David Scott from Georgia took the floor and attacked what he called the "food police."[20] Preventing SNAP recipients from using their food stamps to pay for Mountain Dew, Coke, and Oreo cookies was not only impossible,[21] he argued, but practically a violation of their constitutional rights as well. He ignored the fact that other government programs enforce nutrition standards without violating constitutional rights, such as school lunches and the aforementioned WIC program.

"Look at the complexity you are going to put into the grocery store. Who is going to pick up that extra cost to have the food police there monitoring, and why?"[22] he barked indignantly. "I mean, the solution here is obvious: We need to educate people, not infringe on their freedoms! You can't force them. You can't deny them their freedoms to be able to make choices without violating their pursuit of happiness." Ah yes, the pursuit of happiness—brought to you by Coca-Cola. Because clearly, nothing says "inalienable rights" quite like a 36-ounce soda. Somehow, I don't think that's what Jefferson envisioned when drafting the Declaration of Independence.

Congressman Scott then made a series of claims even though decades of research on diet and exercise contradicted him. "Sodas, candy, sweet things—that's not what makes us obese. It is the lack of our children exercising," he insisted. "Look at the history of this country. Look at us thirty years ago, twenty years ago. What has happened? Our children, and us, we don't exercise. We don't have physical education in the schools anymore."

Scott's argument was a masterful attempt to distract attention from the real issue, America's diet, and shift the blame onto exercise. Of course, exercise is part of the obesity problem and is an integral component in the whole health picture, but as I've shouted for years, you simply cannot exercise your way out of a bad diet. It sounded as if Scott's statements had been taken straight from the food industry's playbook—and that was no coincidence. Lobbying reports show that Big Food companies and their deep-pocketed trade groups routinely shower the members of the House Agriculture Committee with campaign contributions and political gifts. Guess who is a top recipient. Congressman Scott.

If lawmakers were required to wear the logos of their corporate sponsors, Scott would look like a NASCAR driver sponsored by Big Food. Since 2006, Coca-Cola has given him more than $42,000 in direct financial donations. The company was his single largest campaign contributor in 2018, followed closely by the National Confectioners Association, the biggest trade and lobbying group for the candy industry.[23] Scott took an additional $105,000 from an influential political action committee, the Blue Dog PAC, which is funded by a roster of food industry giants that includes Coke, Pepsi, the American Beverage Association, Dunkin' Brands (the parent company of Dunkin' Donuts), and the Grocery Manufacturers Association, the largest food industry lobbying group (now relaunched as the Consumer Brands Association).

Scott wasn't the only one at the hearing who benefited. Top contributors to Congressman Roger Marshall were sugar industry giants Archer Daniels Midland and American Crystal Sugar, two of the country's largest sugar producers.[24] (In an interesting plot twist, however, Roger Marshall is now the senator who heads up the MAHA Caucus in the Senate, which indicates that he's changed his tune. The tide has started to shift in Congress as legislators heed public pressure to address our broken food system.) The sugar industry was a top contributor to both the chair of the House Agriculture Committee, Frank Lucas, and the committee's ranking member, Collin Peterson.[25] In total, the forty-six members of Congress who make up the House Agriculture Committee took roughly $1.2 million in campaign contributions from the soda and sugar industries between 2015 and 2018.[26] While the hearing was full of theatrics, it ended with a collective shrug from Congressman Scott and the other members of the committee, who decided not to implement any junk-food restrictions on SNAP. Congress: bought and sold. Government of the corporations, by the corporations, and for the corporations.

The food industry is no fool. Junk-food companies are acutely aware that sugary-drink restrictions on SNAP would wipe away billions of dollars of their annual revenue. So behind closed doors, their lobbyists have worked closely with lawmakers and government officials to stop that from ever happening. Many anti-hunger groups (which are funded in large part by the food industry) and national food banks, like the Food Research and Action Center, have also used their political influence to resist efforts to ban sugary drinks from SNAP.[27] SNAP is just one of many government food policies that suffer from a systemic problem. Instead of prioritizing public health and the interests of society, lawmakers and government agencies are often forced to do the bidding of Big Food. That explains why the $7 billion question at the heart of that 2017 hearing on SNAP and sugary drinks was decided long before the hearing even began.

Big corporate lobbying is so effective in part because it fills a gap in Congress's bandwidth. Lawmakers juggle countless issues across diverse sectors, leaving them (understandably) too distracted to dive deep into the weeds of every piece of legislation. Lobbyists step in, offering ready-made research, expertise, and even language for bills, which can seem like a lifeline to overworked congressional staff.

The problem? These "helpful" resources are written with corporate interests in mind, often prioritizing profits over public health. In theory, the health movement could provide a counterbalance, offering the same level of guidance and advocacy for policies that benefit people, not corporations. But unlike promoting Big Food or Big Pharma, promoting public health isn't lucrative—there's little profit in pushing for broccoli subsidies or banning junk-food ads. And without those counterforces, corporate lobbyists dominate the narrative, steering policy away from what's truly best for the public.

The truth is, Big Food wields so much power that even a modest attempt to improve public health through SNAP reform has been swiftly crushed. Through my advocacy in Washington, I have supported Republican Congressman Andy Harris in an effort to introduce a simple pilot program to address the glaring health crisis among SNAP recipients—40 percent of whom are obese,[28] and nearly 45 percent of whom suffer from diet-related diseases,[29] rates far higher than are found in the general population. The proposal was straightforward: limit SNAP purchases of junk food like soda and candy, and incentivize healthier options like fruits and vegetables.

As chairman of the House Appropriations Subcommittee on Agriculture, Harris championed this effort,[30] pushing for measures to ensure SNAP funds were used for nutrient-dense foods rather than disease-driving processed products. A small-scale trial,[31] involving just one hundred participants in five states, was proposed to evaluate the impact. But before it even began, the food and beverage industry unleashed its lobbying machine to kill the initiative. What's striking is that this trial wasn't even designed to change policy; it was simply to *study* the impact in a small group of people to inform future policy. The good news is that as of 2025, many states[32] have asked for SNAP waivers to implement reforms to SNAP to incentivize healthier food purchases and disincentivize the purchase of soda and ultraprocessed foods.

Coca-Cola, PepsiCo, Keurig, Dr Pepper, and other corporate giants fiercely opposed the plan, flooding lawmakers with arguments about personal freedom and the administrative challenges of defining "healthy" foods. These companies cynically pointed to their low- and zero-sugar options, claiming they were already offering healthier choices—while their profits from sugary beverages continued to soar. Under the guise of protecting consumer choice, Big Food ensured the pilot program never got off the ground. It was also blocked by all the Democrats on the committee who rationalized their opposition under the pretense of protecting choice for the poor, all the while pocketing massive donations from the food industry.

This isn't just bureaucratic inefficiency; it's corruption cloaked in the language of "freedom" and "choice." The very companies profiting from America's diet-driven health crisis have positioned themselves as defenders of the underserved, while actively undermining efforts to provide healthier food options. Until we break the stranglehold of corporate lobbying on food policy, SNAP will remain a tool for Big Food's profits, not public health.

What's worse is that this pattern of subverting public health and the interests of the American people at the behest of Big Ag continues into the present day.

In response to the Make America Healthy Again Commission report, which is tasked with producing an analysis of the causes of the chronic disease epidemic in the nation, the commission received the letter shown on pages 98–99 from a group of senators and congresspersons, initially leaked from inside the rotunda (though now published publicly on Senator Chuck Grassley's website[33]).

Let's unpack their strategy, one line at a time:

Step 1: Flatter the Regulator, Then Undermine Reform
"We write to express our strong appreciation for your leadership.... It is essential that policies supported by sound science and risk-based analyses are used."

Translation: Start with compliments. Signal alignment with science and leadership to create the illusion of partnership. But make no mistake—this is a prelude to discrediting any policy that threatens the industry status quo.

Congress of the United States
Washington, DC 20510

April 11, 2025

The Honorable Robert F. Kennedy, Jr.
Secretary
U.S. Department of Health and Human Services
200 Independence Ave SW
Washington, D.C., 20201

The Honorable Brooke Rollins
Secretary
U.S. Department of Agriculture
1400 Independence Ave SW
Washington, D.C., 20250

The Honorable Lee Zeldin
Administrator
U.S. Environmental Protection Agency
1200 Pennsylvania Ave NW
Washington, D.C., 20004

Dear Secretary Kennedy, Secretary Rollins, and Administrator Zeldin:

We write to express our strong appreciation for your leadership and interest in working with each of you to ensure America has the healthiest people in the world. In recent decades, chronic illness rates have risen. This warrants our careful scrutiny to support better health outcomes. It is essential that policies supported by sound science and risk-based analyses are used to accomplish this goal.

We also urge you to safeguard the work of the Make America Healthy Again Commission (Commission) from activist groups promoting misguided and sometimes even malicious policies masquerading as health solutions. The influence of these groups in the Commission would result in shoddy science; a less abundant, less affordable food supply; greater reliance on foreign adversaries for our food; diminished U.S. agricultural production and manufacturing; and, ultimately, poorer health outcomes.

President Trump recently stated environmental activists were holding the economic prosperity of our country hostage. We now have concerns that they are seeking to influence the work of the Commission to advance their agenda.[1] For decades activist groups have tried to ban safe, well-regulated

---

[1] Center for Biological Diversity. February 18, 2025. *A Petition to Make America Healthy Again.* https://biologicaldiversity.org/programs/environmental_health/pdfs/FINAL-MAHA-Petition-2.18.25.pdf

Step 2: Frame Public Health Advocates as Dangerous Extremists

"Safeguard the work of the MAHA Commission from activist groups promoting misguided and sometimes even malicious policies masquerading as health solutions."

---

agricultural inputs by any means necessary. Without these products, yields and quality are negatively impacted by otherwise avoidable insects, fungus, weeds, and other pest pressures. This drives up food prices for American consumers and forces reliance of food imports.

The same groups have seized upon the Commission's work as an opportunity to misrepresent the science on common food and feed categories or ingredients, such as plant-based oils. These inputs are subject to robust, risk-based regulatory system which focuses on protecting human health. Unfounded accusations harm the U.S. farmers who grow our food, upend food and feed supply chains, and significantly increase grocery food prices – all without public health benefit.

We have concerns that environmentalists are advancing harmful health, economic, or food security policies under the guise of human health. Despite insinuations to the contrary, regular testing by FDA and USDA finds that more than 99% of all pesticide residues meet extremely conservative limits established by EPA according to the best available science.

We applaud the Commission's desire to improve the health and wellbeing of Americans. We implore you to ensure policy decisions are grounded in sound science and risk-based analyses. With unity, we can protect American agricultural produces form environmental activists' attacks on proven-safe inputs critical to their profitability and long-term viability while promoting positive health outcomes.

Sincerely,

Pete Ricketts
United States Senator

Deb Fischer
United States Senator

Randy Feenstra
Member of Congress

Mark Alford
Member of Congress

Joni K. Ernst
United States Senator

James C. Justice
United States Senator

James E. Risch
United States Senator

Steve Daines
United States Senator

Translation: Label anyone challenging the industry as dangerous. Use fear-based rhetoric to equate science-backed reforms with radical activism, while painting the chemical-laden, ultraprocessed status quo as "safe and proven."

Step 3: Equate Regulation with Economic Collapse
"a less abundant, less affordable food supply; greater reliance on foreign adversaries for our food; diminished U.S. agricultural production"

Translation: Push the panic button. Imply that regulating harmful food additives or fertilizers will somehow cripple the food system, raise prices, and make America dependent on foreign nations—a fearmongering tactic straight from the industrial playbook.

Step 4: Defend the Chemical Tool Kit
"Activist groups have tried to ban safe, well-regulated agricultural inputs by any means necessary."

Translation: Normalize chemical dependency. Frame pesticides, synthetic fertilizers, and hormone-disrupting additives as essential for food security, ignoring mounting evidence of their harm.

Step 5: Weaponize "Science" as a Smokescreen
"a robust, risk-based regulatory system . . . according to the best available science"

Translation: Co-opt the language of science to defend the interests of corporations, not public health. Never mind that much of the science cited by industry is funded, manipulated, or selectively presented to maintain regulatory approval.

Step 6: Paint Reform as Costly and Unnecessary
"significantly increase grocery food prices—all without public health benefit."

Translation: Claim reforms are expensive and useless. Downplay decades of research linking ultraprocessed foods, additives, and pesticides to chronic disease. Instead, suggest that doing nothing is the safer path.

Step 7: Applaud the Commission—As Long as It Stays in Its Lane

"We applaud the Commission's desire to improve health...ensure policy decisions are grounded in sound science"

Translation: We support your work—so long as it doesn't interfere with our profits. We'll praise you, but we're watching closely, and any threat to our inputs, ingredients, or margins will be met with "concern."

The letter is a textbook example of how industry-friendly legislators use polite language and "pro-science" framing to derail meaningful public health policy. It defends a system in which a handful of mega-corporations control the food supply, pump billions into lobbying, and resist change that might jeopardize their ability to sell cheap, harmful, chemical-laced products at maximum profit.

The fight for health isn't just about science; it's about power. And letters like this show exactly where that power wants to stay.

And as expected, when we ran the signatories through the Open-Secrets website, we discovered that many of the senators and congress-persons listed in that letter have clear and documented financial ties to the very industries they are tasked with regulating. These include substantial contributions from agricultural PACs, food-processing companies, and chemical agriculture giants. For example, as of the writing of this, OpenSecrets noted that Senator Deb Fischer (R-NE) received more than $220,000 from the agriculture sector, while Senator Steve Daines (R-MT) accepted nearly $66,000 from food-processing interests during just one election cycle. Congressman Randy Feenstra (R-IA) received $134,635 and $122,000 from PACs associated with agricultural producers, and Senators Joni Ernst and Chuck Grassley, both from Iowa, a state deeply entrenched in industrial agriculture, have long-standing financial backing from Big Ag. Frank Lucas (R-OK) has received more than $758,001 throughout his career from the crop and food production sector. Dan Newhouse (R-WA) maintains significant agricultural holdings, including the James & Daniel Newhouse Partnership, valued between $250,000 and $500,000. Other signers, such as Senators Cindy Hyde-Smith, Thom Tillis, John Cornyn, and Roger Wicker, have similarly benefited from donations tied to major agricultural players like Tyson Foods and the South Dakota Farm Bureau. These contributions raise serious conflict-of-interest concerns, especially when these lawmakers publicly support policies that align with corporate interests rather than public health or environmental safety.

FOOD FIX: PRIORITIZE NUTRITION—PUT THE "N" BACK IN SNAP

Every semester, Pamela Koch, a professor at Columbia University who researches the connections between a sustainable food system and healthy eating, gives the students in her community nutrition class a fascinating assignment. She makes them eat on a $40 budget for exactly one week, so they see what life is like for the average low-income SNAP recipient. Students have to buy all their food from SNAP-eligible locations, like supermarkets and small grocery stores. That means there's no stopping and picking up a $15 salad and a $4 bottle of kombucha from Whole Foods. Often, they can't even afford to buy lunch. "It's an eye-opening experience for them," Koch says. "Truthfully, the amount that people are given for SNAP is based on what's called the thrifty food plan, which is unrealistic in a lot of ways."

The assignment shows her students why SNAP is so vital for people who are food insecure—people who often have no idea where their next meal is coming from. It also makes it crystal clear why food insecurity and obesity go hand in hand. When you only have $40 a week for food, you have to buy cheap food that comes in large quantities: big bottles of soda, boxes of cookies, bags of potato chips, processed meats, sugary breakfast cereals, Wonder Bread, and so on. Since people on

SNAP are not allowed to buy hot foods, you can't go to your grocery store and buy a $5 rotisserie chicken, but you can stock up on 2-liter bottles of 7Up and frozen chicken nuggets. Is it any surprise that these toxic foods are the most popular purchases for people on SNAP?

How do we make sure that SNAP recipients have access to nutritious and affordable foods? While it's a step in the right direction, we can't just eliminate soda and expect that the program will be fixed.

Koch and other experts say the real way to fix SNAP is to combine junk-food restrictions with incentives to buy healthy foods. A study published in *JAMA Internal Medicine* in 2016 shows how this would work. Researchers recruited adults in the Minneapolis area who were living below the federal poverty line and were not already on SNAP. Then they split them into groups and gave them debit cards with money for food—the same way SNAP benefits work. One group was not allowed to buy sugary drinks, candy, and other junk foods. Another group was told they would receive a 30 percent financial incentive to buy fruits and vegetables. In other words, their money would go much further if they spent it on fresh produce. A third group got both the junk-food restrictions and the healthy food incentives. The fourth group, which served as the control, just received the standard SNAP benefits.

After three months, the group that ate the smallest amount of junk food and the largest amount of fresh produce was the group that had both the healthy-food incentives and the junk-food prohibition. Even more interesting was that the incentive-only and the prohibition-only groups didn't see much of a difference in their diets. That is pretty solid evidence that the best way to reform SNAP is to eliminate the worst foods while making the best foods more affordable and accessible.[34]

FOOD FIX: OFFER INCENTIVES FOR HEALTHY FOODS

Some successful real-world experiments are finding ways to enable and encourage SNAP participants to eat healthy, whole food. The USDA makes fresh vegetables and other healthy ingredients at farmers' markets more affordable for SNAP participants through its Gus Schumacher Nutrition Incentive Program.

Many states are also starting to step up to the plate with their own healthy food programs for SNAP participants. In 2017, Massachusetts launched a program[35] that gives SNAP recipients extra money for every dollar they spend on fruits and vegetables grown by local farmers. More than 90,000 SNAP recipients[36] in Massachusetts have taken advantage of the program.

At the popular Birdhouse Farmers Market in Richmond, Virginia, SNAP participants can stock up on locally grown mushrooms, apples, kale, and other fresh veggies while participating in family activities like cooking demos and classes that teach them how to compost. More than half of the roughly 225 farmers' markets[37] in Virginia are authorized to accept SNAP benefits. Thanks to a statewide program called Virginia Fresh Match, Birdhouse is among the farmers' markets where SNAP dollars are worth double their value when they're used to buy fruits and vegetables.[38]

Across the country in Michigan, another program has found a way to give incentives to SNAP recipients to eat healthier: For every $10 in food stamps they spend on locally grown produce, they receive a $10 coupon[39] that enables them to buy additional fruits and vegetables of any kind. The program, called Double Up Food Bucks, was such a hit that it has spread to more than twenty-five other states, including Alabama, Arkansas, California, and North Carolina.[40]

All these programs serve a double purpose. They encourage low-income Americans to use their SNAP benefits for healthy foods instead of junk foods, and they increase business for America's small farmers, who need all the support they can get (more on this in Chapter 16). Unfortunately, healthy incentives have not been a priority for the federal government, though. The 2014 Farm Bill, for example, contained just $100 million in funding over 5 years[41] (out of $956 billion)[42] for these healthy-incentives programs. While that may sound like a lot, it's insignificant compared to everything else in the Farm Bill, like the billions in supports to grow and insure commodity crops and animal feed. It's also a drop in the bucket compared to the billions in SNAP money that pay for soft drinks and junk foods.

Imagine if all the supports the government poured into commodity crops and soft drinks were used to ensure that every city and town in America could provide locally grown produce to low-income families at little or no cost.

Thankfully a group of experts at Tufts' Friedman School of Nutrition Science and Policy (among other institutions) did the math,[43] and they found that providing a 30 percent incentive for fruit and vegetable purchases to Medicaid and Medicare beneficiaries would prevent at least 1.93 million cardiovascular disease events and result in a net savings of $40 billion in health care costs. An even broader 30 percent incentive for nuts, fish, whole grains, and olive oil would prevent 3.28 million cardiovascular events and yield a net savings of $100.2 billion in health care costs after the cost of the healthy food incentives.[44] Not bad for a bit of fresh food.

WANT TO GET INVOLVED?

On a more personal level of action, I urge you to ask your elected leaders about this. These are *your* tax dollars at work. Find out where your local member of Congress stands on SNAP reform. Find out if they have the courage to stand up to the big moneyed interests. And if they are failing on this issue, write to them or tell them about it at your next town hall. Tell them you want your tax dollars to be better spent. Reforming SNAP will improve the health of millions of Americans, and it will help reduce the enormous strain on our health care system.

For a quick reference guide on the Food Fixes and resources on how to demand clean food, go to www.foodfixuncensored.com.

CHAPTER 6

THE POWER OF FOOD INDUSTRY LOBBYISTS

Many of Big Food's tactics, like the widespread marketing of ultraprocessed foods, are plain and easy to see. You practically cannot watch television, flip open a magazine, or drive down a highway without seeing an ad for Coca-Cola, McDonald's, or Burger King. But the dirty politics of food often play out behind closed doors in the halls of Congress, far from public view. As we saw in the SNAP hearing in Chapter 5, government lobbying is arguably the food industry's most effective strategy. Armies of high-powered lobbyists have long occupied Capitol Hill to promote the interests of Big Food, pushing multibillion-dollar efforts to influence our laws, politicians, and government programs and agencies.

FOLLOW THE MONEY

The voices shaping our laws aren't those of citizens—they belong to industry. While we like to imagine that our democracy prioritizes the needs of the people, the truth is starkly different: We operate more like a corporate kleptocracy, where Big Food, Big Ag, and Big Pharma hold the reins. In 2014 alone, food industry lobbyists spent a staggering $500 million to influence the Farm Bill alone.[1] Over the past decade, these industries have poured hundreds of millions more into shaping policies across Congress, the White House, the USDA, and the FDA—not to protect public health but to safeguard their profits.

Lobbying by these industries is pervasive, operating at every level of government, from city halls to Capitol Hill, and even extending globally. Like Big Pharma and Big Oil, Big Food and Big Ag wield an unmatched advantage: bottomless pockets and direct access to the lawmakers and agencies tasked with regulating them. Their primary goal is to capture those institutions and bend them to their will.

So how do they do it? By drowning politicians in campaign contributions—funding that studies have shown directly shapes legislation—changing language, altering provisions, and inserting benefits that serve their donors. Lobbyists also wield influence with lavish perks, from golf outings and Super Bowl tickets to luxury trips and high-priced concert seats. While gift restrictions have been in place since 1995, loopholes are easily exploited. In Utah, for example, lobbyists gave lawmakers more than $250,000 in gifts in a single year, including vacation trips, Utah Jazz game tickets, and even American Express gift cards.[2]

Even our esteemed judiciary isn't immune. Recent reports[3] reveal that Supreme Court justices have accepted more than $3 million in gifts over the past two decades, including luxury trips and private jet travel, often from individuals with interests before the court.

Another lobbying tactic that has fundamentally corrupted American democracy is the use of PACs and super PACs—political action committees that pool money from corporations and wealthy donors to bankroll candidates, attack opponents, and influence elections. Super PACs have transformed the role of money in politics, creating a system where financial clout routinely outweighs the voices of everyday citizens.

The seismic shift that unleashed these lobbying practices onto American politics began with the *Citizens United v. FEC* ruling in 2010, a Supreme Court decision that declared spending on political campaigns a form of free speech protected under the First Amendment. By equating money with speech, the court removed most limits on how much corporations, unions, and individuals could donate to influence elections. The result was an avalanche of dark money—untraceable funds funneled through super PACs—flowing into campaigns. Congressman Tim Ryan has warned that "dark money"—untraceable donations to super PACs—allows millions of dollars to influence elections without the public ever knowing who's behind it.

This influx of corporate and special interest cash isn't just about free speech—it's about buying influence. Super PACs empower industries and billionaires to inject unlimited funds into public discourse, drowning out the voices of ordinary voters. Whether it's Big Coal donating millions to weaken environmental regulations, Big Pharma fighting drug price reforms, or unions securing favorable policies, the result is the same: Legislators shape laws that benefit their biggest donors, not the people they represent. While technically not quid pro quo, the intent is obvious. These donations aren't acts of charity—they're investments in political outcomes. In many cases these super PACs undermine fair elections by providing outsized funding for candidates in primary elections that challenge incumbents unfavorable to industry's agenda, and then fund their general election campaigns. This occurs from the bottom up starting with local, then state, then federal elections.

Harvard Law professor Lawrence Lessig's central thesis is that money from super PACs corrupts elections not through outright bribery, but via a more insidious process he labels "dependence corruption." Here's a concise summary of how this works:

1. **Super PACs concentrate spending power.** They enable a tiny fraction of wealthy donors to exert *outsized influence* on elections—Lessig noted that as few as 196 individuals funded 80 percent of super PAC expenditures in 2012.

2. **This generates political dependence.** Elected officials must devote an increasing portion of their time to fundraising, creating a structural reliance on major financiers rather than voters.

3. **Results are subtle but systemic.** It's not explicit quid pro quo, but a quiet distortion: Politicians shape policies to appease their financial backers—a form of legal corruption.

4. **Democracy suffers.** The outcome is a widening disconnect between public will and legislative action—a government that serves moneyed interests over the majority.

Lessig argues that super PACs perpetuate a cycle of influence: Wealthy donors bankroll campaigns, politicians rely on them to stay competitive, and democratic representation erodes. His book *Republic, Lost* and his activism (e.g., Mayday PAC, Rootstrikers) propose structural solutions like public funding, democracy vouchers, and constitutional amendments to break this cycle.

But *Citizens United* opened the floodgates, turning elections into auctions and creating a political system where money talks—and everyone else gets silenced. Everyday Americans are left watching from the sidelines as corporations and the ultra-wealthy steer public policy in their favor, while systemic issues like health care, education, and environmental sustainability remain unaddressed. This isn't democracy—it's oligarchy by another name. If we don't rein in this corrosive influence, the voices of ordinary citizens will continue to be drowned out by the deafening roar of corporate cash.

This is the reality of America's food policy: not written by or for the people but dictated by industries that use their immense wealth to corrupt the very system meant to hold them accountable.

A CORRUPTION CAROUSEL: THE "REVOLVING DOOR"

The "revolving door" between government and industry continues to spin unabated, with corporate lobbyists—often former politicians and aides—leveraging their insider status to influence policy for private gain. This practice, whereby individuals oscillate between the private sector and roles in government intended to regulate said sector, perpetuates a system in which corporate interests overshadow public welfare.

In 2009, President Obama attempted to address this issue by signing an executive order[4] imposing a two-year "cooling-off" period, preventing lobbyists from joining agencies they had recently lobbied. Despite this initiative,[5] his administration still appointed several industry lobbyists to key positions and similarly, while President Trump's first administration campaigned on promises to "drain the swamp," his tenure actually saw a relaxation of these restrictions; waivers allowing lobbyists to transition seamlessly into government roles (the revolving door) were regularly granted. A report by Public Citizen identified at least 133 registered lobbyists appointed within Trump's first six months, with 36 lobbying on issues directly related to their new government roles.[6]

Under President Biden, the revolving door persisted still. According to OpenSecrets, as of 2021, 139 individuals in the Biden administration held a prior role in lobbying or the private sector, indicating a continuation of the revolving door phenomenon.[7] Notably, his treasury secretary, Janet Yellen, received more than $7 million in speaking fees from major financial firms and tech giants, including Citigroup, Goldman Sachs, and Google, in the two years prior to her nomination.[8] Similarly, his secretary of state, Antony Blinken,[9] and national security adviser, Jake Sullivan,[10] provided consulting services to firms such as Microsoft before their appointments. Even Democratic National Committee heavyweights like Nancy Pelosi have come under fire for their cozy ties to corporate interests, including her well-timed investments in tech companies poised to benefit from legislation she helped shape. Somehow, she's managed to become one of the most prolific investors in history, regularly outpacing the S&P 500.[11] Funny, I must've missed the part where "shrewd stock trader" was in a lawmaker's job description.

The agency where the revolving door spins fastest is the USDA. In a move that raised eyebrows, the agency hired former sugar lobbyist Kailee Tkacz[12] to advise on its 2020 dietary guidelines. Before her cushy government gig, Tkacz worked for the Corn Refiners Association,[13] the PR machine behind high-fructose corn syrup, and SNAC International,[14] alarmingly nicknamed "Washington's voice for sugar, fat, and salt" (representing Kraft, PepsiCo Frito-Lay, and other snack titans). Despite a glaring conflict of interest, the White House greenlit her appointment, claiming she was "uniquely qualified"[15] to help craft America's nutrition policies—because who better to write the rules than Big Food's biggest cheerleader? Revolving doors abound:

Mark McClellan
On the left is the former FDA commissioner in charge of regulating Johnson & Johnson. On the right is a current member of the Board of Directors of Johnson & Johnson.

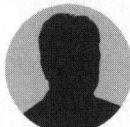

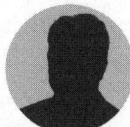

FDA Johnson&Johnson

Scott Gottlieb
On the left is the former FDA commissioner in charge of regulating Pfizer. On the right is a current member of the Board of Directors of Pfizer.

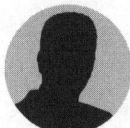

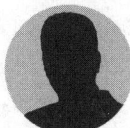

FDA Pfizer

Stephen Hahn
On the left is the former FDA commissioner in charge of regulating Moderna. On the right is the current Chief Medical Officer of Flagship Pioneering — the venture capital firm behind Moderna.

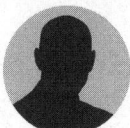

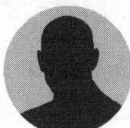

FDA moderna

James C. Smith
On the left is the CEO of Reuters in charge of informing people about the COVID-19 vaccines. On the right is a current member of the Board of Directors of Pfizer.

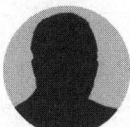

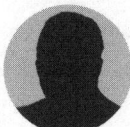

REUTERS Pfizer

Anthony Fauci
On the left is the NIAID Director under the National Institutes of Health. On the right is the funder of bioweapons research on gain-of-function bat coronaviruses at the Wuhan Institute of Virology.

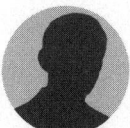

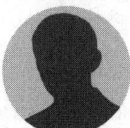

NIH

Fast-forward to January 2025, and Tkacz—now Kailee Tkacz Buller—has now been appointed the USDA's chief of staff,[16] holding one of the agency's most powerful roles. Before this, she headed the National Oilseed Processors Association and the Edible Oil Producers Association, two groups with massive stakes in agricultural policy. If her résumé sounds like a greatest hits album of processed-food lobbying, that's because it is.

Her appointment cements the USDA's reputation as a playground for industry insiders. The same person who once fought for the interests of high-fructose corn syrup and ultraprocessed snacks is now shaping the nation's agricultural and dietary policies. It's less "serving the public" and more "serving seconds of Big Food's agenda."

And not long after Tkacz Buller was appointed initially, the agency plucked three other lobbyists from the food industry to help shape policy:

- Maggie Lyons[17] was hired to advise the head of the USDA and other senior officials on SNAP, WIC (the Special Supplemental Nutrition Program for Women, Infants, and Children), and the school lunch program—the very issues she lobbied the agency on while working for the National Grocers Association only a few months earlier.[18]
- Brooke Appleton, a corn and wheat lobbyist[19] who spent years lobbying the USDA on elements of the Farm Bill, was hired by the agency to advise it on elements of the 2018 Farm Bill.[20]
- Kristi Boswell had lobbied[21] Congress on behalf of the Farm Bureau in support of legislation that would have made it easier for agribusinesses to deny health care coverage to seasonal farmworkers. Boswell was hired by the USDA to work on the same issues that she lobbied on: regulations involving seasonal farmworkers.[22]

The food industry contends that hiring lobbyists for government positions makes political sense because lobbyists often have unique insights and expertise on obscure regulatory issues. To some extent that might be true. But it's also naïve to believe that a former sugar lobbyist would advocate for sugar restrictions in the dietary guidelines. Or that a lobbyist who spent years opposing mandatory health care coverage for seasonal farmworkers would suddenly fight to protect farmworkers' rights. Not to mention that these men and women know that, once they leave their government roles, they can walk through Washington's revolving door and immediately return to their lucrative lobbying positions.

This pattern of appointing individuals with deep industry ties to key regulatory positions raises significant concerns about conflicts of interest and the potential for policies that favor corporate interests over public health. The revolving door between industry and government not only undermines public trust but also poses a threat to the integrity of our food and agricultural systems. Despite efforts across administrations to implement ethics rules, the influence of corporate interests remains deeply entrenched in American governance.

PROTECTING PROFITS IN THE SHADOWS

Louis Brandeis, the Supreme Court justice, once quipped[23] that sunlight was the greatest disinfectant — a poetic nod to the idea that transparency can cure social ills. And yet, more than a century later, the food industry lobbyists seem to have taken that wisdom as a warning, not advice. After all, why let in sunlight when you can thrive in the shadows? These masters of disguise work tirelessly to ensure their lobbying magic happens far away from prying eyes, where public scrutiny can't disinfect their agenda. For them, darkness isn't a problem — it's a strategy.

As of 2023, the number of registered lobbyists in the United States had ballooned to 13,037,[24] which equates to approximately 24 lobbyists for each member of Congress! Some of the biggest corporations, like Walmart, have as many as 100 lobbyists working for them at any given time.[25] No wonder our elected officials struggle under the weight of corporate interests.

But even that is just the tip of the iceberg. Studies show that thousands of unregistered lobbyists — so-called shadow lobbyists — work off the books thanks to obscure loopholes and lax enforcement. James

Thurber, a professor at American University who studies the issue, has found that the true number of lobbyists working in Washington is hovering close to 100,000.[26] That is enough lobbyists to fill two Yankee Stadiums, or enough to have 187 lobbyists for every member of Congress. According to OpenSecrets, total lobbying spending reached approximately $4.4 billion in 2024.[27]

It should not surprise you to learn that many of the biggest names in the food industry deploy sophisticated lobbying operations to protect their profits. According to the Center for Responsive Politics (now OpenSecrets), a nonprofit that tracks special interest spending, the food companies and trade groups that lobby the government the most are Coke, Pepsi, Monsanto, the American Beverage Association, Nestlé, General Mills, McDonald's, Kellogg's, the candy and dairy industries, and the Grocery Manufacturers Association (GMA), renamed the Consumer Brands Association,[28] which collectively spend literally hundreds of millions of dollars to influence lawmakers.

While Big Food companies like to position themselves as champions of public health, their actions tell a different story. The billions the whole industry spends lobbying in Washington aren't about improving health—they're about protecting their coffers. Their primary allegiance and legal accountability is to shareholders, and because their products are often at odds with our health, it's fairly predictable that their lobbying efforts will undermine public health initiatives. Notably, something like 97 percent of the soda industry lobbying is focused on opposing commonsense public health measures, including limits on marketing junk food to children and policies aimed at improving child nutrition. For Big Food, profits trump public health nearly every time.[29]

What exactly is Big Food lobbying against? Here are just a few examples:

Protections from Dangerous Chemicals

In 2009, the American Beverage Association filed eighty different lobbying reports related to twenty-four bills in Congress. Among the legislation it sought to influence was the Ban Poisonous Additives (BPA)

Act of 2009,[30] which would have ended the use of bisphenol-A (coincidentally also known as BPA) in children's food and drink containers. BPA is a synthetic chemical used in various consumer products, including food and beverage containers. It is an endocrine disruptor that can mimic estrogen and has been shown to cause negative health effects, including obesity, in animal studies.[31] Why would anyone want to keep these chemicals in children's food and beverage containers? It's simple: For many in the food industry, including soft drink companies, profit trumps public health, and replacing BPA costs money. The American Beverage Association filed more than a dozen lobbying reports documenting its efforts to scuttle the BPA Act. They were ultimately successful. The bill failed,[32] never making it out of committee for a vote.[33]

Despite the fact that the FDA still declares it "safe,"[34] international actions reflect growing apprehension about BPA's safety. In December 2024, the European Commission adopted a comprehensive ban on the use of BPA in all food contact materials due to its potential harms to human health, followed by Canada, which recently qualified BPA as a dangerous substance, leading to considerations for its banning.[35] These international measures underscore the global recognition of BPA's potential health risks and the need for regulatory action to protect public health. This is a substance with well-researched harms to human health including, but not limited to, endocrine disruption; impaired thyroid function; behavioral changes including depression, anxiety, and hyperactivity; obesity; type 2 diabetes; heart disease; breast, endometrial, ovarian, and prostate cancers; impaired fertility; and even autism. Why is it still allowed in US food products?

Fast-Food Lawsuits

Tobacco companies have been sued for giving people lung cancer. Oil companies have been sued for polluting the environment. Fast-food companies do not want to be sued for making people fat, sick, and diabetic. For more than a decade, they have spent millions trying to get politicians to pass laws shielding them from obesity-related lawsuits. As of 2018, at least twenty-six states have passed these so-called commonsense consumption measures, colloquially known as "cheeseburger laws."[36] These laws are designed to shield the food and beverage industry, including fast-food restaurants, from liability in lawsuits where individuals claim that consuming their products caused obesity or related health issues. Sort of like the implicit acknowledgment of guilt that may be revealed in a president's preemptive pardon, these laws make it difficult or impossible for individuals to sue food companies for damages related to weight gain or health problems stemming from the consumption of their products. Pesticide manufacturers have employed similar tactics. Pesticide manufacturers have, at various points, lobbied Congress to secure legal indemnity—or at least liability protection—for the health and environmental harms caused by their products. These efforts have taken several forms, most notably around glyphosate and PFAS-contaminated pesticides, and often mirror tactics used by Big Tobacco, Big Oil, and pharmaceutical companies seeking to limit future legal exposure.

The food-related laws explicitly bar individuals from suing food manufacturers, distributors, or sellers for claims alleging that their products led to weight gain, obesity, or associated health conditions (e.g., diabetes, heart disease). They protect companies from liability related to marketing practices, even when products are perceived as unhealthy or misleadingly marketed.

But it's not just Big Food that's anti–consumer protection. Federal lawmakers have tried to enact these laws too. The biggest proponent of these measures was Ric Keller, a Republican congressman from Florida who sponsored two separate bills[37] protecting fast-food makers from obesity-related lawsuits.[38] The Personal Responsibility in Food Consumption Act passed in the House but not in the Senate. Why would Keller sponsor these ridiculous bills? Could it be that he took hundreds of thousands of dollars in donations from a PAC representing McDonald's, Wendy's, and Burger King? He also took roughly $60,000 from Darden Restaurants, the parent company of Olive Garden, as well as $50,000 from the National Beer Wholesalers Association and more than $30,000 from the National Restaurant Association, which represents Taco Bell, Dunkin', and Domino's Pizza.

While fast-food lawsuits might strike some as frivolous, there is a reason Big Food companies are so desperate to stop them. As Michele Simon, a public health lawyer and food industry expert, argued in her book *Appetite for Profit,* the food industry is terrified of forced disclosure: "What scares food companies even more than costly jury verdicts is the prospect of the discovery process — when lawyers are allowed access to the defendant's documents and other inside information — unearthing damning data about dishonest industry practices, including in many cases, deliberate obfuscation of public health implications necessary for informed consent. This in turn, can open the door to a plethora of new government regulation." Illustratively, an avalanche of incriminating documents discovered through litigation against the tobacco industry revealed so much information that an entire research group at the University of California was deployed to its study.[39]

The food industry has learned from tobacco that litigation is a powerful public interest tool.[40] The buried information includes acknowledgment of the addictive nature of processed food, the specific and deliberate targeting of children, minorities, and people with low income, and the strategic manipulation of science and scientists to influence policy and public opinion, among other revealing information.

As health activist Calley Means writes,[41] "Americans are being crushed by the devil's bargain between the $6 trillion food industry, which wants to make food cheap and addictive, and the $4 trillion healthcare industry, which profits off interventions on sick patients and stays silent about the reasons they are getting sick. Every institution that impacts your health makes more money when you are sick and less when you are healthy — from hospitals to pharma to medical schools, and even insurance companies."[42] And Big Food doesn't want you to know that.

All of that said, a tsunami of class action suits is soon to be unleashed on the Big Food frauds. As recently as December 2024, legal actions targeting major food corporations over the production and marketing of ultraprocessed foods have kicked off in full force. These lawsuits primarily allege that companies have deliberately engineered these products to be addictive, leading to severe health issues, particularly among children.

A significant lawsuit[43] was filed in the Philadelphia Court of Common Pleas by plaintiff Bryce Martinez against major food companies, including Kraft Heinz, Mondelēz, and Coca-Cola, claiming[44] that these corporations designed and marketed ultraprocessed foods to be addictive to children, resulting in chronic diseases such as type 2 diabetes and non-alcoholic fatty liver disease. Martinez, diagnosed with these conditions at age sixteen, claims that the companies employed tactics similar to those used by tobacco firms to enhance product addictiveness, including allegations of conspiracy, negligence, fraudulent misrepresentation, and unfair business practices.

As you consider your personal experience with these predatory practices, look out for the following:

1. **Deliberate Engineering for Addictiveness:** Companies are accused of formulating products to be hyper-palatable, exploiting human psychology to encourage overconsumption by manipulating levels of sugar, fat, and salt to create a heightened sensory experience.

2. **Aggressive Marketing to Children:** By utilizing colorful packaging, cartoon characters, and promotional toys, these companies allegedly target children, fostering brand identification and loyalty from a young age, encouraging unhealthy eating habits during development.

3. **Failure to Warn About Health Risks:** Despite awareness of the potential health consequences associated with consuming ultraprocessed foods, companies are accused of neglecting to inform consumers adequately, prioritizing profits over public health.

4. **Comparison to Tobacco Industry Practices:** The lawsuits draw parallels between the strategies used by food companies and those historically employed by tobacco firms, suggesting a deliberate effort to create dependency and downplay health risks.

GMO Label Transparency

When it comes to your health, nothing is more important than what you put in your mouth. As I always say: Food isn't just calories; it's information, like computer code that programs your biology with every bite—for better or worse. It provides the raw materials that make up every cell, muscle, tissue, organ, and bone in your body, so each bite of food you take can either support... or damage your health.

That's why the more we know about our food—what's in it, where it's from, and how it was grown or raised—the better. But the food industry would rather keep you in the dark. The most damaging result of Big Food's battle against transparency was a bill passed in 2016[45] that limited your right to know whether GMOs lurk in your food. This is an issue that should be concerning to everyone.

A brief history lesson on GMOs: Genetically modified organisms (GMOs) were introduced with grand promises of agricultural revolution. These engineered crops were heralded as the solution to global hunger, praised for their resistance to pests and herbicides while allegedly boosting crop yields.

The narrative was one of scientific ingenuity overcoming nature's limitations; however, decades later, reality tells a starkly different story. Recent studies have revealed that genetically modified crops have provided little to no improvement in crop yields and, instead of alleviating the burdens of agriculture, they have potentially contributed to an alarming array of environmental and health crises. The widespread adoption of GMO crops has given rise to herbicide-resistant "superweeds," which now infest more than 60 million acres of American farmland. These invasive weeds have forced farmers into an arms race with nature, leading to increased reliance on potent chemical herbicides like Monsanto's Roundup (Monsanto is now Bayer)—a pesticide laden with glyphosate, a known carcinogen. Over the last 5 years Bayer has had to pay $19 billion in settlements, jury verdicts, and damages because of the harms of glyphosate.

The environmental consequences are profound and far-reaching; these toxic chemicals leach into the soil, seep into rivers and streams, and infiltrate our water supply, creating a cascade of contamination. Aquatic ecosystems are disrupted, biodiversity declines, and the very foundations of sustainable farming practices are undermined. Far from the promise of reducing chemical usage, GMO crops are now among the most pesticide- and herbicide-saturated crops in modern agriculture.

The push for genetically modified crops has also centralized control of the food supply into the hands of a few multinational corporations, exacerbating economic disparities for small-scale farmers and threatening global food sovereignty.

Today, an estimated three-quarters of the food found on American supermarket shelves contains genetically modified ingredients. This means that, unknowingly, consumers are regularly exposed to crops that not only carry high levels of chemical residues but also present unknown long-term health risks. Enter: the movement for GMO labeling.

The fight for GMO labeling in the United States has been fiercely opposed by Big Food and Big Agriculture. These industries claimed that requiring labels for genetically modified foods would increase production costs, resulting in higher prices for consumers[46]—a claim repeatedly refuted by independent studies.[47] Despite the evidence, the food industry leveraged its considerable influence in Congress to overturn state laws mandating GMO labeling, culminating in the passage of the so-called DARK (Denying Americans the Right to Know) Act. Its official but strangely Orwellian name: the Safe and Accurate Food Labeling Act of 2015.[48]

Big Food's lobbying efforts to block mandatory GMO labeling were extraordinary. According to an analysis by the Environmental Working Group, food companies spent more than $50 million in just the first half of 2015[49] to lobby for the legislation, a staggering sum that could have easily been directed toward improving product labeling or ingredient quality. The major players, including Coca-Cola, PepsiCo, Kraft, Kellogg's, Land O'Lakes, and General Mills—which rely heavily on GMO ingredients such as high-fructose corn syrup and vegetable oils—were among the biggest spenders, collectively funneling at least $20.6 million into lobbying efforts. The aforementioned GMA hired 34 lobbyists and contributed more than $10 million to the fight. Between 2013 and 2015, the combined spending by the food and biotech industries on lobbying and public campaigns opposing GMO labeling reached a mind-blowing $192.8 million.

The industry's efforts were not limited to lobbying. They launched a sophisticated nationwide, omnichannel media campaign, saturating the public with billboards, commercials, flyers, and social media ads aimed at convincing Americans that GMO labeling would drive up food prices. Yet these claims failed to convince savvy consumers. A *New York Times* survey[50] found that three-quarters of Americans expressed concern about GMO ingredients, and 93 percent supported mandatory labeling. Yet, despite the overwhelming public support, the food industry continued to wield its political clout to subvert the will of the people.

The DARK Act ended up nullifying labeling laws in Vermont[51] and other progressive states, replacing them with a watered-down federal standard. Instead of requiring clear GMO identifiers on packaging, the act made labeling voluntary and gave companies the option to include QR codes or 800 numbers for consumers to access ingredient information.[52] This "compromise" placed the burden on consumers to scan products or call helplines—an unrealistic process for most busy shoppers, and obviously inaccessible for vulnerable populations, such as those without smartphones or internet access. The DARK Act effectively deprived Americans of straightforward and easily accessible information about their food.

Nonetheless, the fight for transparency continued. On January 1, 2022, the United States implemented the National Bioengineered Food Disclosure Standard,[53] making GMO labeling mandatory and joining 64 other countries[54] in adopting such measures. These nations had already established comprehensive GMO labeling laws, reflecting a global consensus on consumers' right to know. Even countries with weaker consumer protections, such as China and Russia, recognized the importance of regulating genetically engineered ingredients.

While the disclosure standard marked a step forward, it has faced significant criticism. Consumer advocates argue that the law's reliance on digital disclosures like QR codes creates barriers for many consumers, especially those in rural or underserved areas. Additionally, certain refined ingredients derived from GMOs may be exempt from labeling if they no longer contain *detectable* genetic material due to their processing,[55] further limiting transparency.

Admittedly, despite these shortcomings, the global adoption of GMO labeling laws underscores a shared understanding of the need for transparency in food systems, which gives me hope for the next generation.

DARK MONEY PROPAGANDA THROUGH FAKE GRASSROOTS EFFORTS

An earlier battle over GMO labeling illustrates one of the most insidious ways that Big Food controls public opinion, through benevolently named front groups that masquerade as promoting the interests of citizens and the science.

Long before the DARK Act was signed into law, food activists like Chris and Leah McManus, a couple of organic-loving vegans from northwest Washington, were doing their part to push for strong GMO labeling laws. Early one Friday morning in the summer of 2012, Chris and Leah walked into the Washington State Capitol building in Olympia with a petition for a statewide referendum. They wanted to launch a state law requiring that all genetically modified foods carry a clear and easy-to-read GMO label.[56]

The couple had a groundswell of grassroots support: about 350,000 people across the state had signed their petition. Supporters of the referendum, called Initiative 522, included some of Washington's most recognizable icons, like the fishmongers who toss freshly caught salmon and halibut at Seattle's famous Pike Place Fish Market,[57] who were worried about genetically modified farmed salmon escaping and interbreeding with wild salmon.

Initiative 522 also attracted the attention of the GMA. Most people have never heard of the GMA (now called the Consumer Brands Association — the food industry's largest and oldest lobbying group) but they most certainly know its 300 or so member companies. A major player in DC, the institution boasts a member list that reads like the Academy Awards of Big Food, including industry titans like General Mills, Hershey, Kellogg's, Procter & Gamble, Welch's, Coca-Cola, PepsiCo, and Kraft Heinz.

Between 2005 and 2016, the GMA spent approximately $50 million lobbying the federal government, with GMO labeling becoming a top priority in 2012. In a speech to the American Soybean Association that year, GMA president Pamela Bailey bluntly declared it "the single-highest priority for GMA this year."[58] And it's no wonder: A mandatory labeling requirement would have been a nightmare for the processed food industry. General Mills would have to slap GMO labels on Cinnamon Toast Crunch and Honey Nut Cheerios. Coke and Pepsi would have to put it on their sodas. Kellogg's would have to label frozen waffles, Pop-Tarts, and cornflakes, and even Welch's fruit juice would face the same fate. The prospect of this level of transparency was enough to send the industry into a frenzy, determined to keep consumers in the dark.

The GMA was prepared to obstruct the Washington State initiative at all costs. The board members hatched a plan to fund an aggressive "No on 522" campaign[59] to discredit the GMO labeling measure, using television, print, radio, and internet ads, aiming to tarnish its credibility by branding it unscientific, costly, and confusing. The resulting ads were blatantly misleading, claiming that "farmers, food producers and scientists" were against the labeling initiative, making it appear to the public that there was grassroots opposition to GMO labeling. This tactic—known as astroturfing—has a long and notorious history. Perfected by Big Tobacco companies, astroturfing—a metaphor for something that looks natural but is actually manufactured—involves creating fake grassroots campaigns against policies and regulations to dupe the public.

There was one problem for the GMA, though: Because it was trying to influence the outcome of an election ballot initiative, it was required under campaign finance laws to disclose that it was funding the "No on 522" campaign.[60] It's tricky to convince Americans that farmers are raising their pitchforks against GMO labeling when your ad has a disclaimer that it was paid for by Coke and Pepsi.

The GMA and its member companies knew this tactic could backfire because they had already used it to discredit a similar labeling initiative in California earlier that year—Prop 37, the California Right to Know Genetically Engineered Food Act[61]—spending more than $30 million on a misinformation campaign. Though Prop 37 narrowly failed at the polls, the ensuing media coverage cast the food companies and their tactics in a harsh light, and heavy pushback from consumers and health advocates soon followed, including threats of boycotts.[62] At a board meeting in January 2013, Pamela Bailey lamented to the board that although their astroturf campaign in California was successful, it carried the costs of heavy criticism and shrinking consumer confidence in all the brands that were involved. That was something they had to avoid in future battles.[63]

Louis Finkel of the GMA realized they would need to develop a covert strategy that shielded the companies from the kind of backlash they got after the mudslinging in California. His idea? A "multiple use fund"—which is essentially a war chest where corporations could secretly funnel money with a dual purpose: to bankroll attacks on state-level GMO labeling measures and to cleverly sidestep campaign finance laws.[64] It wasn't just about strategy; it was about staying in the shadows while waging a long-term war on transparency.

Altogether the GMA member companies spent more than $15 million[65] on "No on 522":

- Pepsi dumped almost $3 million into the war chest.[66]
- Coke and Nestlé each poured $1.7 million into it.
- General Mills contributed $1 million, as did Conagra Brands, and so on.

This time, the GMA took it a step further, acting as a shield for its member companies to secretly bankroll the "No on 522" campaign without revealing their direct involvement. The audacity was staggering. Internal documents revealed that the GMA coached companies on how to dodge reporters' questions, scripting responses like an outright "No" to deny funding the campaign[67]—an unapologetic lie. To keep the cover-up intact, the GMA warned them to say nothing further, fearing any additional comments could tip off journalists or NGOs to the existence of their covert "secret" fund designed to avoid public scrutiny.

In mid-2013, as the campaign blanketed the Washington State airwaves with attacks on the labeling measure, the GMA's plan seemed to be working flawlessly, but for one minor snag: It was illegal. Fortunately, the state's attorney general, Bob Ferguson, noticed that the campaign was identical to Big Food tactics employed in other states. As Washington voters prepared to cast their ballots, Ferguson filed a restraining order in October 2013, demanding that the GMA publicly disclose who was funding the campaign.[68]

In November, the initiative narrowly failed, with 51 percent of voters opposing it and 49 percent supporting it—the same slim margin that took down the California proposition.[69] Big Food and its deep pockets once again made the difference, and in the process helped to set a new record for money spent against a Washington State initiative.

Ferguson and his office dug deeper into Big Food's web of deception, discovering blatant campaign finance violations in an attempt to mislead the public. They filed suit against the GMA. Finkel and Bailey both testified that their intentions were not to hide the sources of the money, that shielding the member companies from public scrutiny was not their goal, and that they had no intention of violating the law. Unfortunately for them, the judge presiding over the case didn't see it that way. In her decision, Judge Anne Hirsch lashed out at Bailey and Finkel for their behavior and said it was simply not believable, arguing that they certainly knew all along that their scheme was not legal.[70] "The totality of the record establishes under a preponderance of the evidence," the judge wrote, "that GMA intentionally violated Washington State public campaign finance laws."[71]

Judge Hirsch slapped the GMA with a record-setting penalty, ordering the group to pay an astounding $18 million[72] for knowingly breaking the law to conceal the identities of the corporations behind its astroturf campaign. It was the largest campaign-finance penalty[73] in American history, and several million more than the $14.6 million penalty the attorney general had requested. On top of that, the GMA was ordered to pay the state's legal fees too.[74] The penalty was later reduced by an appeals court to $6 million, but the Washington attorney general said in 2018 that he would fight that decision.[75] It was a good day for the law and for integrity, and a bad day for Big Food and its playbook of dirty tricks. "It's one of my happiest days as attorney general," Ferguson told reporters. "GMA's conduct was just so egregious."[76]

Still, what's a few million in fines compared to hundreds of billions in profit? They might have lost the lawsuit, but they are still ahead in the war. Today, there remain no GMO labels in Washington State.

As outlined above, the GMA, recently rebranded the Consumer Brands Association,[77] is a formidable force against any regulation or legislation that might improve the food system. But encouragingly, their resistance to progress is so egregious that even corporate giants like Nestlé, Unilever, Danone, and Mars have come out against them, publicly quitting the GMA[78] to form the Sustainable Food Policy Alliance,[79] citing the "need for a better approach to food policy." While the effectiveness of their alliance remains to be seen, the departure was a clear acknowledgment of consumer demand for healthier food and better policies.

And as recently as March 2025, troubling reports have surfaced alleging that the American Beverage Association may have orchestrated a covert campaign to influence public opinion against the proposed removal of sugary sodas from SNAP. According to social media statements made by influencer and whistle-blower Riley Gaines,[80] the American Beverage Association was allegedly behind a disinformation push aimed at shaping the public narrative and socializing opposition to soda restrictions within SNAP.

The strategy, Gaines claims, involved enlisting social media influencers to promote industry-aligned talking points, apparently creating the appearance of grassroots resistance to what many public health advocates view as essential reform. These influencers, many of whom have large online followings, suspiciously posted nearly identical messages criticizing the proposed restrictions as government overreach and invoking "consumer choice" as a rallying cry. This coordinated messaging effort appears to fit the classic profile of an astroturf campaign — an orchestrated attempt to simulate organic public opposition, most likely to shield corporate interests.

While the American Beverage Association has publicly denied involvement, several reports suggest that public relations firms, possibly connected to industry stakeholders, approached influencers with compensation offers for content opposing the SNAP changes. If true, this would raise serious concerns about transparency, ethics, and the tactics being used to influence policy debates that affect millions of vulnerable Americans.

Though many of the details remain unconfirmed, and more investigation is needed, the incident highlights the *alleged* extent to which powerful food and beverage interests may go to protect profits — even if it means undermining public health policy aimed at reducing diet-related diseases among low-income communities.

MORE ADDICTIVE THAN COCAINE? NOT BY ACCIDENT

The very same food industry funding manipulation campaigns in public politics has also "invested" in manipulating us on an individual level.

Big Food has unlocked the secret to making you crave more — and it's all by design. Their nutritionally bankrupt ultraprocessed products are crafted with scientific precision to exploit your brain's reward mechanisms, ensuring you crave more with every bite. They are not merely meals; they are engineered to stimulate your senses and override your body's natural satiety signals, keeping you in an endless cycle of consumption.

Central to this process is the "bliss point," a calculated balance of sugar, salt, and fat that creates an irresistible allure. This is not a lucky accident, but a deliberate design rooted in decades of food science research. By hitting this perfect sensory combination, these ingredients deliver a powerful dopamine release that makes the eating experience intensely rewarding. This flood of dopamine keeps you reaching for more, long after you've had enough, transforming food into a product of addiction rather than sustenance.

To achieve this level of manipulation, companies employ advanced technologies like functional magnetic resonance imaging (fMRI) scans to study how their formulations activate the brain's pleasure centers, even in children as young as two! These scans track blood flow to core regions in the brain, helping to provide insight into how ingredient combinations trigger craving cycles, enabling manufacturers to refine their products for maximum appeal.

Beyond flavor, the industry has also invested millions into understanding the neuroscience behind texture and mouthfeel (how food feels as you chew it, how it breaks down, and how it triggers pleasure signals in the brain). Seeking enhancements in these foods with carefully optimized textures and sensations—whether it's the crunch of a chip, the creaminess of a dessert, or the fizz of a carbonated drink—these tactile elements are engineered to amplify enjoyment. Food developers meticulously test and refine these sensory cues to deliver maximum pleasure to ensure you continue consuming, often without realizing the extent of your intake. It's a methodical exploitation of human biology designed to benefit corporate profits at the expense of public health.

The impact of these engineered foods goes beyond individual choice. By creating products that are almost impossible to resist, the food industry has contributed to widespread health issues like obesity, diabetes, and metabolic disorders. Critics argue that this is not just a matter of personal responsibility, but a systemic issue driven by deliberate corporate strategies to prioritize profit over public well-being.

In his book *Ultra-Processed People,* Dr. Chris van Tulleken emphasizes that these foods are engineered to be hyper-palatable, leading to overconsumption and associated health issues. He states, "With a physiological confusion that barely makes it to the surface of our conscious experience, we find ourselves reaching for another—searching for that nutrition that never arrived." Most ultraprocessed food is not food; it's an industrially produced edible substance.

Clearly, the food industry's use of advanced science and psychology to manipulate cravings is not about feeding you—it's about controlling your consumption patterns. These ultraprocessed foods are designed to hack your biology, keeping you trapped in a cycle of overindulgence. The result is a public health crisis that benefits corporate bottom lines while leaving consumers to bear the consequences, one bite at a time.

Don't believe me? You might be surprised to learn that Cargill—one of the world's top producers of high-fructose corn syrup (HFCS)[81]—stands as the world's most successful privately held company,[82] topping annual revenue charts with figures recently reaching $165 billion[83]—an unmatched achievement in the private sector. Founded in 1865, the company remains family-owned and tightly controlled, with the Cargill–MacMillan clan boasting 14 billionaires,[84] *more than any other family on Earth.*

As a global agribusiness titan, Cargill is deeply embedded in the modern food system—managing everything from grain trading and meatpacking to seed oils and industrial sweeteners, especially the cheap and abundant sweetener that is now ubiquitous in ultraprocessed foods, high-fructose corn syrup (HFCS).

HIGH-FRUCTOSE CORN SYRUP (HFCS)

HFCS is a cheap, highly processed sweetener derived from corn starch. Its use skyrocketed in the 1970s and '80s, fueled by US corn subsidies and soaring demand from soda, snack, and fast-food companies.[85] Cargill, one of the world's largest producers, played a central role in flooding the global food supply with HFCS.

But the public health costs have been profound. Unlike naturally-occurring glucose, which is metabolized throughout the body, fructose is processed almost entirely by the liver, where it is rapidly converted to fat. This metabolic pathway drives a cascade of chronic health issues: it promotes visceral fat accumulation[86] and insulin resistance[87] (a key driver of obesity and pretty much every other chronic health disease), fuels non-alcoholic fatty liver disease[88] and metabolic dysfunction[89] (contributing to type 2 diabetes), and elevates inflammation and LDL cholesterol (increasing cardiovascular risk). Some studies even suggest that fructose may hijack brain reward pathways, encouraging addictive patterns of overconsumption.

In short, HFCS is not just a cheap sugar substitute, it is a foundational ingredient in the modern ultraprocessed diet, and a major contributor to the global epidemic of chronic disease.

THE TALKING POINTS OF BIG FOOD

Big Food has mastered the art of using manipulative talking points to defend ultraprocessed foods and GMOs and to deflect criticism of their role in the global health crisis. By framing these products as essential for food security, affordability, and safety, they distort the narrative to justify the continued dominance of highly profitable, unhealthy food systems. They claim ultraprocessed foods are indispensable, invigorating fears of hunger and food scarcity while ignoring the root causes of these issues, like inequitable food systems and unsustainable farming practices. They cloak their arguments in the language of personal choice, framing any criticism as an attack on consumer freedom, and even weaponize identity politics by labeling efforts to reduce ultraprocessed food consumption as classist or racist. These tactics shift blame from corporations to individuals, obscuring the public health consequences of their products and perpetuating the very inequities they claim to address.

Here are some of the common talking points of Big Food and their cronies to keep an ear out for next time you're reading the mainstream media (much of which is funded by them or their health care counterparts: Big Pharma). While not unreasonable on the surface, these arguments are carefully crafted to deny, deflect, and defend the obvious health consequences of their fake foods. The following quotes are general talking point examples, commonly represented by Big Food parrots.

1. **"We Can't Define Ultraprocessed Foods"**
   "The term 'ultraprocessed foods' is vague, subjective, and lacks a universally accepted definition. Foods are processed to varying degrees for countless reasons, and lumping them together under an ill-defined term risks oversimplifying a complex food system. This kind of language unfairly targets popular and convenient products that millions of people rely on every day."

2. **"We Need Ultraprocessed Foods for Food Security"**
   "Ultraprocessed foods play a vital role in ensuring food security for a growing global population. These products are designed to be

shelf-stable and widely distributed, which means they can reach areas where fresh produce or minimally processed foods are scarce or unavailable. In regions with limited agricultural infrastructure or inadequate refrigeration or sanitation practices, ultraprocessed foods provide essential calories and nutrients, helping to prevent hunger and malnutrition on a massive scale. Without these innovations, many communities would face critical food shortages."

3. **"We Need Ultraprocessed Foods for Affordability"**

"Ultraprocessed foods are affordable and accessible, which is why they are a staple for millions of families, especially those on tight budgets. Fresh and organic foods are simply out of reach for many consumers due to their higher cost and perishability. Ultraprocessed foods offer a practical alternative, providing calories, flavor, and essential nutrients at a fraction of the price. Demonizing these products ignores the financial realities faced by low-income households and unfairly stigmatizes their choices."

4. **"We Need Ultraprocessed Foods for Food Safety"**

"Ultraprocessed foods undergo rigorous processing methods designed to ensure food safety. Techniques like pasteurization, fortification, and vacuum sealing protect against foodborne illnesses and contamination, especially in vulnerable communities. These measures make ultraprocessed foods some of the safest products on the market, offering peace of mind to consumers who prioritize health and safety. Without these technological advances, many food products would be far less reliable and pose greater health risks."

5. **"We Need Ultraprocessed Foods for the Right of Choice"**

"Everyone has the right to choose the foods they want to eat. Ultraprocessed foods are just one of many options available to consumers, and restricting access to them infringes on personal freedom and autonomy. People value convenience, flavor, and variety, and ultraprocessed foods deliver all of these qualities. Trying to dictate what people can or can't eat is paternalistic and undermines the basic principle of consumer choice."

6. "It Is Racist to Deny People the Choice"

"Restricting access to ultraprocessed foods disproportionately impacts marginalized communities and people of color, many of whom rely on these products due to economic and systemic barriers to fresh, minimally processed alternatives. Labeling these foods as inherently 'bad' or promoting bans perpetuates classist and racist stereotypes about what different communities 'should' eat. Everyone deserves the dignity of making their own choices without judgment or restriction, and attempts to limit ultraprocessed foods unfairly target vulnerable populations under the guise of health advocacy."

Don't be fooled by these talking points. Big Food and its defenders may frame ultraprocessed foods as essential for addressing practical concerns like food security, affordability, and safety, while positioning criticisms as elitist or even discriminatory, but they are just distractions. The focus on personal choice and consumer rights to deflect attention from broader public health critiques, portraying ultraprocessed foods as indispensable rather than addressing systemic issues in the food system, is strictly a PR game.

FOOD FIX: FIGHT THE FOOD LOBBYISTS WITH REAL GRASSROOTS EFFORTS

Microplastics in food and beverage containers. Roundup in your morning oatmeal. Hormones in the beef at your local grocery store. These may seem like health hazards to you and me. But to Big Food they are business as usual. These practices are big moneymakers, which is why the food industry is willing to spend billions lobbying against regulations designed to rein them in.

We often feel powerless against the overwhelming influence of big corporations. What we fail to realize sometimes, though, is that we hold significant power as consumers to challenge their predatory practices by wielding our purchasing decisions strategically. When we disapprove of a company's actions, we can drive change by voting with our dollars. This means actively supporting and investing in companies that demonstrate social, environmental, and nutritional responsibility. At the same time, we can leverage the megaphone of social media to organize mass boycotts of companies that perpetuate harmful practices, sending a clear message that unethical behavior will not be rewarded. Corporations ultimately depend on consumer demand—a business requires customers, after all. We have the power to choose to determine what they can sell, if we organize it well.

Think this kind of public pressure won't work? Plenty of grassroots efforts have spurred food industry changes. Though we've seen a few examples of how Big Food has overcome attempts at GMO labeling laws, they are a great example of how public sentiment can be as important as legislation. Some big companies saw the writing on the wall when Vermont's law was on the verge of taking effect in 2016 and decided to accommodate consumers instead of fighting them. Several big companies, led by Campbell Soup Company, announced that they would start disclosing GMO ingredients on all of their packages nationwide—not just in Vermont.[90] Many of these companies received widespread praise from non-GMO activists and applause from consumers. Walk into any big-box supermarket and you will now see that a lot of companies use GMO labels that go above and beyond what the law requires. Even better, an increasing number of companies are deciding to avoid GMOs entirely. They recognize not only that it's better for their products and the environment, but also that it's a smart business move.

Other giant food corporations are evolving in response to grassroots consumer campaigns. Take a look at the dairy industry. Sales of cows' milk have been plunging for years over concerns about hormones, antibiotics, animal welfare, and the environmental impact of dairy farms. Plant-based alternative milks like almond, macadamia, coconut, and cashew milk have quickly become a billion-dollar industry as consumers reach for more ethical and sustainable alternatives.

Let's all work together to send a message to Big Food.

FOOD FIX: SHUT THE REVOLVING DOOR AND ENFORCE LOBBYING RESTRICTIONS

The federal government can start by making the lobbying system more transparent. The more we know, the more we can change. Right now, lobbyists are held to weak disclosure laws. They're required to file quarterly reports listing their clients, their compensation, and the agencies or branches of government they're targeting. The nonpartisan Center for Responsive Politics (now OpenSecrets) does an excellent job of tracking this information and making it available to the public online. But the disclosure system doesn't go far enough. All it tells us is that corporations spend a ton of money lobbying the government, which we already knew.

The public deserves to know, in a timely manner, exactly who in the government is being lobbied and why. Some research groups like the Brookings Institution have proposed a more transparent system that would involve the federal government creating an online portal where every piece of legislation is posted before it is voted on or signed into law. There, under each bill, lobbyists would be required to state who their clients are, which members of Congress or agencies they lobbied, and their positions on that bill or its amendments. This site could also serve as a forum for the public to weigh in on proposed legislation. The Library of Congress had a website where it made legislation available online, called the THOMAS system (http://thomas.loc.gov) that has become Congress.gov. Now we just need to update this system to make it more democratic and useful for the public.[91]

Government can and should be a tremendous force for good, not for powerful special interest groups and their well-connected lobbyists. That's why the revolving door between industry and the government should be closed and locked for good. For starters, here are the changes we need to see:

- Elected and appointed government officials should ideally be banned from becoming lobbyists when they leave office, or at least face an extensive "cooling-off" period of five years or longer.

- At the same time, people who worked as corporate lobbyists should be restricted from taking jobs in the federal government. If you worked as a lobbyist for the sugar industry or McDonald's, you should not be allowed to take a job at the USDA as an adviser on the dietary guidelines. If you worked for the FDA, you should be banned from taking a corporate job in the fast-food or pharmaceutical industry lobbying the very agency you just left.

- A windfall tax could be imposed on excessive lobbying to clamp down on any one corporation's or union's ability to spend unlimited sums of money lobbying against the greater good of society. Controversial senator Elizabeth Warren has proposed[92] a tax of 35 percent on lobbying expenditures between $0.5 million and $1 million, 60 percent between $1 million and $5 million, and 75 percent on expenditures over $5 million. I tend to agree with her here.

- Restrictions should be enforced and loopholes that permit personal gifts to public officials should be closed.

While changing the lobbying laws and regulations may seem far out of our realm of influence, we can vote with our dollars on the local level and pressure our senators and congresspeople to support reform at the national level. Let's speak up and put an end to the politics of bad food.

For a quick reference guide on the Food Fixes and resources on how to demand clean food, go to www.foodfixuncensored.com.

HOW THE US GOVERNMENT SUBSIDIZES DISEASE, POVERTY, AND ENVIRONMENTAL DESTRUCTION

By now, we've seen many ways in which junk-food companies prioritize their profits over the health of their customers—and frankly, I don't think it surprises many. They do what they are designed to do: chase profits. But what you might not fully grasp is how complicit Uncle Sam is in it all.

Big Food's lobbyists have wormed their way into Congress, the White House, and basically every government agency that's supposed to protect you from, well, them. And what's the result? Policies that don't just allow ultraprocessed foods to dominate your grocery store— they actively *promote* their production, sale, and marketing. These foods are the fuel behind the diabesity epidemic (that not-so-fun mix of obesity and type 2 diabetes), chronic diseases, and environmental destruction on a grand scale. The government doesn't just turn a blind eye to this; it actually lends a helping hand. Here are just a few examples.

The US Food and Drug Administration (FDA) bows down to the companies it's supposed to regulate, allowing them to churn out Frankenfoods even when they're found to contain toxic chemicals like glyphosate, BPA, and hydrogenated oils. The whole system is confusingly designed to protect companies at the expense of their consumers.

Another pernicious example is how the Federal Trade Commission (FTC) implicitly gives Big Food permission to prey on children, paving the way for the food industry to market billions of dollars' worth of junk foods that cause weight gain, diabetes, and fatty liver in kids. Meanwhile the Centers for Disease Control and Prevention (CDC) takes millions of dollars[1] in funding from the soft drink industry[2] to launch obesity campaigns[3] that ignore nutrition while focusing exclusively on physical activity.

But no agency has been more critical to Big Food's profiteering than the U.S Department of Agriculture (USDA). To understand this, look no further than the one piece of legislation that is the single most important component of our food system: the Farm Bill.[4] As I outlined earlier, the Farm Bill (implemented by the USDA) designates funding for SNAP and other government food programs, but it *also* doles out billions of dollars' worth of subsidies and crop insurance for farmers. These subsidies have been in place in some form or another since the Great Depression, when the government began providing aid to farmers to ensure that the country had a steady food supply. Fast-forward to almost a century later, and the Farm Bill that passed in 2014 authorized nearly $1 trillion in spending—$956 billion to be exact—through 2024.[5] Those expenditures were largely reauthorized by Congress in the 2018 Farm Bill and then signed into law[6] by President Trump 1.0.

Whether you realize it or not, the Farm Bill plays a direct role in agriculture and your diet. The Farm Bill determines which crops farmers choose to grow. It influences the cost of groceries and the foods we eat. And it has enormous health consequences for the entire nation.

Before we get into how farm subsidies shape what American farmers grow, let's take a look at another important task of the USDA (along with the Department of Health and Human Services, HHS): establishing the country's dietary guidelines.

DIETARY GUIDELINES: THE FOOD INDUSTRY'S UNDUE INFLUENCE

The USDA and HHS collaborate to update the Dietary Guidelines for Americans. Revised every five years,[7] the Dietary Guidelines for Americans are intended to synthesize the latest nutrition science into simple guidelines that then form the foundation of all government food programs and are followed by almost all health care institutions and public health and professional societies. These guidelines serve as the foundation for federal nutrition programs, public health initiatives, and dietary recommendations, with which you are probably familiar—the Food Pyramid and MyPlate recommendations fall under their purview. They are a pretty big deal for American health, because their recommendations also guide food procurement in prisons, schools, and federal agencies and for veterans, as well as shaping food assistance programs like SNAP and the National School Lunch Program, *and* they influence food-labeling regulations, public health messaging, and industry practices. Not insignificant.

But the USDA's dual mandate to promote agricultural industries while also guiding public health has led to accusations of conflicts of interest. Critics argue that the USDA's ties to agribusiness may prioritize industry profits over evidence-based health recommendations. Hence the following contradiction: The Dietary Guidelines Advisory Committee, a group of independent nutrition experts, reviews scientific evidence and submits recommendations to the USDA and HHS.

The recommendation process makes sense, but what many fail to recognize is that the final guidelines are determined by government agencies with competing agendas, not the advisory committee (which is actually qualified to make these recommendations). Instead, these agencies, most of which are bought and paid for by Big Business, get the final say. Food and agriculture industry lobbying holds a tight grip on shaping the final dietary guidelines, often twisting the narrative to downplay the health risks of certain foods. Instead of prioritizing public health, these industries leverage their influence to protect their profits, ensuring the guidelines reflect their interests rather than the latest science.

Here's what most of you don't know: Since the very first Dietary Guidelines for Americans were drafted in the late 1970s,[8] lobbyists representing different industries have been deeply embedded in the process. For example, the guidelines committee wanted to advise Americans to cut back on their meat consumption, but meat industry lobbyists, unhappy about this, pressured the guidelines committee to soften their language. So instead of issuing recommendations to reduce meat consumption, the guidelines committee reached something of a compromise, recommending that Americans cut back on "saturated fat" (coded language for red meat). The advice to cut back on eggs was changed to a recommendation to cut back on cholesterol. And instead of urging Americans to limit sugar because of its emerging link to heart disease, the guidelines mentioned that Americans might want to go easy on sugar for a less urgent reason: dental cavities.

But let's rewind a second to understand how we got here. The very first guidelines were already based on a set of poor epidemiological research from the 1960s that blamed fat and exonerated sugar for heart disease. Mark Hegsted, a Harvard physician, was an author on a 1967 *New England Journal of Medicine* paper[9] that accused fat but gave sugar a pass for a role in the development of heart disease. He headed up George McGovern's Senate commission on the first Dietary Guidelines for Americans in 1977.[10] Turns out the sugar lobby paid him the equivalent of close to $50,000[11] in today's dollars to write that article, even though studies showed that inflammation, abnormal cholesterol, and other heart disease biomarkers were driven by sugar and starch.[12] The original guidelines evolved for the worse, piling on the low-fat bandwagon and culminating in the 1992 Food Guide Pyramid advising us to eat six to eleven servings of bread, rice, cereal, and pasta a day and to eat fat only sparingly.[13] This led to the worst public health disaster in the history of humankind, driving a global epidemic of obesity and type 2 diabetes. Finally, in 2015, after decades of overwhelming evidence that fat was not the enemy, the US Dietary Guidelines removed any limits on dietary fat,[14] declaring that eating fat didn't cause weight gain or heart disease. To get the full story you can read my book *Eat Fat, Get Thin*.

In 2005 George W. Bush made the guidelines fully political[15] when the final guidelines had to be approved by politicians, not scientists. The last advisory group recommended including sustainability in the guidelines, but the factory-farmed meat industry went up in arms over it, and of course, the policymakers ended up removing environmental considerations from the final guidelines.

Through the efforts of the Nutrition Coalition, a nonprofit advocacy group, in 2015 Congress mandated that the National Academy of Sciences (NAS) review the process by which the dietary guidelines are developed.[16] The NAS found that many members of the advisory committee had consistently published work in favor of low-animal-fat vegetarian diets. It was revealed that several members had consulting agreements with or were funded by the food industry. I wonder if that might have had anything to do with why they ignored huge swaths of science on meat and low-carb diets.[17]

For a while the recommendations from the NAS offered a hopeful vision for reforming the US Dietary Guidelines, but under the Trump administration, the process became even more politicized and less grounded in science. For the first time, HHS and the USDA imposed strict limits on the research that could be reviewed.[18] They allowed only internal government studies vetted by agency officials, excluded any data prior to 2000 (which is when much of the foundational research was conducted), and prohibited consideration of outside research, data on ultraprocessed foods, feedlot meat, sodium, or the environmental impacts of the food system. These restrictions starkly contradicted the NAS recommendations, making it clear that transparency and comprehensive scientific review were not priorities.

As a result, the Trump administration's 2020 Dietary Guidelines Advisory Committee was riddled with conflicts of interest:[19] Thirteen of its twenty members had strong ties to the food industry, including organizations like the National Potato Council and the snack food trade association. Unsurprisingly, the final guidelines largely ignored research that implicated Big Food or Big Ag in public health or environmental crises, effectively shielding corporate interests.

The Biden administration, despite its posturing as a champion of public health advocacy, similarly struggled to confront the deeply entrenched corporate influence in the dietary guidelines process. While there were token gestures toward acknowledging sustainability and environmental impacts, insiders know that the 2025 Dietary Guidelines Advisory Committee remains a revolving door for agricultural and food industry insiders.

Members with clear ties to Big Ag and Big Food continued to shape policies under the guise of impartiality, raising serious doubts about the administration's alleged commitment to transparency and scientific integrity.

Despite promises of inclusivity and public health focus, the Biden administration failed to dismantle the structural flaws that allow corporations to dictate the narrative. Instead of restoring scientific independence, the process remains riddled with conflicts of interest, shielding powerful industries from accountability. The result? Dietary guidelines that still prioritize corporate profits over public health and environmental sustainability, leaving the systemic harms of the food system unchecked and the American public paying the price.

It remains to be seen whether the influence of MAHA will move the needle for Trump's second administration. I truly hope for the sake of the American people that he gets better advice this time around.

FOOD POLICIES AT ODDS WITH ONE ANOTHER

Today, the dietary guidelines may have taken a step toward healthier recommendations, but the USDA's advice to eat better is directly undermined by its own actions, leaving consumers caught in the contradiction. It's like the USDA is trying to plant a garden while simultaneously salting the earth. While the dietary guidelines encourage Americans to fill half their plates with fruits and vegetables to prevent obesity, the agency stacks the deck against consumers by making junk foods cheaper and easier to buy than nutritious foods. Government subsidies enable lower prices for processed food by encouraging the growing of food surpluses, while not supporting farming of fruits and vegetables, even though the very same agency tells us to eat five to nine servings of fruits and vegetables a day. Basic laws of markets and economics show how challenging this would be.

According to data collected by the federal government, the foods that make up the top sources of calories in the American diet are grain- and sugar-based snacks such as cakes, cookies, doughnuts, and cereal.

Top Sources of Calories in the US Diet	
Cakes, cookies, doughnuts, granola	138 kcal
Breads	129
Chicken dishes	121
Soda, energy and sports drinks	114
Pizza	98
Alcohol	82
Pasta	81
Tortillas, burritos, tacos	80
Beef dishes	64
Dairy desserts	62
Chips	56
Burgers	53

Source: USDA Dietary Guidelines.[20]

Not far behind them are bread, sugary drinks, pizza, pasta, and "dairy-based desserts" (in other words, ice cream). All of these are the products of just a handful of crops and farm foods — corn, soybeans, wheat, rice, sorghum, milk, and meat — that your tax dollars heavily subsidize.

Between 1995 and 2013, the Farm Bill doled out more than $550 billion to farmers and large agribusinesses to finance the production of these foods.[21] Farmers were motivated not only to produce these foods but also to *overproduce* them. The laws of supply and demand no longer apply in an arbitrarily manipulated market economy. Those subsidies work like a floodgate, driving down the prices of commodities like wheat, corn, and soy and flooding the market with cheap, abundant ingredients. The effect is that fast food, soft drinks, and junk food became as plentiful as weeds in an untended garden—growing everywhere; cheap and impossible to avoid. During this period, the price of sugary drinks sweetened with high-fructose corn syrup fell nearly 25 percent, and American children increased their consumption of soft drinks by 130 calories a day. At the same time, the cost of fruits and vegetables rose almost 40 percent.[22]

PROCESSED CORN AND SOY HIDDEN IN EVERYTHING

When hearing about the most heavily subsidized foods, like corn and soybeans, you might think that those plants are not inherently unhealthy. But the vast majority of these crops are not consumed in their natural, whole state. Only 1 percent of American-grown corn is sold and eaten whole as corn on the cob. [23] Much of the rest is either fed to factory-farmed livestock to fatten them up before being slaughtered, or converted into biofuels. As for what does hit your plate, America's heavily subsidized bounty of corn and soy may start out as whole foods, but by the time you eat them, they've been overwhelmingly adulterated into ultraprocessed oils and sweeteners and food additives.

Corn is processed into cornstarch and high-fructose corn syrup, which are some of the most prevalent additives in the food supply, found in everything from applesauce to breakfast cereals to baby food, baked goods, bread, ketchup, frozen dinners, soft drinks, and yogurt. Soybeans are broken down into refined soybean oil (also a foundation of processed foods) and meal that is fed to livestock and pets. Soybean oil, until very recently, was then further processed into partially hydrogenated cooking oils, also known as trans fats, which increase the risk of heart attacks and strokes.[24] Refined soybean oil alone accounts for 55–60 percent of all the oil that Americans consume,[25] up from virtually none in 1900, which represents a thousandfold increase over the twentieth century. Most of that is hidden in processed or fried foods. Wheat and other grains are ground into flour and refined carbs, which are worse for your body than natural sugar (even whole wheat bread has a higher glycemic index than table sugar).

So how does all this impact the American diet? Marion Nestle, a professor of nutrition, food studies, and public health at New York University, did the calculations. She found that if you designed your meals to match the way the government funnels its subsidies, "You'd get a lecture from your doctor."

"More than three-quarters of your plate would be taken up by a massive corn fritter (80 percent of benefits go to corn, grains, and soy oil). You'd have a Dixie cup of milk (dairy gets 3 percent), a hamburger the size of a half dollar (livestock: 2 percent), two peas (fruits and vegetables: 0.45 percent), and an after-dinner cigarette (tobacco: 2 percent). Oh, and a really big linen napkin (cotton: 13 percent) to dab your lips."[26]

According to Dr. Nestle, here's what the USDA's MyPlate advice would look like if it reflected what the USDA supports with subsidies.

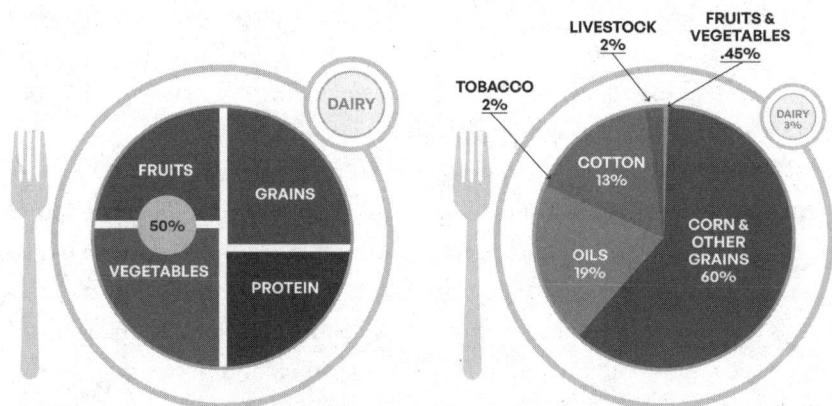

As evidence of this trend, Big Ag grows 500 more calories per person per day than it did just 25 years ago,[27] most of it made up of corn and soy in the form of ultraprocessed food. That's because farmers get paid to grow extra food even when it's not needed. Our McGovernment provides them with billions of dollars' worth of crop insurance, so there's no risk of losing money if they have a bad season, and they are incentivized to grow crops on marginal land they know will fail. A lot of the crop insurance helps farmers pay for the seeds and nitrogen fertilizer used to grow crops on marginal land. Koch Fertilizer,[28] founded by major political donors the Koch Brothers, provides much of the fertilizer and receives big benefits from current agricultural policies. Even worse: If those farmers want to diversify and grow tomatoes and broccoli on their farms, they automatically lose their government support. Talk about an ultimatum game.

These government supports are essential to protect farmers (many are one bad season away from bankruptcy), but they are concurrently hamstringing their potential for innovation and regeneration.

As a result of farm subsidies, taxpayers are footing the bill for the chronic disease epidemic on the back end of our destructive diet, while simultaneously underwriting the production (and consumption via SNAP) of the very foods that are causing it. With the money used to subsidize corn- and soy-based junk-food ingredients, the government could buy almost 52 billion Twinkies—enough to circle the Earth 132 times when placed end to end or meet the caloric needs of the entire US population for twelve days.[29] Not coincidentally, the Twinkie offers an illustration of the degree to which government subsidies favor junk-food production. "Of the 37 ingredients in a Twinkie, taxpayers subsidize at least 17, including corn syrup, high-fructose corn syrup, vegetable shortening, and corn starch."[30] Speaking of a Twinkie, back in the 1950s, the treat was made with about eight or nine simple, recognizable ingredients—things you might have in your own kitchen. Today, the ingredients list has snowballed, including many added items that you can't even pronounce, let alone cook with. What changed along the way? It seems like the result of some questionable priorities, don't you think?

In 2016, researchers at the CDC published a study that examined the direct impact that these subsidies have on America's health. They analyzed more than 10,000 adults and split them into groups according to the proportion of foods they ate that were derived from the most heavily subsidized commodities. They found that people who had the highest intake of federally subsidized foods had a nearly 40 percent greater likelihood of being obese. They were also significantly more likely to have metabolic disease, with higher levels of belly fat, blood sugar, cholesterol, and C-reactive protein, a marker of inflammation. The CDC researchers concluded their paper with a thinly veiled rebuke of the USDA and its contradictory policies and nutrition advice, stating that "nutritional guidelines are focused on the population's needs for healthier foods, but to date, food and agricultural policies that influence food production and availability have not yet done the same."[31] (Of course, the CDC has had its own conflicted positions.)

FRUITS AND VEGETABLES: TOO FEW AND TOO EXPENSIVE

In contrast to huge subsidies on the crops that will end up in junk food, the percentage of federal subsidies that are actually allocated for nutritious foods is trivial. Apples are the only fruit or vegetable that receive significant subsidies (other than corn), and the amount allocated for apples between 1995 and 2013 was just $689 million[32]—less than 1 percent of total government subsidies for food. Even still, those subsidies aren't likely to enhance nutrition; much like corn, a lot of the apples grown in America are not eaten as whole foods. They are processed into anti-nutritious junk foods masquerading as health foods like apple juice and applesauce, which are often sweetened with another subsidy staple, high-fructose corn syrup.

Behind the scenes of America's agricultural policy lies an increasingly obvious reality: The system gives farmers almost no incentive to grow the very foods that form the foundation of a healthy diet. In fact, the government has actively discouraged the production of fruits, nuts, and vegetables for decades.

Buried within versions of the Farm Bill, fruits and vegetables—astonishingly labeled as "specialty crops"—are treated as second-class citizens of agriculture. The legislation has long stipulated that farmers receiving subsidies for commodity crops like corn, wheat, and soybeans are prohibited from growing these "specialty" foods. If they dare to do so, they risk facing severe penalties, effectively turning fruits and vegetables into a risky venture for subsidized farmers.

As a result, today, only about 2 percent of farmland in the United States is dedicated to growing fruits and vegetables,[33] while a staggering 59 percent is allocated to commodity crops. These crops aren't destined for your dinner plate but are instead funneled into processed foods, animal feed, and biofuels—far removed from the fresh produce Americans are urged to consume.

This policy, rooted in outdated priorities, highlights a glaring disconnect: While public health experts emphasize the importance of fruits and vegetables, government policies continue to favor crops that contribute to the nation's overproduction of cheap, calorie-dense, and nutrient-poor foods. The consequences ripple through both our diets and our agricultural landscape, raising critical questions about whom the system truly serves.

This begs the question: Is our subsidy system designed to support farmers—or an agenda that prioritizes profits over public health? Let's unpack it a bit.

The way the subsidy program is structured to favor large agribusinesses is no accident. Archer Daniels Midland, Bayer (which purchased Monsanto), Cargill, DuPont, Tyson, Syngenta, and other Big Food and Big Ag corporations have the lobbying power to mold the Farm Bill to their liking. As Marion Nestle at NYU points out,

> If you examine how its incentives are structured, you quickly see that they strongly favor industrial agriculture in the Midwest and South over that in the Northeast and West. Methods that require chemical fertilizers, pesticides, and herbicides are prioritized over those that are organic and sustainable, and commodity crops for animal feed, vegetable oils, and ethanol take precedence over so-called "specialty" crops—translation: fruits and vegetables for human consumption.[34]

This makes food hugely competitive and forces the manufacturers of processed foods and drinks to do everything possible to encourage sales of their products. The result is a food environment that encourages overeating of highly caloric, highly processed foods, but discourages consumption of healthier, relatively unprocessed foods.[35]

Legendary investor Charlie Munger's famous line "Show me the incentive, and I'll show you the outcome" is no truer than in American agriculture.

Who Influences What Goes On Your Plate?

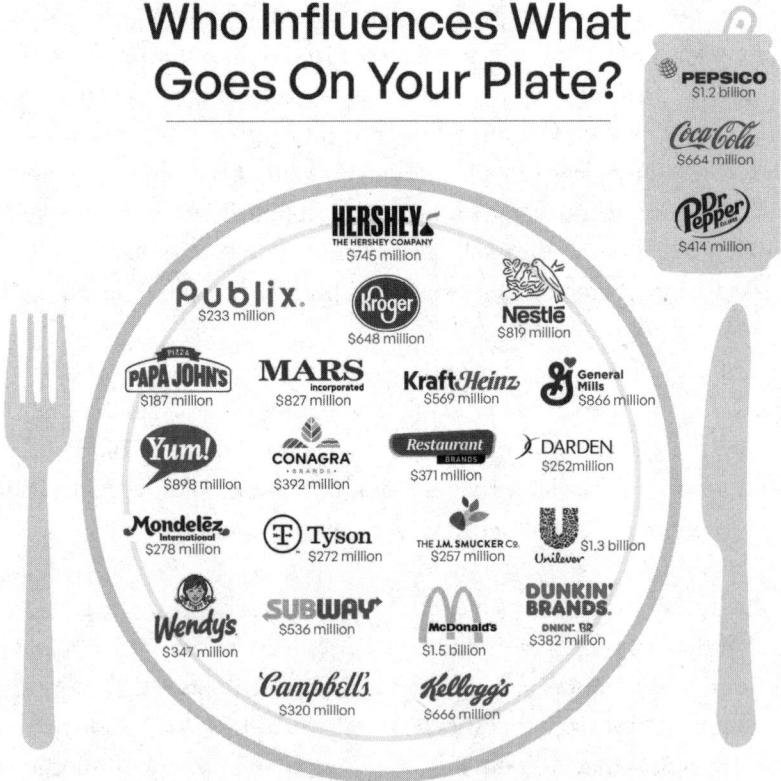

Brand	Amount
PEPSICO	$1.2 billion
Coca-Cola	$664 million
Dr Pepper	$414 million
HERSHEY, THE HERSHEY COMPANY	$745 million
Publix	$233 million
Kroger	$648 million
Nestlé	$819 million
PAPA JOHN'S PIZZA	$187 million
MARS incorporated	$827 million
Kraft Heinz	$569 million
General Mills	$866 million
Yum!	$898 million
CONAGRA BRANDS	$392 million
Restaurant BRANDS	$371 million
DARDEN	$252 million
Mondelēz International	$278 million
Tyson	$272 million
THE J.M. SMUCKER CO.	$257 million
Unilever	$1.3 billion
Wendy's	$347 million
SUBWAY	$536 million
McDonald's	$1.5 billion
DUNKIN' BRANDS DNKN: BR	$382 million
Campbell's	$320 million
Kellogg's	$666 million

In 2014, the top 25 food industry advertisers spent $14.9 billion advertising* their products.

Source: Ad Age. 200 Leading Advertisers 2015.
*Spending on measured and unmeasured advertising
by 25 top food industry advertisers

FOOD FIX: THE NEED FOR A NATIONAL FOOD POLICY

Since the food and agriculture industry is the biggest business in America and affects every single American, it is surprising that we actually don't have a national food policy. Our federal government has multiple agencies governing various aspects of food and agriculture, all acting independently, mostly without coordination, supporting a food and agricultural system that creates disease and endless human suffering and is bankrupting our economy while devastating the environment and driving climate change. We need a comprehensive reform of food policy in America (and globally) at the national and local levels, governed and administered by an accountable food czar.

Countries like Brazil and Norway have taken the lead on creating national food policies. Their dietary guidelines recommend eating whole foods and their federal governments levy taxes on soft drinks and other junk food, as well as provide assistance to farmers who grow nutritious foods. Brazil's national food policy, implemented in 2004, has already helped to reduce poverty and child mortality rates while boosting business for farmers.[36]

What would such a policy look like in America? The Union of Concerned Scientists did the research[37] and concluded that a national food policy would ensure the following goals:

- That all Americans have access to healthy food;
- That farm policies are designed to support public health and environmental objectives;
- That our food supply is free of toxic bacteria, chemicals, and drugs;
- That the production and marketing of food are done transparently;
- That the food industry pays a fair wage to people it employs (see Part 4);
- That the food system's carbon footprint is reduced and the amount of carbon sequestered on farmland is increased (see Part 5).

So how would this actually work in practice? For starters, the government has to reform its subsidies system. Farmers need incentives to grow more nutritious foods using regenerative practices. The government needs to restructure the Farm Bill so that subsidies are used to increase the production of "specialty crops" such as fruits, vegetables, and nuts and shift away from corn, soy, wheat, animal feed, and biofuels (which paradoxically require lots of fossil fuels to grow). The process of creating nitrogen fertilizer is energy intensive, releasing a ton of CO_2 and methane in the process, and when synthetic nitrogen is applied as fertilizer to fields, it emits N_2O, another potent greenhouse gas.[38] Whether you care about climate change or not, this should appeal to your self-interest, because these chemicals are not just harming animals and plants—they're poisoning you too. As these toxins devastate the natural world, they work their way up the chain and into our bodies, something you *definitely* do not want. Finally, we are all aligned.

Beyond subsidies, as one of the largest food procurement entities in the country, the government wields immense purchasing power—feeding millions every day in schools, hospitals, prisons, the military, and even government offices. With such enormous influence, the government could be a driving force for healthier, more sustainable food systems. Instead, it often reinforces the dominance of commodity crops and ultraprocessed foods, perpetuating a cycle that prioritizes cheap calories over nutritional quality.

The government can promote healthy eating and create markets for farmers by requiring that schools, prisons, and military bases use a percentage of their budgets to buy locally sourced food from nearby farms and, at the very least, purchase healthy whole foods that promote health rather than disease. As Congressman Ryan explained it, "How do we get military bases healthy? How do we get processed food out of the bases and more healthy food in? We get the bases to buy local, support the local farmers and the local area. A lot of times you'll have a military base and surrounding it will be a lot of farmland." The same goes for schools, prisons, hospitals, and other government-funded institutions. We should be making use of that.

The choices the government makes in its purchasing decisions ripple across the entire agricultural sector, influencing what is grown, how it's produced, and ultimately, what ends up on your plate. A national food policy would transform our broken food system into one that aligns public health objectives with economic and environmental goals. It would make healthful choices the default option for Americans while slashing health care costs and helping farmers, protecting the environment, and reversing climate change.

FOOD FIX: FOOD-AS-MEDICINE INNOVATIONS

Instead of being the country with one of the worst chronic disease epidemics, we could become a model for health. While there are many ideas proposed by many groups, here are a few that could make a big impact in addressing the burden of chronic disease. Many of these have been outlined in a key paper published in *BMJ* in 2018 entitled "Role of Government Policy in Nutrition—Barriers to and Opportunities for Healthier Eating."[39]

- **Reimburse food as medicine.** Change medical reimbursement to pay for food as medicine through all federal and state health insurance programs such as Medicare and Medicaid for at-risk populations. The data is clear: Giving people food instead of drugs saves money. A new study[40] providing medically tailored meals to sick patients was shown to reduce hospital and nursing home admissions, saving about $9,000 per person per year after providing free food.

  Pilot projects include the $25 million Produce Prescription Program in the 2018 Farm Bill[41] to test how doctors' prescriptions of fruit and vegetables bundled with financial incentives, education, and better access can improve health outcomes and reduce the use of health care services. California provided $6 million in support of food prescriptions and medically tailored meals for chronic disease.

Similar programs have found that health care costs are reduced by 55 percent and hospital and long-term-care admissions are reduced.[42]

In 2018, John Hancock turned life insurance upside down by making all its policies part of the John Hancock Vitality Program,[43] which provides financial incentives for healthier lifestyles, including $600 a year for purchasing healthy food.[44] These types of business innovations will inspire other businesses, proving that it's possible to increase profits while promoting social good. We have now partnered with John Hancock (one of the most proactive employers in the country) at the lab testing company I co-founded, Function Health, to activate an employee-wide focus on prevention and early intervention.

Geisinger's Fresh Food Farmacy provided $2,400 in food to food-insecure diabetics with education and social support and reduced costs by 80 percent while improving health care outcomes.[45] Participants receive enough food to prepare ten healthy meals per week, along with education and support from a dedicated care team.

The Food Is Medicine Coalition, an association of twenty-eight member organizations in eighteen states and Washington, DC, that provides medically tailored food to people with serious or long-term illnesses, helps advance this strategy. There is even a bipartisan Food Is Medicine Working Group in Congress today.[46] It's a start. And the return on investment is dramatic. Here are some other ways you can get involved:

- **Create a food savings account, like a health savings account (HSA),** where people can save money (tax-free) in an account that can only be used to buy whole, real, health-promoting foods. It could ultimately save billions in downstream health care costs. Check out Truemed (https://www.truemed.com), a platform that enables consumers to utilize their health savings accounts (HSAs) and flexible spending accounts (FSAs) for a broader range of health-related products and services, including fitness equipment, supplements, and health technology. By partnering with various merchants, for example, Truemed allows users to purchase health and wellness products using pre-tax dollars, potentially saving an average of 30 percent on eligible items.

- **Fund research and change reimbursement to pay for functional medicine,** a systems approach to addressing the root cause of chronic disease. Imagine scaling an approach that changes both the medicine we do and the way we do medicine:

  o Addressing root causes
  o Using food as medicine
  o Treating the body as a system rather than a set of isolated symptoms
  o Shifting delivery of care in the community, putting patients and communities at the center of health care, not doctors and hospitals
  o Using proven behavioral change strategies such as peer support models, group visits, and health coaching to change people's lifestyle

- **Integrate nutrition into health care** because currently, most medical doctors are still not required to take a single nutrition course in their entire education. How could they possibly learn to evaluate cause and effect when it comes to diet, if they aren't even trained in it? Support for nutrition education in medical schools and changing licensing exams to include nutrition would change what doctors have to study, thus forcing medical school curricula to change. Robert F. Kennedy Jr. suggested that the government tie any funding to academic medical centers to mandatory nutrition education for physicians.
- **Reimburse nutrition visits for chronic disease and obesity.** Integrate nutrition into electronic health records. Develop reimbursement and quality metrics, which will incentivize the integration of nutrition into medical practice. In other words, if doctors don't document nutrition status and use food as medicine, they don't get

paid! Invert the incentives. Develop quality metrics and payment reform that support community-based programs to address the upstream causes of poor health. Integrate public health and health care.

For a quick reference guide on the Food Fixes and resources on how to support a national food policy, go to www.foodfixuncensored.com.

CHAPTER 8

How the Food Industry Preys on Our Children

Kids today are fatter than ever. Obesity rates in children have nearly quadrupled[1] since the 1970s with now 36 percent being overweight or obese.[2] In fact, one in four teenagers now has type 2 diabetes or pre-diabetes—a condition we used to call "adult-onset diabetes" (this was something I never saw in a young person during my medical school training 40 years ago).[3]

If I sound like I'm obsessing over obesity and weight, it's because I am—and with good reason. Over the past decade or so, and in the name of political correctness and feel-good rhetoric, we've created a culture that glorifies ignorance under the guise of body positivity. As a doctor, I would be betraying my Hippocratic oath by pandering to this "healthy at any size" narrative. It is simply not scientifically accurate: Clinically speaking, if a child is overweight, his or her life expectancy may be reduced by *10 to 20 years!*[4]

So let's be clear: Ignoring this critical medical fact isn't compassion—it's negligence. Worse, it's a form of societal child abuse, trading long-term health for short-term comfort. We owe our children better than this dangerous delusion. As you can see on the next page, numerous health conditions are likely to result from being overweight or obese.

One of the biggest culprits behind childhood and teenage obesity is the food served in schools—a problem our government has a direct hand in. School meals are often a toxic mix of sugar, processed carbs, industrial fats, and excess salt masquerading as "nutrition." In some

Relative Risk and Impact of Being Overweight or Obese on Health

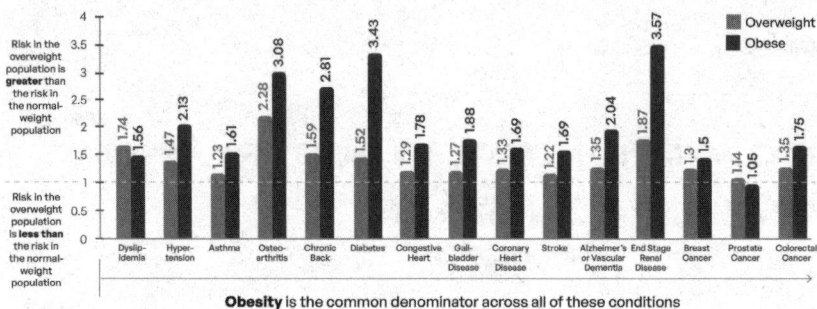

Obesity is the common denominator across all of these conditions

cases, schools don't even bother pretending. Fast-food chains like Domino's and McDonald's are given free rein to sell pizza and cheeseburgers on campus, slapping their logos on cafeterias and gym walls like a corporate sponsorship deal for junk food.

Schools are supposed to be a sanctuary for learning and growth, but instead, they've become ground zero for poor dietary habits. The Institute of Medicine calls schools "the heart of health" for a reason: They play a central role in shaping children's well-being. Close to 30 million kids rely on school meals every day, and for many low-income families, these meals are the bulk of a child's daily calories. This makes school food one of the most critical weapons in the fight against childhood obesity — yet we continue to allow it to be weaponized against children's health. It's time to demand better. Schools should set the highest standard for nutrition, not bow to the profit-driven interests of Big Food.

As you might expect, public health officials have long tried to make school meals more nutritious, but an enormous (and familiar) obstacle stands in the way: the food industry. In 2010, President Obama signed into law the Healthy, Hunger-Free Kids Act,[5] a signature piece of legislation that Michelle Obama championed as part of her effort to make a dent in child obesity rates. The law mandated that 100,000 public schools[6] provide healthier foods to their students, by granting the USDA the power to create new nutrition standards for school lunches for the first time in decades.

The law accomplished some good: It essentially banned much of the obvious junk foods from school vending machines,[7] like soft drinks, cookies, gummy bears, and sugar-laden sports drinks such as Gatorade. It created standards for school meals that prioritized whole grains over heavily processed carbs, lowered sodium, and required at least a *minimal* amount of vegetables per meal. But that's about all the legislation got right.

Its passage and implementation faced considerable opposition from various industry groups and lobbyists concerned about the potential impact on their products and profits. Sadly, it was fatally flawed from its inception because food industry lobbyists were intimately involved in shaping it.[8] Indeed, more than 111 food companies, trade groups, and industry organizations registered to lobby on the bill.[9] They were led by the misleadingly named School Nutrition Association, a leading industry-funded lobbying organization. About half of the association's $10 million budget comes from Big Food companies,[10] among them Kraft, Coke, Conagra, and Domino's Pizza. The association watered down the legislation's criteria for what could qualify as nutritious and pushed for a clause that allowed schools to opt out of the standards. The school lunch lobby fought to ensure that tomato paste would count as a vegetable,[11] tragicomically making pizza legally a vegetable, and that starchy potatoes—code word for French fries—would be favored in the standards. Case in point: The two most commonly eaten vegetables in America are officially potatoes and tomatoes—eaten in the form of French fries, ketchup, and pizza. Ah, the pinnacle of modern nutrition. Minnesota Democratic senator Amy Klobuchar lobbied hard for this because the nation's largest pizza provider to schools, Schwan Food Co., is in her native state (sadly this is indeed how Washington works).[12]

When the dust settled and the USDA finalized its nutrition standards for schools, the menu looked less like a plan to combat childhood obesity and more like the lineup at a state fair. Because what better way to nourish young minds than with a culinary parade of syrup-drenched waffles, deep-fried tater tots, and sugar-laden Slush Puppies? "Truly, a triumph of public health," said no doctor ever.

With assistance from the food industry, the USDA also created a Trojan horse policy it called Smart Snacks in School.[13] The idea was to hold snack foods to higher nutrition standards. But ultimately it allowed branded junk foods to sneak into schools.[14] While it sounded like a good idea in theory, the nutrition criteria for the Smart Snacks program provided an easy workaround for the industry, which reformulated their products into slightly different junk foods.

Potato chip makers created "reduced fat" versions of their chips that met the Smart Snacks criteria. Cookie companies created "whole grain" cookies and crackers (essentially junk food with a few flakes of whole grain sprinkled in). And instead of offering sugary soda, soft drink makers met the Smart Snacks criteria by offering "100% fruit juice," which typically contains just as much sugar as soda. To meet the Smart Snacks standards, PepsiCo offered schools reduced-fat Nacho Cheese and Cool Ranch Doritos, Flamin' Hot Cheetos, and oatmeal raisin Quaker Breakfast Cookies.[15] Pepperidge Farm introduced lower-fat chocolate, vanilla, and "whole grain" Goldfish crackers.[16] General Mills created reduced-fat strawberry-yogurt-flavored Chex[17] and a line of Fruit Roll-Ups.[18]

BIG FOOD'S FAVORITE WEAPON: NUTRITIONISM

A quick sidebar on Big Food's tactic of moderately adjusting their ingredients to reflect a different health profile. Leveraging the nutrition science concept called "nutritionism"—obsessing over isolated nutrients while ignoring the whole food health profile—Big Food obscures the fact that their products are ultraprocessed health bombs. It's a brilliant sleight of hand, really. Instead of asking whether the food itself is good for us, nutritionism convinces us to fixate on one or two ingredients. Is your cereal packed with fiber? Does your soda have added vitamins? Does that candy bar boast about its protein content? Congratulations! You're now the proud consumer of what is essentially edible marketing, wrapped up in pseudoscience and buzzwords.

Big Food has mastered the art of deflection. Their sugary, salty, fatty concoctions are bad for us? No problem. Just slap "low-fat" on the label, pump it full of sugar, and call it a day. People catching on that soda is liquid diabetes? Roll out a new line of vitamin-enhanced beverages, because nothing says "health" like carbonated sugar water with a splash of vitamin C. Nutritionism lets Big Food dodge accountability by turning their products into Frankenfoods — built to check one "healthy" box while actively harming you in every other way. It's like a get-out-of-jail-free card for Big Food.

The marketing genius of nutritionism is that it makes us complicit. Suddenly, we're walking down the grocery aisle, analyzing grams of protein and omega-3s while ignoring the mile-long ingredients list of chemicals and preservatives. We feel like health experts while we're being sold food that barely qualifies as edible. It shifts the blame, too. If you're unhealthy, it's not because the food system is engineered to push cheap, nutrient-poor calories at you. No, it's because *you* didn't eat enough whole grains or *you* didn't buy the yogurt with probiotics.

As Dr. Chris van Tulleken sardonically states,[19] "If emulsifiers damage the microbiome, let's add some probiotics. If the food's too soft, add more gum. If it's too dense in energy, add artificial sweeteners. Their solution to ultraprocessing is hyper-processing, also known as reformulation. We undermine 'em with one hand and build 'em with the other. The vitamins we destroy in the canning, we restore in Revito…By forcing the damn-fool public to pay twice over…we keep the wheels of commerce turning."[20]

Nutritionism is Big Food's Trojan horse — a shiny, health-conscious facade that distracts us from the undeniable truth: The vast majority of their products are designed for profit, not health. And as long as we keep falling for the nutrient-of-the-month game, they'll keep cranking out ultraprocessed junk with just enough "added benefits" to keep us hooked — and sicker than ever.

All these junk foods carry the same brand names, logos, and characters as their traditional versions—and all of them were allowed into schools with the USDA's blessing. What's bizarre and contradictory is the mandate to lower fat in school lunches but allow increased starch and sugar while the US Dietary Guidelines recommend removing any limits on total fat and reducing starch and sugar. No wonder we are all confused. At the USDA, it would be generous to conclude that the right hand doesn't know what the left hand is doing.

In perhaps the most flagrant example of all, in 2018 the largest public school system in Texas—the Houston Independent School District—entered into a four-year deal with Domino's to market its Smart Slice pizza in Houston schools.[21] Even though they look and taste like any ordinary pizza, the company claimed its Smart Slice pies were healthful because they contained less fat and sodium[22] than regular pies. The crust is 51 percent whole wheat (just sneaking in at the standards for "whole grain"), and they have low-fat cheese and low-fat pepperoni. Hardly good for you, but enough to meet the government's anemic standards for "healthy." Domino's gave the Houston school district $8 million in exchange for the right to sell these branded pizzas[23]—served in Domino's-emblazoned cardboard boxes and sleeves—in school cafeterias. The company claims it sells its Smart Slice branded pizza in more than 6,000 school districts in forty-seven states.[24] But I guess that's okay because...pizza is a vegetable?

In distorting this initially high-minded legislation to improve the quality of school food, the USDA effectively gift wrapped a present for Big Food. What started as an effort to improve school nutrition devolved into a corporate free-for-all, with watered-down standards crafted by armies of lobbyists. The result? "Copycat" snacks flooding school cafeterias, offering kids the illusion of health while delivering the same candy bars, potato chips, and fast food they'd find at the corner store—just with a slightly more acceptable label.

Instead of providing real nourishment, the school menu reads like a Frankenfood lab. Removing these ultraprocessed "healthified" junk foods from school cafeterias wouldn't just be a win—it could be a game changer for children's health. Too bad the USDA seems more interested in protecting corporate profits than kids' well-being.

BIG FOOD DELIBERATELY TARGETS OUR CHILDREN

The government also allows unregulated food marketing in schools. Studies[25] show that 70 percent of elementary and middle school students in America see ads and product placements[26] for fast food, candy, and soft drinks in their schools—and those ads have a direct impact, leading children to consume more junk-food-laden diets. Food companies pimp their junk via direct advertising in classrooms, such as advertiser-sponsored video and audio programming; indirect advertising by corporate-sponsored educational materials; product sales contracts for soda and snack foods; ads in gyms and school buses and on book covers and bathroom stalls; and "educational TV" such as Channel One. Channel One was available in 12,000 schools and provided ten minutes of current events with two minutes of commercials that went for $200,000 each and reach 40 percent of America's teenagers.[27] We don't let tobacco makers market their products in schools; why do we let processed-food companies, given that those foods kill more people than cigarettes?[28]

Junk-food companies engage in this type of predatory marketing because it's hugely profitable. An Institute of Medicine (IOM) study, *Food Marketing to Children and Youth: Threat or Opportunity?*, which analyzed 123 peer-reviewed research papers, outlines in frightening detail the methods and practices used by the food industry to target youth through conventional TV, billboards, advertising, and stealth marketing.[29] They pay steep bucks to advertising executives to develop commercials specifically designed to entice children, and they've even been known to employ brain-imaging studies to learn how to elicit the desired neural responses from the marketing, as well as hire sophisticated psychographic (read: manipulative) research firms to learn how to influence preschoolers. This *Brave New World*–esque use of neuroscience to manipulate our children is effective. According to the IOM, the most widely employed strategy is to deliberately target children who are too young to distinguish ads from the truth, encouraging them to eat high-calorie, low-nutrient (but highly profitable) junk foods and to demand these foods from their parents. Data shows that kids under age three recognize food brands even before they can read (and sometimes even before they can walk).[30]

Every year, companies such as Coke and McDonald's spend $1.8 billion marketing their products to children as young as two years old.[31] The average child between two and eleven years of age sees ten to eleven of these ads per day.[32] That's roughly 4,000 ads every year! As you might imagine, the majority of these ads aren't for apple slices and sweet potato snacks. They're for products like Cocoa Puffs, Gatorade, and McDonald's Happy Meals that star SpongeBob SquarePants and the Minions.

Most adults can see a television ad for McDonald's and pay it little mind. But according to the American Psychological Association,[33] children under the age of eight don't instinctively recognize the difference between TV commercials and the programs they're watching, which makes them particularly vulnerable to persuasive subliminal messaging. The food industry understands this, and it is why they spend $11 billion[34] just on television ads marketing junk food to our kids every year.[35] That's just on television. Now kids consume most of their media online or on smartphones, where they are not just passive recipients for the big brands but are uniquely, individually targeted, based on their personal preferences and browsing behaviors.

Even scarier, the IOM report was published in 2006, before the arrival of Facebook, Instagram, Twitter/X, Snapchat, TikTok, and other smartphone apps. Now the problem of insidious marketing is much worse. The average kid now spends forty-two to forty-nine hours a week[36] in front of screens and is subject to intense and manipulative stealth marketing.[37] Stealth marketing is harder to track and includes embedded advertising in movies and television, toys, games, educational materials, songs, and movies; character licensing and celebrity endorsements; and less visible campaigns involving word of mouth, text messages, and exposure to products on the internet and social media.

A new subversive and powerful model for marketing junk food to children is "advergames," "free" social media games and apps that integrate junk food into games for little children.[38] These games are almost exclusively marketing obesogenic foods: that is, metabolism-disrupting foods that can lead to obesity.[39] Online marketing is simply more pervasive, pernicious, and effective. In 2001 McDonald's alone spent $635 million on marketing, much of it targeted at children.[40] All of which drives kids to eat more junk and more food overall.

Even our athletics aren't immune to this nonsense. Watching the Super Bowl commercials last year, I was horrified to count eleven junk food and fast food commercials in just the first half. Here we are watching a pinnacle of human athleticism — a testament to peak physical performance — only to be bombarded with commercials glorifying ultraprocessed, artery-clogging, metabolic land mines. Big Food, in all its insidious brilliance, has once again managed to co-opt A-list celebrities, world-class athletes, and even politicians, the very people who should be championing health, to peddle the products that are fueling America's chronic disease crisis.

Imagine if instead of pushing sugar-laden sodas, they promoted hydration, real electrolytes, and, I don't know, maybe health food companies? Imagine if instead of glorifying deep-fried mystery meat, they championed real protein sources and whole foods; if instead of marketing ultraprocessed slop, they invested in making nutritious, accessible meals as desirable as their junk-food counterparts. But that's just not as profitable. These corporations know exactly what they're doing, leveraging people of influence and stardom to associate glamour and success with that triple bacon cheeseburger.

"Advertising directed at children this young is by its very nature exploitative," the American Psychological Association says. Food companies target children because they know that the way to hook them is to reach them early, when they're most impressionable. As the adage goes, a customer created early is a customer for life.

These tactics work. Studies show that children have an uncanny ability to remember the food ads they've seen. Exposure to just a single thirty-second fast-food commercial is enough to instill brand and product preferences in a child,[41] and repeated exposure can set the stage for that child to become a lifelong customer.[42] Fast food and the marketing behind it can lead to detrimental changes in the adolescent brain associated with dysfunctional eating and impulsive behaviors.[43] It can also thwart parents' efforts to instill healthy eating habits in their kids. Teaching your kids to appreciate real food is a herculean task when they're besieged with ads for Frosted Flakes and Pizza Hut.

Fast-food ads don't just play with a child's psyche but also have a direct impact on their weight and long-term health. Scientists have repeatedly shown in studies that even slight increases in the amount of time kids spend viewing junk-food ads can increase their odds of becoming obese by about 20 percent.[44] Teenagers are twice as likely to become obese if they can recall at least one junk-food ad daily.[45] One large study of thousands of teens found that 40 percent of them felt "pressured" to consume unhealthy diets by fast-food and soft drink ads. The more familiar they were with these ads, the more junk food they ate, and that was linked to a higher body weight regardless of their age or gender.[46] In short, the more fast-food ads kids see, the fatter they become.

Make no mistake: Chuck E. Cheese and Ronald McDonald are manipulating children just as Joe Camel did for decades. Only now, the consequences are more devastating. The obesity rate in kids shows no signs of slowing down. In some states, like West Viriginia, almost two-thirds (66 percent) of children are either overweight or obese. The CDC has even begun to document a new category of severely obese kids that it euphemistically calls Class 3 obesity—more commonly known as "morbid obesity."[47]

Even in kids who are not obese, doctors are discovering horrifying metabolic conditions driven by their junk-food diets. Ten percent of children in the United States have fatty liver disease,[48] a condition that was unheard of in youth just 20 years ago and that is now the fastest growing indication for liver transplants nationwide.[49] Liver centers across the country now have teenage patients on their transplant waiting lists—all because their livers can't keep up with the sugar, starch, and heavily processed food they're consuming.

Shouldn't we be outraged? Don't we care to protect our children?

Ultraprocessed Foods on Your Kid's Brain

For the parents reading this, it's crucial to understand just how toxic fast, ultraprocessed foods are for your child's cognitive development. These ingredients don't just flood their small bodies with synthetic, often untested chemicals—they also deprive their developing brains of the essential nutrients needed for learning, focus, and emotional regulation.

Studies have shown that diets high in ultraprocessed foods are linked to lower IQ scores, reduced attention spans, and increased behavioral issues in children. One study[50] published in *The Journal of Epidemiology* found that children who consumed high amounts of processed foods by age three had lower cognitive test scores by age eight. Research has linked children's diets rich in sugar, artificial additives, and refined carbohydrates with higher rates of ADHD symptoms and impaired executive function—skills crucial for reasoning, problem-solving, and impulse control.

Beyond immediate cognitive effects, poor childhood nutrition has long-term consequences. A diet heavy in ultraprocessed foods increases the risk of early-onset metabolic disorders, insulin resistance, and inflammation, all of which are now being linked to neurodegenerative diseases later in life. Simply put: What your child eats today could shape their brain health for decades to come.

And yet, Big Food spends billions ensuring these very products are the easiest, cheapest, and most appealing choices on grocery store shelves and school menus. This isn't just a public health crisis—it's an assault on our children's future.

GOVERNMENT: ON TASK OR FOOD INDUSTRY SERVANT?

With obesity rates soaring and our children's health under constant threat from an assault of sophisticated ads and marketing, a coalition of public health groups, medical experts, and children's health advocates came together to demand that the government take action on food marketing to children. In 2009,[51] Congress ordered the FTC to work with the FDA, CDC, and USDA to recommend standards for food marketing (one of the few times these agencies collaborated). Two years later, the agencies, collectively known as the Interagency Working Group, issued a report that proposed a set of nutrition standards for foods that could be marketed to children. The proposed standards called for the food industry to market foods that were reasonably nutritious—like fruits, vegetables, whole grains, and low-fat dairy products—or products that minimized things like salt, saturated fat, sugar, and sodium.

But like most of our hallowed guidelines, the standards were completely voluntary. The food industry was under no obligation to abide by them at all. Still, the mere proposition of nutrition standards sent the industry into a frenzy. Food companies realized that under the voluntary guidelines, which were fairly lax, they would not be able to market their most profitable soft drinks, breakfast cereals, and junk foods to little children. General Mills, Kellogg's, Pepsi, and an array of other corporate food giants got together and formed a lobbying group to block the nutrition standards. Calling themselves the Sensible Food Policy Coalition (quite the euphemism, I think) the group plowed almost $7 million into their lobbying efforts. Another corporation that joined the fight against the standards was Viacom,[52] which owns Nickelodeon, the kids network whose cartoon characters—such as Sponge-Bob and Dora the Explorer—star in many ads for junk foods targeting kids. The company poured millions of dollars into the effort.[53]

Together the companies pressured the government to drop the voluntary restrictions, saying they were unfair and would harm their business.

Their lobbying coalition even released a dubious report claiming that the voluntary standards would cause $28 billion in lost sales and revenue and ultimately spur the loss of 74,000 jobs (another major industry talking point).[54] As extreme and predictable as it was, the pushback worked. The then head of the FTC, David Vladeck, issued public statements reassuring companies that the proposed standards were toothless and that the FTC had no plans to regulate them. "The proposal doesn't ban any marketing or any foods at all," he told them. "Companies can continue to market and sell the same products they do now. The proposal simply recommends that the products companies choose to market directly to kids—as opposed to the products marketed to their parents—meet the nutrition principles outlined in the report."[55] Good luck with that!

Through its intense lobbying efforts, Big Food effectively neutered the already anemic marketing guidelines. As a gesture, the industry formed its own organization, the Children's Food and Beverage Advertising Initiative,[56] through which each company set their own nutrition criteria[57] and pledged to market only healthy foods during kids' programming, like Saturday morning cartoons.

The criteria were so absurd they bordered on satire. Under Kellogg's own standards, the company was still free to market Froot Loops and Frosted Flakes—both drowning in sugar—to children. Even more egregious, they could promote Yogos, a so-called snack whose primary ingredients were little more than sugar and trans fats masquerading as something remotely nutritious. If this was their idea of responsible advertising, it was a master class in corporate doublespeak.

ONLINE TARGETING OF CHILDREN

In 2016, fifty-six of the biggest food companies placed 509 million banner ads and impressions on CartoonNetwork.com, Nick.com, and other kids' websites. They also placed 3.4 billion ads on Facebook and YouTube alone.[58] In 2016 the World Health Organization issued a report[59] warning that food companies were targeting kids on the internet using powerful ads and extremely effective digital marketing tactics like heavily branded online video games, known as "advergames." The agency warned that fast-food chains were hooking kids in clever ways. One technique involved making McDonald's restaurants important locations in augmented-reality games like the wildly popular Pokémon GO.[60] Pokémon's maker, which signed a sponsorship deal with McDonald's, said it had driven millions of visitors to the chain's restaurants.[61] The WHO warned that parents and public health experts needed to take aggressive steps to counter this new style of marketing.

"The food, marketing and digital industries have access to extremely fine-grained analyses of children's behavior," the agency said in its report. "Children have the right to participate in digital media; and, when they are participating, they have the right to protection of their health and privacy and not to be economically exploited."[62]

FOOD FIX: KICK JUNK FOOD OUT OF SCHOOLS

The Boston public school system was once a model of terrible food. Historically most of the 126 public schools in Boston, which serve 56,000 kids a day, didn't even have real kitchens. They used "satellite kitchens" that consisted of just a freezer and a warming oven. School meals were produced out of state and shipped to Boston schools, where they were heated up in the satellite kitchens—still wrapped in their plastic—and then served to students. In other words, kids were handed TV dinners for breakfast and lunch.[63] When Jill Shah, an entrepreneur and philanthropist whose husband founded the e-commerce website Wayfair, saw how Boston Public Schools was feeding its students, she was horrified.

Shah looked into what it would take for Boston to create full-service kitchens and was told it would cost more than the city was willing to spend: at least $1 million. Shah was undeterred. She came up with a brilliant plan that she called the "Hub and Spoke" model. Rather than ship prepackaged meals from out of state, the schools that already had full-service kitchens would prep food for nearby schools, whose kitchens would be retrofitted with special "combi-ovens" that could steam, roast, and even fry multiple types of food simultaneously without cross-contamination. Shah brought in a well-known local chef, Ken Oringer, to teach food service workers how to prepare meals that were healthier but still delicious. The cost of all this was far less than the city had anticipated: just $65,000 to get the program started, much less than the cost of creating brand-new full-service kitchens for every underprivileged school. In fact, the city ultimately ended up saving substantial money per student meal.

The program, called My Way Café, began as a pilot program at four schools in East Boston in 2017. Prepackaged meals were eliminated. Schools were provided full salad bars and freshly prepared breakfast items — eggs, fruit, turkey, yogurt, and homemade granola. The food was healthier, and students were allowed to choose their own meals. That meant that for the first time they had options. Obviously, the students loved it. The rate of students eating school meals increased by about 15 percent. As a bonus, the program created more jobs for local Boston residents. Shah's program was so successful that in 2018 the mayor of Boston, Martin Walsh, announced he was expanding it to all of Boston's public schools. "Boston is leading the way in making sure our students have access to fresh, healthy food," he proclaimed.[64]

Boston Public Schools, once a model of poor nutrition, is now a model for how every school district should feed its students. It is a travesty that public schools often don't even have real kitchens. Most have only deep fryers, microwaves, and displays for candy and junk food at the cafeteria checkout counters. But Shah's program and others like it are having a huge impact on children's health. They're models for how other school districts can save money, serve better food, and improve the health and well-being of their students.

FOOD FIX: BAN JUNK-FOOD MARKETING THAT PREYS ON KIDS

Unfortunately, some problems only the government can fix. At local and state levels, we also need to limit the reach of fast food—enacting zoning restrictions on fast-food outlets near schools and instituting levies or taxes on fast-food outlets to support community programs for health, education, and so on. On a federal level, we need the FTC to get strict.

The First Amendment doesn't stop us from protecting children from harmful marketing and advertising. Over fifty countries have already taken steps to regulate food marketing aimed at kids—yet the United States remains glaringly absent from that list. Even we managed to get rid of Joe Camel, recognizing the damage of targeting children with tobacco ads. Imagine if a foreign country were harming our children the way Big Food does today. We would go to war to protect them. So why are we allowing this assault on our kids' health to continue unchecked?

The FTC could use its authority to rein in the industry's out-of-control marketing tactics, and lawmakers should enact legislation to protect the most vulnerable. It has the power (but not yet the will) to do the following:

1. **End junk-food advertising to children.** The IOM report advises Congress to act to limit food marketing to kids, including bans of cartoon characters, celebrity endorsements, health claims on food packaging, stealth marketing, and marketing in schools, and to provide support for healthier foods. The IOM advises. Congress ignores. Why? Congress is funded by food lobbyists. Congress and the FTC *should* ban all junk-food ads from airing during children's programming, as recommended by the American Academy of Pediatrics. According to studies[65] referenced by the Academy of Pediatrics, a ban on fast-food ads aimed at kids would reduce the number of overweight children and adolescents in America by an estimated 14 to 18 percent. Meanwhile,

eliminating federal tax deductions for junk-food ads that target children would reduce childhood obesity by up to 7 percent.[66] Why should Big Food get a tax break for manipulating our kids into getting fat and sick?

2. **End predatory digital ads.** In addition to television ads, Congress needs to ban online, digital, and other forms of interactive junk-food and fast-food ads aimed at kids. In many ways these ads are even more harmful because children today spend increasing amounts of time on social media, where regulations are especially lax. In the meantime, pediatricians and family practitioners should discuss food advertising with their patients, encouraging parents to monitor children's exposure. Medical professionals could also emphasize the importance of good nutrition to help counteract the weekly blitz of junk-food advertising most kids are forced to endure.

More than fifty countries regulate food marketing to kids.[67] Following are just a few of the governments that have taken aggressive regulatory steps. When will the United States join them?

- The **Quebec** government was the first to forbid predatory marketing, banning fast-food advertising to kids in electronic and print media way back in 1980.[68] This one aggressive measure has had an impact that still resonates today. A study published in 2011[69] found that the advertising ban led to a 13 percent reduction in fast-food expenditures and an estimated 3.4 billion fewer calories consumed by Quebec's children.[70] Quebec has the lowest childhood obesity rate in Canada.[71]
- Not far behind Quebec is **Sweden**. In 1991 the country instituted a ban on all toy and junk-food commercials aimed at children under the age of twelve. To this day, the law remains very popular in Sweden. Sweden has one of the lowest childhood obesity rates in Europe.[72]
- The **United Kingdom** has one of the highest rates of childhood obesity in Europe (about 40 percent of children ages ten

and eleven in London are overweight or obese),[73] but British public health officials have begun to take action in recent years. About a decade ago the government implemented a ban on junk-food TV ads aimed at children under the age of sixteen.[74] The impact was so striking that some cities decided to go further. In 2018 the city decided to ban all junk-food ads from its public transport system. That meant no more ads for candy bars, soft drinks, and potato chips on its iconic double-decker buses or the Tube. The United Kingdom now has some of the strictest standards in the world. In 2018,[75] its Advertising Standards Authority pulled several online ads created by Cadbury and other candy companies because they did not do enough to prevent adolescents from viewing them.[76]

3. **Parents: Limit your children's screen time.** If you have a child under two years of age, make sure he or she does not watch television or use technology. Studies have shown that it can be detrimental to their brains. Why do you think so many Silicon Valley tech executives—the guys behind the forever scroll—don't let their children use technology such as smartphones, iPads, or computers?[77] They know that they are designed to be addictive. Similarly, many Big Food company executives don't let their kids use their own products (or eat or drink them themselves). For older children, the best thing you can do is tightly monitor their screen time and filter out the programs or channels with harmful ads. Look for programs you can download that are free of junk-food commercials and other predatory ads. Select programs for kids to watch on PBS, which tends to restrict junk-food ads, or Netflix so they won't be bombarded with food commercials every five minutes. Limit their amount of screen time to an hour or less each day. Strong evidence also exists that screen time is linked to attention deficit disorder in children and is the second-biggest driver of obesity after sugar-sweetened beverages.[78]

We don't have to sit idly by letting Big Food prey on our children. Let's protect them at home and in school with nutritious foods and education that builds the foundation for a healthy life. And let's support organizations and leaders who want to do the same.

> For a quick reference guide on the Food Fixes and resources on how to protect your children, go to www.foodfixuncensored.com.

CHAPTER 9

HOW THE FDA FAILS TO PROTECT US

The average American eats a junk-food diet; about 60 percent of adult calories,[1] and close to 70 percent of kids' calories,[2] come from ultraprocessed foods. But even if you're trying to eat "healthy," you've probably struggled trying to make sense of food labels. Which is fair because many of them might as well be written in a foreign language. You practically need a nutritional biochemistry degree to decipher the ingredients label on a protein bar or a cup of yogurt. Have you ever read a food label and wondered what the heck mono- and diglycerides are? Or why carrageenan, maltodextrin, and soy lecithins are in so many processed foods? I certainly don't recall finding any of those ingredients in my grandma's cupboard, do you?

Spoiler alert: These ingredients are emulsifiers and chemical additives that warrant a "drop the package and run" response. As a rule of thumb, if you can't pronounce an ingredient, it's probably not something you want to put in your body.

Unfortunately, most people don't know to read the ingredients labels, which, admittedly, are usually buried on the back of food packages and written in print that requires a magnifying glass. It certainly doesn't help that the other essential source of health information, the "nutrition facts" panel, is often just as confusing. Most people don't know what a "percent daily value" is or whether the serving sizes listed under the nutrition facts are realistic (they are not).

How to Make
Canola Oil

Shelf-life: 2+ years

- Collect GMO canola seed from rapeseed
- Clean seed and perform flaking
- Cook and press seeds
- Use chemical solvent on press cake (hexane)

RBD Process:

- Refined (mixing oil with chemicals)
- Bleach (filtering through bleaching clay
- De-gum (heating oil with water + acid)
- Deodorize (oxidizing oils at 440-485°)

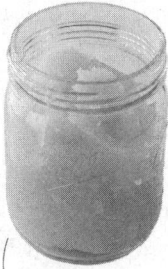

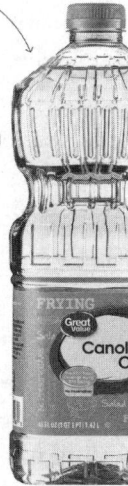

How to Make
Tallow
(Beef Fat)

Shelf-life: 1-3 months

- Cook meat or bones (bone broth)
- Collect fat and cool

Dr. Marty Makary, a surgeon and public health researcher who was recently appointed commissioner of the FDA, has been critical of the US food supply, describing it as "poisoned" due to the prevalence of unhealthy additives and processing methods. He has expressed concerns about the influence of Big Food companies and the widespread use of pesticides, advocating for a reevaluation of dietary guidelines and food safety regulations to prioritize public health. To understand my point about processing methods, see the image above for the differences between a naturally occurring fat (tallow) versus a highly processed fat (canola oil).

The FDA regulates food labels—a prime example of how the agency is failing the public. Allowing them to be deliberately misleading and confusing only serves the interests of Big Food, not those of the consumers they are supposed to protect. As Jerold Mande, a nutrition expert who worked on food labels[3] at the FDA and the USDA, explained it to me, many food companies do not want you to know what's in their products, so they deliberately make their ingredients hard to read. "A lot of companies use all capital letters and they squish them together and use a super small font, about 1/16-of-an-inch letter," he said. It is not an accident.

In a similarly egregious obfuscation, companies cheat the requirement to list ingredients in the order of their predominance (how much of each ingredient is in the product). While they are *technically* required to list ingredients in order of their predominance by weight, this rule is deliberately vague and leaves out critical context. It doesn't tell you how much of each ingredient is actually in the product. For instance, if sugar is listed as the second ingredient, it could make up a staggering 30 percent of the product—or a relatively smaller 5 percent. Without a volume or ratio requirement, the label provides no way to tell the difference, allowing manufacturers to hide just how much of the unhealthy stuff you're consuming.

The situation becomes even murkier when companies use ingredient splitting to game the system further. By breaking down sugar into multiple forms—like cane sugar, high-fructose corn syrup, dextrose, or malt syrup—they can list each one separately in smaller amounts, pushing them lower on the ingredients list. This allows ingredients like sugar to appear scattered across the label, making it look less prominent than it actually is, even if it's the single largest component of the food. This tactic not only deceives consumers but also undermines the spirit of transparency the labeling rules are supposed to enforce.

Have you ever picked up Nutella, one of America's favorite "healthy" breakfast staples, or a jar of strawberry jam at the supermar-

What's *really* in Nutella?

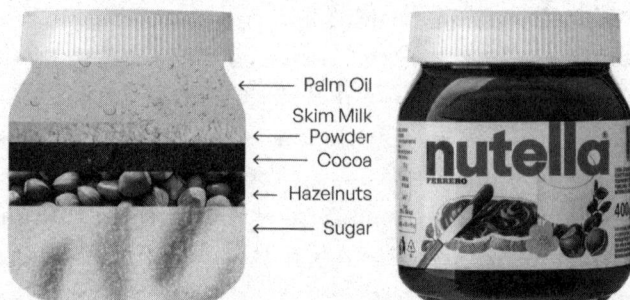

- Palm Oil
- Skim Milk Powder
- Cocoa
- Hazelnuts
- Sugar

ket, and looked at the ingredients list? A jar of Smucker's strawberry jam lists strawberries as the first ingredient, and then the second, third, and fourth ingredients are as follows: high-fructose corn syrup, corn syrup, and sugar.[4] This tactic is very common. The reason companies often use several sweeteners in one product is so they don't have to list "sugar" as the first ingredient. As Mande explained, "What we know from some investigations is that companies often use five different sugars in their products so that they don't show up high on the list."

THE FDA ALLOWS HARMFUL INGREDIENTS IN OUR FOOD

In addition to regulating food labels, one of the FDA's top responsibilities is ensuring the safety of the food supply. Under a federal regulation passed in 1958 called the Food Additives Amendment, any substance that the food industry intentionally adds to its products is considered a food additive.[5] All food additives are theoretically subject to premarket review and FDA approval (similar to how pharmaceuticals work). Food additives are only exempted from this rule if they are GRAS, or *generally recognized as safe*. The GRAS system was designed to apply to ingredients that have been dietary staples for generations, like cinnamon, vanilla, baking powder, salt, pepper, olive oil, vinegar, caffeine, butter, and a variety of natural extracts and flavorings.[6] In other words, things our forefathers would recognize.

But thanks to aggressive industry lobbying and systemic under-resourcing for the agency, the FDA has ceded much of its regulatory power over food additives to food manufacturers. In a blatant case of the fox guarding the henhouse, the FDA has allowed chemical industry trade groups like the Flavor and Extract Manufacturers Association to declare new food chemicals as GRAS without any scientific explanation at all.[7]

In 2013, a study published in *JAMA Internal Medicine* found that the GRAS review process lacked integrity because many of the GRAS committee members who make safety determinations have strong industry ties. "Between 1997 and 2012," the authors concluded, "we found that financial conflicts of interest were ubiquitous in determinations that an additive to food was GRAS. The lack of independent review in GRAS determinations raises concerns about the integrity of the process and whether it ensures the safety of the food supply."[8]

Today more than 10,000 additives are allowed in food with 43 percent of them alleging to be GRAS,[9] while the majority have never actually been tested for safety(!).[10] The average American consumes six to nine pounds[11] of these chemical additives every year.

Consumer watchdog groups have repeatedly urged the FDA to step up its oversight of these additives. In 2015, the Natural Resources Defense Council, the Center for Science in the Public Interest, the Environmental Working Group, and other organizations filed an eighty-page report[12] with the FDA, laying out exactly how its failure to vet new chemicals violates the law. The report listed a number of additives that cause cancer. In a very strange statement, the FDA said those additives were not harmful even if they caused cancer in animals, but they were removing them anyway because of the law.[13]

Even more alarming is the fact that many chemicals and agricultural drugs banned in Europe and other countries remain perfectly legal in the United States. Why? Because our regulatory system operates under a "prove it's dangerous first" model, rather than a "prove it's safe first" approach. Innocent until proven guilty works in our judicial system, but not when it comes to potentially harmful chemical food additives. Here, chemicals are considered innocent until they've caused enough damage to warrant regulation—often after years of widespread exposure and harm to our population. Trans fats were created in 1911 and not ruled as harmful by the FDA until 2015 despite decades of evidence showing harm! In contrast, the European Union follows the precautionary principle, restricting or banning substances until they are proven safe. Meanwhile, we wait for the body count to stack up before taking action. Call me crazy, but Europe's system seems like the smarter bet.

In early 2025, seeing the writing on the wall, the Consumer Brands Association (CBA)—formerly known as the Grocery Manufacturers Association—scrambled to meet with the newly appointed Health and Human Services Secretary Robert F. Kennedy Jr. to discuss his "Make America

Healthy Again" (MAHA) agenda, which has publicly announced its priority to eliminate harmful chemicals from the American food supply.

While the CBA publicly framed the meeting as "constructive"[14] and claimed to be open to collaboration on public health initiatives, behind closed doors, private intel indicates that their strategy is nothing more than a PR ploy to maintain their grip on a broken system. For decades, these corporations have fought tooth and nail against meaningful reform, prioritizing cost-cutting measures and shareholder profits over the well-being of American families. Their history is littered with efforts to stonewall regulation, gaslight consumers, and deceive the public into believing their chemical-laden products are "safe."

The CBA's insistence on preserving the outdated and corrupt GRAS standard—which allows companies to unilaterally decide the safety of food additives with zero meaningful oversight—exposes their true agenda. This self-regulatory sham has given the food industry carte blanche to flood the US market with synthetic dyes, harmful preservatives, and untested chemicals, many of which are banned in other countries. Their playbook? Exploit regulatory loopholes, flood legislative channels with industry-backed studies, and ensure that American consumers remain in the dark about the toxic cocktail hidden in their food.

Moreover, the CBA's relentless push to block state-led food safety initiatives under the guise of avoiding a "patchwork" of regulations is nothing more than an attempt to consolidate power at the federal level—where their lobbying machine can wield the most influence. They fear stricter state-level protections that could set a precedent for real accountability, so instead, they lobby for weak, industry-friendly national standards that leave consumers unprotected.

The American public has been manipulated, misled, and fed lies for far too long. The CBA and its corporate cronies are not allies in the fight for public health—they are the very entities blocking the long-overdue progress. As the adage goes: Don't judge people based on what they promise; judge them based on what they *actually* do.

It is imperative that consumers, lawmakers, and health advocates remain vigilant, demand transparency, and hold these corporations accountable. The time for half measures and empty promises is over. The era of unchecked industry dominance over America's food supply must come to an end.

CORPORATE HYPOCRISY: WHY DO AMERICAN FAMILIES GET THE SHORT END OF THE STICK?

Now let's talk about corporate hypocrisy: The same American food companies that fill grocery store aisles with dyes, fillers, and chemicals linked to cancer, hyperactivity, and metabolic dysfunction have no problem removing those same ingredients when selling their products in Europe, the United Kingdom, and even China.

Let that sink in.

The food your children eat every day—cereal, snacks, soda, and even so-called healthy convenience foods—contains ingredients that wouldn't even be legal in other countries. And in some cases, using these ingredients could result in jail time.

Take Kraft Mac & Cheese. In the United States, it has been made with yellow dyes no. 5 and no. 6,[15] both of which are banned or restricted in the European Union due to health concerns. But in Europe? The same product is colored with the natural spice paprika and beta-carotene (found in carrots)—because regulators there actually hold companies accountable. Or consider Fanta Orange soda—in the United Kingdom, it contains real orange juice, no artificial dyes, and far less sugar. In the United States? Fanta has been a chemical cocktail of high-fructose corn syrup, artificial flavors, and petroleum-based dyes like red dye no. 40 and yellow dye no. 6[16]—ingredients that are restricted abroad because of their links to hyperactivity in children and potential carcinogenic effects.[17]

And it's not just those products. Kellogg's cereals[18]—like Froot Loops and Frosted Flakes—have been packed with synthetic dyes (red dye no. 40, blue dye no. 1, yellow dye no. 6) and the preservative BHT, a chemical banned in Japan and the European Union due to safety concerns. But in Europe, Kellogg's uses natural alternatives and removes BHT entirely.

Why does this happen?

Because these companies can get away with it. Instead of following one global standard based on health and safety, they exploit the weakest regulations of each country—maximizing profit at the expense of public health. If American companies are already making cleaner, safer versions of their products for other nations, why are we still eating the chemical-laden versions here? Because they know US regulatory agencies won't stop them. And as long as their profit margins stay high, they have zero incentive to change.

U.S. Version

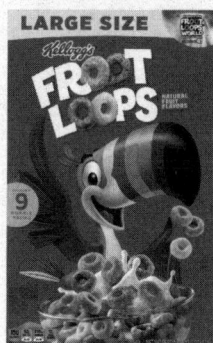

Froot Loops: Corn Flour Blend (Whole Grain Yellow Corn Flour, Degerminated Yellow Corn Flour), Sugar, Wheat Flour, Whole Grain Oat Flour, Modified Food Starch, Contains 2% or Less of Vegetable Oil (Hydrogenated Coconut, Soybean and/or Cottonseed), Oat Fiber, Maltodextrin, Salt, Soluble Corn Fiber, Natural Flavor, **Red 40, Yellow 5, Blue 1, Yellow 6, BHT for Freshness.** Vitamins and Minerals: Vitamin C (Ascorbic Acid), Reduced Iron, Niacinamide, Vitamin B6 (Pyridoxine Hydrochloride), Vitamin B2 (Riboflavin), Vitamin B1 (Thiamin Hydrochloride), Folic Acid, Vitamin D3, Vitamin B12.

Canada Version

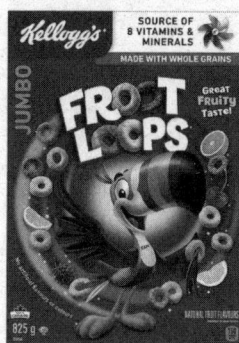

Froot Loops: Sugars (Sugar, Maltodextrin), Whole Grain Corn Flour, Wheat Flour, Whole Grain Oat Flour, Degerminated Corn Flour, Corn Bran, Oat Hull Fibre, Hydrogenated Coconut and Vegetable Oil, Salt, Concentrated Carrot Juice (for colour), Anthocyanin, Annatto, Turmeric, Natural Flavour, Concentrated Watermelon Juice (for colour), Concentrated Blueberry Juice (for colour), Concentrated Huito Juice (for colour), Stevia Leaf Extract. Vitamins and Minerals: Iron, Niacinamide, Zinc Oxide, Thiamine Hydrochloride, D-Calcium Pantothenate, Cholecalciferol (Vitamin D), Pyridoxine Hydrochloride, Folic Acid.

The good news? Consumers are waking up, and influencers with massive platforms are amplifying the issue.

In October 2024, food activist Vani Hari (the Food Babe) launched a petition[19] against Kellogg's, calling out their refusal to clean up their ingredients in the United States despite doing so overseas. The campaign gained massive traction, forcing Kellogg's to respond publicly.[20] Her viral videos exposing synthetic food dyes and chemical-laden American cereals juxtaposed against other developed nations' cleaner versions of the same products have been shared millions of times, with everyday consumers flooding comment sections, demanding change.

Meanwhile, the grassroots group Moms for MAHA (Moms Against Harmful Additives)[21] has gained momentum, rallying parents to push for food safety reforms and urging school districts to ban artificially dyed and processed foods. A recent viral parody video,[22] distributed by the White House, featured moms, Congress members, and even RFK Jr. humorously struggling to pronounce complex food ingredient names—highlighting the prevalence of questionable additives in everyday products. While comically mocking US food companies for using dangerous ingredients here but not abroad, the video sparked outrage online, with millions sharing their disgust at Big Food's exploitation.

This initiative is part of Kennedy's broader MAHA agenda, which seeks to align US food safety standards with stricter European regulations within four years. The agenda has garnered support from President Trump and aims to eliminate artificial dyes and reassess the GRAS standard that allows many additives into the food supply without rigorous oversight.

The pressure is mounting. The public is demanding better, and companies can no longer hide behind regulatory loopholes and deceptive marketing. The question now is: Will they clean up their act, or will consumers (or legislation) force their hand?

In response, some food companies are proactively adjusting their products. For instance, several restaurant chains like Steak 'n Shake have begun replacing seed oils in their cooking processes, influenced by recent advocacy and consumer demand for healthier options.

FROM SNACK TO SCIENCE EXPERIMENT: HOW BIG FOOD TURNED JUNK FOOD INTO CHEMICAL WARFARE

It's bad enough that American food companies sell cleaner versions of their products overseas while pumping the US market full of chemicals. But what's even worse? Over the last few decades, they've systematically transformed junk food from simple, indulgent treats into ultraprocessed, lab-engineered Frankenfoods.

Let's take a simple cookie from the 1970s. A homemade version back then might have been made with flour, sugar, butter, eggs, vanilla, and maybe a little baking soda—ingredients your grandmother would recognize. Even the processed store-bought version had relatively straightforward ingredients.

Now? The modern equivalent is a science experiment loaded with artificial preservatives, emulsifiers, seed oils, synthetic flavors, and chemical dyes—most of which are linked to gut inflammation, metabolic dysfunction, and neurological issues. Take a look at what's happened to some of America's most iconic junk foods:

Product	Then	Now
Wonder Bread	1921: Flour, water, yeast, salt, milk, and eggs	2025: Enriched bleached flour (wheat flour stripped of nutrients, then artificially "enriched" with niacin, reduced iron, thiamine mononitrate, riboflavin, and folic acid), water, high-fructose corn syrup, soybean oil, wheat gluten, and yeast; it also includes less than 2% of salt, calcium carbonate, dough conditioners (which may contain mono- and diglycerides, ethoxylated mono- and diglycerides, sodium stearoyl lactylate, calcium peroxide, calcium iodate, DATEM, azodicarbonamide), yeast nutrients (calcium sulfate, ammonium sulfate), calcium propionate (a preservative to retain freshness), monocalcium phosphate, and soy lecithin

Product	Then	Now
Gatorade	1965: Water, sugar, salt, potassium, and lemon juice	2025: Water, sugar, dextrose, citric acid, salt, sodium citrate, monopotassium phosphate, modified food starch, natural and artificial flavors, sucrose acetate isobutyrate, glycerol ester of rosin, and color additives such as red dye no. 40, yellow dye no. 5, or blue dye no. 1, depending on the flavor; these ingredients are used to enhance flavor, improve texture, and extend shelf life, with artificial colors and stabilizers giving Gatorade its signature bright appearance.
Twinkies	1930: Flour, eggs, sugar, butter, and vanilla	2025: Enriched bleached wheat flour (niacin, ferrous sulfate, thiamine mononitrate, riboflavin, folic acid), sugar, corn syrup, high fructose corn syrup, tallow, hydrogenated tallow, soybean oil, cottonseed oil, eggs, water, dextrose, corn starch, modified corn starch, whey, glycerin, salt, sodium acid pyrophosphate, baking soda, monocalcium phosphate, mono- and diglycerides, polysorbate 60, sodium stearoyl lactylate, soy lecithin, cellulose gum, xanthan gum, sorbic acid, potassium sorbate, natural and artificial flavors, and color additives yellow dye no. 5 and red dye no. 40; these ingredients include preservatives, emulsifiers, stabilizers, and artificial colors, ensuring Twinkies remain soft, flavorful, and shelf-stable for extended periods

What was once real bread is now a chemical mystery that never molds and barely qualifies as food. What started as a hydration tool for athletes is now a sugar-laden chemical cocktail that's marketed as a health drink. And a simple sponge cake became an industrialized science project with a shelf life longer than the lives of some small animals.

And it's not just snack food. Even seemingly "healthy" items like granola bars, yogurt, and protein shakes have become ultraprocessed, packed with fillers and synthetic additives.

"It's fine, I ate that when I was a kid."
(no you didn't)

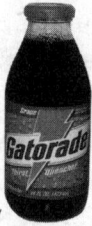

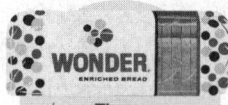

"It's fine, I ate that when I was a kid."
(no you didn't)

Then:
Glass
Container

Water, Sugar
Potassium,
Lemon Juice

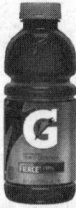

Now: Plastic Container
Water, Sugar, Dextrose
Citric Acid, Natural Flavor,
Sodium Citrate, Salt,
Monopotassium Phosphate,
Modified Food Starch,
Glycerol Ester of Rosin,
Blue 1, Red 40

Then:
Wheat Flour,
Water, Sugar,
Yeast, Salt,
Milk, Butter

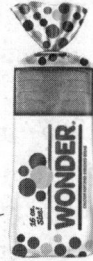

Now:
Enriched Bleach Flour, Water, **High Fructose Corn**
Syrup, Yeast, **Soybean Oil,** Salt, Wheat Gluten,
Vinegar, and **Calcium Propionate** as a Preservative
Monoglycerides, Dicalcium Phosphate, Calcium
Sulfate, Ammonium Sulfate, Sodium Stearoyl
Lactylate, Calcium Carbonate, DATEM (a dough
conditioner), Soy Lecithin (an emulsifier)

Why did this happen? Because it's cheaper, extends shelf life, and makes food more addictive (in other words: repeat customers). The food industry isn't just feeding us—they're engineering products designed to keep us hooked, eating more, and getting sicker.

The real question is: If Big Food was once capable of making simpler versions of these products, why have they turned them into chemical-laden junk? The answer is clear: because it maximizes profit at the expense of our health. It's time we stop accepting Frankenfood as normal—and start demanding real food again.

Here's the question we should all be asking: Why do these companies treat American consumers as second-class citizens? And more importantly, when are we going to stop letting them get away with it?

Here are just a few of the many examples of the food toxins compromising our health that are banned abroad but fully legal in the United States:

- **Potassium bromate and azodicarbonamide,** used in baked goods to make flour rise faster and look pretty, and also used ubiquitously in home goods like yoga mats (raising an eyebrow yet?). In 1999, potassium bromate was labeled as a potential human carcinogen[23] by the International Agency for Research on Cancer; it causes cancer in animals, and in Singapore azodicarbonamide use carries a fine of

$450,000 and 15 years in jail![24] Petitions to ban it have been at the FDA for years, but so far, only public pressure—led by Vani Hari's campaign against Subway—has pushed fast-food chains like McDonald's, Chick-fil-A, and Wendy's to remove it, while the FDA still permits its use under GRAS regulations.

- **Brominated vegetable oil (BVO).** If you have ever had Mountain Dew or sports drinks, you have had BVO. Bromine is a flame retardant that causes memory loss, nerve damage, and skin problems. Used in some soda and sports drinks as an emulsifier, BVO is banned in the European Union, Canada, Japan, and India, but until recently, allowed in the United States.[25]
- **Farm animal drugs.** Drugs used in raising livestock, including bovine growth hormone to promote milk production and ractopamine to make animals fat, are also harmful to humans. Used to increase milk production in dairy cows, recombinant bovine somatotropin (rBST) and recombinant bovine growth hormone (rBGH) are banned in Canada, the European Union, Australia, New Zealand, and Japan, but allowed in the United States.
- **Yellow food dyes no. 5 and no. 6 and red dye no. 40.** If any of these dyes are used in Europe, the foods are slapped with a warning label that says "may have an adverse effect on activity and attention in children."[26] Studies have clearly shown that these dyes cause hyperactivity and behavior changes in children.[27] Yet in America, they are everywhere—candy, icing, cereal, mustard, ketchup, breakfast bars, and other foods. Yellow dye no. 5 is known to cause allergies, hives, and asthma. Notably, following a major protest of Kellogg's Froot Loops in the autumn of 2024—organized by my friends and fellow nutrition warriors Vani Hari and Jason Karp—red dye no. 3 (erythrosine) was banned by the FDA on January 15, 2025,[28] citing health concerns, leaving eight synthetic dyes currently approved for general use in the US food supply.
- **BHA and BHT.** BHA and BHT are used in many processed-food products as preservatives and flavor enhancers. They're even in our children's cereals. These additives are severely restricted in Europe.

BHA is actually listed by our own government as "reasonably anticipated" to be a human carcinogen.[29] But that's not a strong enough association for the FDA to protect us, or could it be the food lobby and the revolving door between the FDA and the food industry? All of the cereals in the following image contain BHT in America. The question is . . . why?

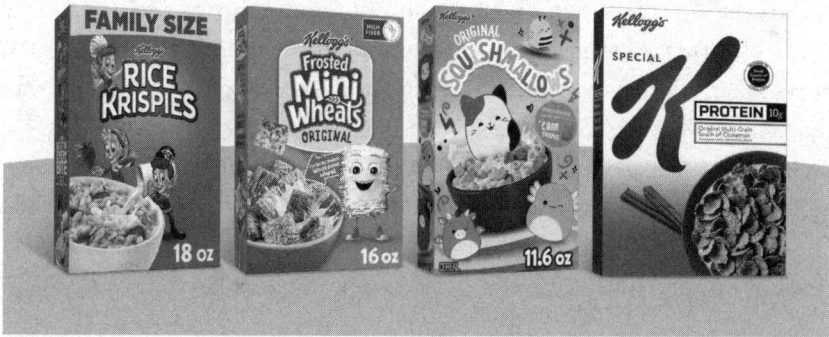

This is just illustrative. I could write an entire book on these ingredients alone. So why are we allowing ourselves to poison our children and our nation?

The FDA is asleep at the wheel, at best. At worst it is doing the bidding of the food industry. And sadly, we have seen this story before. The most striking example of this is trans fats, a man-made additive that persisted in the food supply for 50 years after it was found harmful and after it was known that it caused millions of heart attacks. Yet because trans fats were designated and promoted as "safe," Americans swapped out their natural butter, tallow, and lard for the synthetic, factory-made margarine and shortening instead. It was only in the 1990s that well-designed studies demonstrated that even slight increases in trans-fat consumption promoted heart disease,[30] giving scientists the smoking gun they needed to wipe it off the market. It took 50 years from the time scientists found that trans fats were harmful for the FDA to remove it from the GRAS list, and even then, it was only after a lawsuit. Why? Trans fats were one of the main building blocks of processed and fast food. The food industry did what it usually does: It downplayed the science and fought against regulations.

But in a plot twist from the rest of this story, the public health community banded together and succeeded in banishing trans fats as a nutrition outcast. The beginning of the end for trans fats came in 2006, when New York City banned trans fats in restaurant food.[31] The food industry aggressively opposed the measure, but other cities and states across the country—from Massachusetts and Vermont to Maryland and California, among others—soon followed suit. Then, finally, after years of dragging its feet, the FDA announced in 2015 that it was removing trans fats from the GRAS list. The FDA ultimately did the right thing. But it should have acted sooner. New York City's bold and early action on trans fats paid dividends: A study of its 2006 trans-fat ban found that in just a few years it led to a nearly 7 percent citywide drop in hospital admissions for heart attacks and strokes.[32]

A DIFFERENT TYPE OF CHEMICAL: ANTIBIOTICS IN ANIMAL FEED

Antibiotics are a multibillion-dollar category of drugs that save many lives. But the majority[33] of antibiotics aren't prescribed by doctors and used by sick patients—they're fed to livestock on factory farms to reduce the spread of nasty infections caused by overcrowding, filth, and other cruel and unsanitary conditions in confined animal feeding operations, or CAFOs. In other words, the drugs are used to address some of the horrific conditions of factory farming, like cows' stomachs exploding as a result of eating corn (which ferments and creates excess gas in the stomach) instead of their natural food, grasses. Without antibiotics, the cows' stomachs would explode. Sounds awfully dystopian to me.

For the food industry, a welcome side effect of stuffing animals with antibiotics is that it makes them bigger and fatter with less food, so they are more profitable.[34] As a result, antibiotics have become a staple in industrial farming. But this comes at a terrible cost to global health (and, obviously, animal welfare).

The spread of antibiotic-resistant diseases is a rapidly growing threat across the globe, contributing to the deaths of 700,000 people worldwide each year, and it's predicted that by 2050 this global epidemic will kill *more people than cancer*.[35] There is little dispute over what is driving this epidemic: It's the overuse of antibiotics. This isn't just because antibiotics are wildly overprescribed in hospital settings (including for viral infections, for which they are useless). It's also because of the excessive use of antibiotics in animal food production. The drugs reduce the infection rate in farm animals, but a small number of bacteria invariably survive and then mutate into drug-resistant germs. Remember how COVID-19 mutated into several more virulent variations once the vaccines came out? It's kind of a similar concept for bacteria.

According to the CDC, "Use of antibiotics on the farm helps to produce antibiotic-resistant germs. Giving antibiotics to animals will kill most bacteria, but resistant bacteria can survive and multiply. When food animals are slaughtered and processed, these bacteria can contaminate the meat or other animal products. These bacteria can also get into the environment and may spread to fruits, vegetables, or other produce that is irrigated with contaminated water."[36] It's a lose-lose-lose situation.

The CDC reports that at least half a dozen multistate outbreaks of food poisoning have been linked to drug-resistant bacteria since 2011, including one that sickened 634 people in 29 states. More than one-third of those people were hospitalized.[37] *Consumer Reports* testing found that meat from conventionally raised animals is twice as likely to contain superbugs as meat from animals that are raised without antibiotics.[38]

It's not just meat eaters who have to worry. One outbreak of E. coli that killed three people in 2006 was linked to spinach that had been contaminated by pig and cow manure from a nearby farm.[39] Experts have found that the drug-resistant bacteria that spawn from the indiscriminate use of antibiotics on farms can spread to people in many ways:

■ Farmworkers can be infected while handling animals and manure and then pass superbugs to other people.

- Superbugs can be spread to crops and groundwater through the use of contaminated fertilizer.
- Manure and urine slurries containing antibiotics are often spread on fields, killing the microbiology of the soil, disrupting ecosystems that support nutrient-dense crops, and allowing antibiotic-resistant bacteria to enter the food chain. This ultimately threatens human gut health, immune function, and our ability to fight infections.[40]
- Drug-resistant bacteria can even be spread throughout communities by the wind. One study of people living near farms in rural Pennsylvania found that they were nearly 40 percent[41] more likely to contract MRSA infections (a bug you definitely don't want) than people who lived farther away.[42]

The economic price of overusing antibiotics is likely to be staggering as well. RAND Europe, a nonprofit research organization, looked at the impact of the overuse of antibiotics in agriculture on labor productivity. Hold on to your hats, ladies and gentlemen: Globally, between now and 2050, the cost of antibiotic resistance is estimated to climb as high as $124.5 trillion!! That doesn't even include any associated health care costs, so this is obviously a massive underestimate.[43] The Union of Concerned Scientists estimates that in the United States alone the public health costs are already more than $2 billion a year.[44]

With so much at stake, you might think that the FDA would take aggressive action to protect the public. The agency has the power to clamp down on the use of antibiotics in animal feed. It can tightly regulate them, forcing drug companies and factory farms to be more circumspect about using antibiotics. And the FDA could track their usage more closely, so that health authorities could prevent drug-resistant outbreaks or contain them more quickly when they occur.

In 2020, the FDA estimated that approximately 10.4 million pounds of antibiotics were sold for use in livestock, primarily to prevent disease in overcrowded conditions.[45] In 2019, health care providers wrote 251.1 million antibiotic prescriptions.[46] While antibiotic use in livestock has declined from its peak in 2015, it still accounts for nearly twice the volume of human antibiotic consumption in the United States.

How could that be? Because, as I elucidated above, the FDA allows the food industry to police itself. Illustratively, in 2013, the FDA announced[47] that it wanted drug companies to change the way veterinary antibiotics were sold and labeled. It asked drug companies to remove indications for weight gain and growth promotion, and said that antibiotics should only be fed to animals with a veterinarian's approval. That means that in theory the drugs should not be prescribed specifically to make animals bigger and fatter.

But the FDA made the plan completely *voluntary*. No regulation, no legislation. It just politely suggested that Big Ag not use antibiotics, advice that was (obviously) promptly ignored. Not a surprise considering that the deputy commissioner of the FDA from 2010 to 2016, Mike Taylor, was the former vice president of public policy for Monsanto. Another major loophole is that the food industry can continue to haphazardly use antibiotics and then claim that they are doing so for reasons other than growth promotion. Even when the FDA placed a "ban"[48] on using antibiotics for growth promotion on factory farms in 2017, it had little impact. Today, the food industry continues to pump animals full of these drugs; it remains the nation's largest procurer of antibiotics. Actually, 70 percent of all antibiotics sold annually are used in food animal production.[49]

FOOD FIX: THE POWER OF ONE PERSON TO CHANGE BIG FOOD

By now, you may be thinking, *What can I really do about any of these problems in the food industry?* Well, in fact, you can do a lot. My friend Vani Hari proves it.

Vani Hari might be the single most influential food activist in America today. She has taken down Big Food companies and spurred more food industry reforms than any other person I know. She's forced multibillion-dollar corporations to remove unhealthy additives and disclose potentially harmful ingredients in their products. Her words and actions are so powerful that in 2015, *Time* magazine named her one of its 30 Most Influential People on the Internet.[50]

Long before she became the self-proclaimed Food Babe and a household name, Hari was just your average person eating a junk-food diet like the vast majority of other people on this planet. As the daughter of Indian immigrants who came to the United States to pursue the American Dream, Hari was raised to believe that the American food system was among the best in the world. But eating the American diet made her sick and fat. She had asthma, eczema, acne, stomach problems, and severe allergies. Then she embarked down a rabbit hole, learning about nutrition (or the anti-nutrition she was used to), and realized her food was making her sick. She changed her diet to whole foods and her health problems and the excess weight disappeared.

She started sharing her experiences on a blog, *Food Babe,* and exposing the chemical and harmful ingredients in most fast and processed foods. She started with Chick-fil-A, which listed one hundred ingredients in a chicken sandwich, including MSG and TBHQ (a derivative of butane, an ingredient in gasoline). In response, Chick-fil-A invited her to their headquarters and not only listened but actually made changes. In 2013, the company announced that it was removing artificial dyes, high-fructose corn syrup, and TBHQ from its products. The company also said it would begin using only antibiotic-free chickens. For Vani, it was a huge victory, and one that would turn out to be the first of many.[51]

She later took on Chipotle, outing them for using trans fats and GMO ingredients while claiming to be a healthy food restaurant. They were forced to be transparent and became the first national chain to remove GMO ingredients from their food after thousands signed Vani's petition.[52] Kraft was next in her sights for using artificial dyes and preservatives in their mac and cheese in the United States but not in the United Kingdom, where they are prohibited. Using her "Food Babe Army" to garner hundreds of thousands of signatures and camping out at their offices, she ultimately forced them to remove the chemicals.[53] Next on her list was Subway, whose slogan "Eat Fresh" was misleading. Why? They used an ingredient called azodicarbonamide—also found in yoga mats—in their bread in the United States but not in other countries, where it was banned. Hari got Subway to stop using it and also agree to source only antibiotic-free meat. Many of the biggest fast-food chains across the globe followed suit. McDonald's, Wendy's, Jack in the Box, Chick-fil-A, and White Castle, among others, all removed azodicarbonamide from their products too![54] Starbucks was called out for using a carcinogenic caramel color in their pumpkin spice latte and removed it. General Mills and Kellogg's agreed to stop using the toxic preservative BHT.

Her latest victory came as recently as 2025, when she reignited her campaign against Kellogg's, focusing on the company's continued use of artificial dyes and the preservative BHT in their US cereals—a practice Kellogg's had pledged to eliminate by 2018. This commitment remained unfulfilled, with products like Froot Loops still containing these additives, despite international versions using natural alternatives.

Hari's renewed efforts included a petition demanding the removal of these artificial ingredients, which garnered over 400,000 signatures. In October 2024, she led a protest at Kellogg's headquarters in Battle Creek, Michigan, delivering the petition alongside more than 1,000 supporters. This demonstration, which aimed to hold Kellogg's accountable for its unkept promise and to advocate for healthier ingredients in their cereals, caught the attention of A-listers such as Eva Mendes and Ellen DeGeneres, further amplifying the conversation.

And while as of January 2025, there has been no official announcement from Kellogg's regarding a comprehensive removal of artificial dyes and BHT from all their US cereals, the campaign led by Hari has intensified public scrutiny on food additives, including the recent ban of red dye no. 3 by the FDA.

Thankfully, Vani Hari lays out a blueprint for how anyone can use food activism to fight for food industry reforms in her latest book, *Feeding You Lies: How to Unravel the Food Industry's Playbook and Reclaim Your Health*. The book exposes the industry's deceptive practices, its manipulation of nutrition science, its misinformation campaigns, and its label and marketing trickery. It's an empowering book that I encourage you

TEAMING WITH THE US PUBLIC INTEREST RESEARCH GROUP

Although I generally recommend avoiding chain restaurants because of their ultraprocessed foods and bad fats, you can check a restaurant's grade in regard to antibiotic-free meat. Find the restaurant scorecard on the Public Interest Research Group's website: uspirg.org/blogs/blog/usp/grades-are-antibiotics-more-top-us-restaurants-receive-passing-grades-year.

Join the fight by going to their website and signing up to support the campaign, called "Stop the Overuse of Antibiotics": https://pirg.org/campaigns/stop-the-overuse-of-antibiotics/.

to check out. She maps out an action plan as someone who has taken on Big Food and won. It will not just open your eyes and educate you; it will also give you tools to follow in Vani's footsteps.

Vani Hari is proof that one person can start a revolution. And now that many of our peer health influencers with major platforms have joined her, we'll be able to turn around these problems in our food system—for everybody's good.

Jason Karp, another food activist, claims his personal health transformation—fueled in part by works of mine—inspired him to cofound Hu Kitchen, aiming to provide unadulterated, sustainable food without compromising on taste. He later founded HumanCo, a mission-driven company investing in brands focused on healthier living and sustainability.

Karp isn't just talking about fixing the food system—he's going to war with Big Food. In March 2024, alongside Vani Hari, he launched a shareholder activist suit against Kellogg's, calling out their use of artificial food dyes linked to hyperactivity, allergies, and cancer. His message? Enough is enough. "We need to expose the cereal killers—the companies that profit off poisoning our children." He's not just fighting for cleaner labels—he's forcing corporations to take responsibility for the toxic ingredients they've been feeding America for decades.

His relentless pursuit of transparency, accountability, and food free from industrial chemicals proves one thing: Big Food's days of unchecked power are numbered.

With enough pressure from citizens and companies that choose to make better decisions about their ingredients, eventually the FDA will have to step up.

FOOD FIX: REFORM AT THE FDA— PREVENTING ANTIBIOTIC OVERUSE AND SUPERBUGS

I once asked Peggy Hamburg, the former FDA commissioner, why the FDA didn't mandate clearer food labels, restrict toxic food additives, and end the use of antibiotics for growth and disease prevention in animal feed. She was honest: Whenever the FDA attempts to implement stricter regulations, Congress—deep in the pockets of Big Food and Big Ag—wields its power to block funding and stifle enforcement efforts. Instead of protecting public health, our own lawmakers have become the hired muscle for the food industry, ensuring that meaningful oversight remains toothless.

The revolving door between the FDA and the industries it's supposed to regulate certainly doesn't help matters. Time and again, key FDA appointees have come straight from the executive suites of Big Food, Big Pharma, and Big Ag, making it painfully obvious where their loyalties lie. When the people writing the rules are the same ones who profit from bending them, the system isn't just broken—it's rigged.

As consumers we have to push for change at the state and local levels. We can support groups like the US Public Interest Research Group (PIRG), a consumer watchdog group that has been leading the charge on this issue. The advocacy group helped California[55] and Maryland[56] pass laws banning their states' factory farms from routinely using medically important antibiotics. Thanks to California and Maryland leading the way on this issue, many more states are now looking to enact similar measures. Doing so will go a long way toward protecting the public from lethal superbugs.

Even the WHO has called on the agriculture industry to stop giving antibiotics to healthy animals.[57] It's important that we all support the following solutions proposed by PIRG, the WHO, and other prominent authorities and health experts:

1. **Implement an outright ban on antibiotics for "disease prevention" in livestock.** The use of antibiotics on factory farms must be limited to cases of animal sickness or direct disease exposure only.

2. **Stop factory farms from using antibiotics that are especially valuable to human medicine,** including fluoroquinolones, glycopeptides, macrolides, and third- and fourth-generation cephalosporins. The WHO describes these antibiotics as critically important for humans.[58]

3. **Bring in qualified veterinarians.** Implement requirements that they oversee the administration of antibiotics to animals on factory farms, and that antibiotics be administered only in cases where these veterinarians have directly assessed the animals.

4. **Promote and apply good practices** at all steps of production and processing of foods from animal and plant sources. Ideally, transitioning from factory farms to regenerative agriculture and practices will solve this problem. (More on this in Part 5.)

5. **Improve biosecurity on farms** and prevent infections through improved hygiene and animal welfare.

6. **Reduce the need for antibiotics altogether by adopting new technologies** (for example, vaccines) to improve animal health and prevent disease.[59]

7. **Track the misuse of antibiotics.** The USDA and FDA don't effectively track the use of antibiotics in livestock production. The drug and agriculture industries refused to release any data until 2003 and now release only limited data. In order to track and regulate the misuse of antibiotics there must be mandatory transparency.

I am fired up, however, that Marty Makary was recently confirmed as the commissioner of the FDA, which means we finally have someone taking the reins at the FDA with the guts to call out the corruption, expose the lies, and take on the giants of Big Food and Big Pharma. For the first time in decades, there's a real disruptor in the system—one who isn't afraid to follow the money, investigate the toxins in our food, and shake the very foundations of the broken health care machine. Buckle up—things are about to get interesting.

FOOD FIX: FDA POLICIES FOR PEOPLE, NOT CORPORATIONS

The FDA has a vital job to do. It's supposed to keep our food supply safe and regulate food. But right now, it gets a grade of D+, just barely passing.

I have proposed a handful of relatively simple fixes that could vastly improve the FDA's handling of our food system that I urge Americans to demand, putting pressure on Congress to make these reforms a reality. The FDA needs to improve in three key areas: It needs to create stronger safety standards for the use of antibiotics in our food, enforce stricter food-labeling standards, and mandate safety testing before products or additives are used in our food supply. Many countries have already shown the way. The FDA just needs to follow suit.

But all is not lost. Senator Cory Booker is leading the fight for safer food—and we are proud to stand with him. A recent video[60] of his went viral on social media in which he castigated our food companies for their artificial dyes:

Red 3. Blue 1. Red 40. No, this isn't a quarterback calling plays—it's a list of chemicals hiding in ultraprocessed foods, many of which are linked to cancer, hormonal disruption, and damage to the immune and nervous systems. Take Red 3, a common food dye found in over 2,900 products, despite research showing it causes cancer in animals. Or Red 40, which has been linked to hyperactivity and attention deficits in children. And this isn't just about food dyes—it's preservatives, emulsifiers, artificial sweeteners—many of which have been banned in other countries but are still pumped into American food unchecked.

Senator Booker isn't letting this slide—and we're proud to see a leader in Washington finally calling this out. As he's pointed out, our food safety system is broken. Right now, the FDA doesn't require food companies to report new chemical additives or submit independent studies proving their safety. Even when evidence mounts that these ingredients are harmful, the FDA drags its feet—red dye no. 3 was banned in cosmetics in 1990, but was still in our food until 2025. Unsafe for your skin, but safe to consume? The logic escapes me...

And back to the conversation on ingredient dosing: Why do nutrition labels report grams of sugar instead of teaspoons, especially in a country that doesn't use the metric system? Simple. The food industry wants us confused. If the nutrition label of a 20-ounce soda said it contained 15 teaspoons of sugar, we might think twice about buying it.

Here's what else the FDA can do to make food labels easier to understand, because now you have to have a PhD in nutrition to make any sense of them.

1. **Use the stoplight system for food labels.** Similar to the GMO-labeling tactics we've discussed, in Chile and many European countries the food labels use a brilliantly simple system. A green logo means the food is good for you: Go ahead and buy it. Yellow means it's essentially neutral: not so good for you, but not necessarily bad for you either. Proceed with caution. And a red logo is the equivalent of a great big stop sign: This food could kill you, so either put it down and back away or be doubly sure that this is what you really want to put in your body or feed to your children. Front-of-package warning labels have been used very successfully in countries such as Chile for foods that are harmful. The industry will fight back, all guns blazing, but it is the right choice. Don't make it hard for consumers; make the right choice the easy choice.

2. **List ingredients by their percentages.** The United States is one of the few developed countries that uses an outdated system. As Jerold Mande explains, "Other countries actually state the percentages of

ingredients. If it's the second ingredient, is it 30 percent or is it 5 percent? You just don't know with our current labels. Other countries require the top ingredients and their percentages [to be] listed." The FDA needs to require food companies to list the percentages of sugar, oil, food coloring, and other ingredients on their labels.

3. **Restrict health claims on package labels.** Food companies have a right to package their products in appealing ways. They can slap pictures of mountain springs and green valleys on their labels if they like. They can come up with clever brand names to entice consumers. But the FDA should put its foot down when companies make unwarranted or misleading health claims. Americans spend billions every year on cereal, bread, yogurt, and other foods that claim to be "all natural" despite containing synthetic and genetically engineered ingredients. Many foods are labeled "whole grain" even though their first ingredient is refined flour. There are foods that claim to "strengthen your immune system"—like Ocean Spray cranberry juice—even though they are loaded with sugar (a known immunosuppressant). And many processed foods claim to be "lightly sweetened" (like Kellogg's Frosted Mini-Wheats) or "a good source of fiber," even though they are nothing of the sort.[61] The FDA allows Froot Loops to be labeled "heart-healthy" because it has no fat or cholesterol (but tons of sugar) but deems KIND bars unhealthy because they contain "fatty" nuts, even though it is now universally accepted that nuts help with weight loss and with preventing heart disease and diabetes.

4. **Strengthen the FDA's regulation of chemical food additives.** Food industry groups should not be allowed to declare new food chemicals and other additives safe without the proper scientific evidence. The FDA must enforce the current standards under the law. The safety of our food supply depends on it. In March 2025,[62] when Robert F. Kennedy Jr. met with the Consumer Brands Association, he urged major food companies, including PepsiCo and Kraft Heinz, to remove artificial dyes from their products by the end of his term. This initiative seeks to improve public health by reducing exposure to potentially harmful additives. As I write this, the FDA plans to collaborate with the

industry to establish a federal framework on food dyes, addressing inconsistencies across state regulations.

5. **Reform the GRAS loophole.** The generally recognized as safe (GRAS) rule permits companies to self-determine the safety of food ingredients without mandatory FDA notification, leading to potential undisclosed additives in the food supply. RFK Jr. has announced that the FDA will explore new rules to eliminate this self-affirmation pathway, aiming to enhance oversight and ensure all new ingredients undergo FDA review before market introduction.

As we'll see in the next chapter, Big Food's influence on the FDA is not the only way we are being deceived. But we will expose their tactics and show you how everyday citizens can lead the way toward transformation.

For a quick reference guide on the Food Fixes and resources on how to demand FDA protection, go to www.foodfixuncensored.com.

PART III

INFORMATION WARFARE

When I was in medical school, I believed science was a pure and noble pursuit, rooted in integrity and truth. I bought into the orthodoxy like a moth circling a porch light, convinced it was the sun. But over time, I realized that the field of nutrition research had been hijacked by the food industry.

Reality check: Big Food and Big Agriculture are not in the business of public health—they're in the business of selling more products. Big Food is aggressively pushing false science, shaping public perception, and influencing policy to protect its profits. Their strategies go beyond clever marketing; they manipulate government policies, infiltrate public health groups, and influence professional societies, all while investing billions in misleading corporate social responsibility campaigns. These efforts don't just promote their products; they buy silence from organizations we trust, obscure scientific truths, and drown out legitimate health research.

The food industry isn't going to change on its own. That's why we have to stay vigilant, questioning the so-called science they fund and recognizing the partnerships they forge to keep us consuming their products. Their ultimate goal isn't your well-being—it's to keep you hooked and buying more. The sooner we see through these tactics, the better we can reclaim our health and make truly informed choices.

Warning: What you're about to learn will shock you.

CHAPTER 10

"Wrongspeak": Challenging the Orthodoxy

The ideal subject of totalitarian rule is not the convinced Nazi or the convinced Communist, but people for whom the distinction between fact and fiction, true and false, no longer exists.

—HANNAH ARENDT

THE DEEP STATE OF FOOD

If it isn't already obvious, the investigative journalism I undertook for this book opened my eyes to the dark underbelly of a corporate kleptocracy that I never really knew existed. I had my suspicions that the data didn't add up, but I didn't really get "red-pilled" until I peeled back the curtain and realized that the deep state is not just a radical, fringe conspiracy theory but a deeply embedded, highly sophisticated layer of society that many elites from both sides of the aisle belong to. The so-called battle between Left and Right is nothing more than political theater: It's a carefully crafted illusion to keep us distracted; meanwhile, behind the curtain, the same few elites pull the strings, ensuring their wealth and power remain untouched at the expense of ordinary Americans.

These unelected bureaucrats, corporate elites, and entrenched institutions exert enormous influence over government policy regardless of which political party is in power. Unlike elected officials who come and go (and at least, in theory, represent the people's interests), the deep state operates in the shadows, exerting alarming influence over key regulatory agencies, trade policies, and economic decisions. It is a system in which government agencies, think tanks, lobbyists, and multinational corporations work together to shape policy in their own interests—not the interests of the American public.

At its core, the deep state thrives on continuity, secrecy, and financial influence. It ensures that massive industries remain profitable, trade agreements favor the global elite, and public perception is carefully managed through media control and academic funding. The food system is one of the deep state's greatest triumphs—a rigged system where Big Food and Big Ag manipulate government policies to serve their bottom line while keeping the public trapped in a cycle of addiction, malnutrition, and dependence.

Food is not just something we eat—it's one of the most powerful tools the deep state can leverage. Those who control the food supply dictate public health, economic stability, and even political power. And make no mistake, the deep state has ensured that Big Food and Big Ag have an iron grip on what we eat, how it's produced, and who profits from it.

The deep state has rigged the game. But the good news is, you don't have to play by their rules.

THE TOXIC TRIAD

Within this shadow network of corporate influence operating behind the scenes of America's food and health care systems lies a web of industry giants pulling the strings on policy, public perception, and scientific research. This unholy alliance of Big Food, Big Agriculture, and Big Pharma—what I call the Toxic Triad—isn't just shaping what we eat and how we're treated when we get sick. It's engineering a system where poor health is inevitable . . . and it's up to us to stop it.

Big Food: Hooking You on Ultraprocessed Junk

The first pillar of the Toxic Triad, Big Food, controls the modern diet with ultraprocessed, addictive, and nutritionally empty products that fuel the obesity and chronic disease epidemic. As I've laid out in earlier chapters, these corporations spend billions lobbying Congress and funding misleading nutritional research, ensuring that government dietary guidelines continue to promote industrialized grains, refined oils, and excessive starch and sugar, all while demonizing real, whole foods like meat, eggs, and butter.

Through deep political ties, these companies have infiltrated school lunch programs, SNAP (food stamps), and hospital meal plans, ensuring that the most destructive foods are also the cheapest and most accessible foods. And when research threatens to expose the dangers of their products? They fund their own "science" to manufacture doubt...just as Big Tobacco did in the past.

Big Ag: The Industrial Engine of Disease

If Big Food is responsible for what we eat, Big Agriculture controls how it's produced. Industrial farming practices have transformed once-nutrient-rich foods into glyphosate-drenched, pesticide-laden, genetically engineered commodities. The same companies that pushed for the Green Revolution—which promised to "feed the world" but instead delivered monocropping, soil depletion, and synthetic fertilizers—are now the architects of modern food production.

It is thanks to their powerful lobbyists that subsidies flow endlessly toward corn, wheat, and soy (the backbone of processed food and factory-farmed livestock) while regenerative, nutrient-dense farming is suffocated under red tape and denied funding. Meanwhile, chemical giants like Monsanto (now Bayer) and Syngenta hold patents[1] on genetically modified seeds, forcing farmers into a system of dependency that prioritizes yield and corporate profits over health and sustainability.

Big Pharma: The Cleanup Crew That Never Cleans Up

The final pillar of the Toxic Triad is Big Pharma—the industry that profits from the destruction caused by the first two. When an ultraprocessed diet drenched in pesticides inevitably leads to obesity, diabetes, autoimmune diseases, and metabolic dysfunction, Big Pharma is right there to sell you the solution. In some cases, the very same companies that produce the chemicals that poison you also sell you the treatment. (Bayer, which makes Roundup, a weed killer that has paid billions in personal claim settlements for its likely cause of non-Hodgkin's lymphoma, conveniently developed a drug called Rituxan, used to treat the very disease Roundup causes.) Instead of addressing the root causes of disease, our medical system funnels patients into a lifelong dependency on medications.

The system isn't designed to cure—it's designed to manage symptoms for profit.

This didn't happen by accident. These corporations fund medical "education" and "research," creating a generation of doctors trained to prescribe drugs to manage and not prevent chronic illness or address its root causes (namely our diet and environmental toxins). Why cure illness when you can manage it for life with medication? The FDA and government, deeply entangled with the pharmaceutical industry, routinely fast-track new drugs while sidelining low-cost, effective preventive therapies or root-cause approaches such as functional medicine.

To understand how we got here, we need to go back to the origins of our pharma-first medical system, specifically to one of America's most infamous robber barons: John D. Rockefeller. Known as the original Big Oil tycoon, Rockefeller played a critical—and controversial—role in reshaping American medicine. In the early twentieth century, he funneled vast sums of his Standard Oil fortune into a new vision of health care: one built around a pharmaceutical-centric, reductionist model that sidelined traditional, holistic, and natural healing practices in favor of what we now know as conventional, allopathic medicine. His influence laid the foundation for the biomedical paradigm that dominates global health care to this day.

After becoming the world's first billionaire, Rockefeller embraced what he called "scientific philanthropy." One of his key vehicles was the Rockefeller Institute for Medical Research (established in 1901, it is now Rockefeller University), which championed lab-based medicine and germ theory—a model that framed disease as something to be attacked with drugs rather than prevented through lifestyle and nutrition.

In 1910, Rockefeller funded *The Flexner Report*,[2] detailing a landmark (and deeply controversial) study conducted by educator Abraham Flexner under the aegis of the Carnegie Foundation but largely backed by Rockefeller money.[3] The report evaluated medical schools across North America and recommended shutting down institutions that did not align with the new scientific model of medicine—particularly those teaching naturopathy, homeopathy, osteopathy, herbalism, and ancient medicine. As a result, more than half of all US medical schools were closed, including many that served women and people of color, and many that taught holistic healing.[4]

With Rockefeller's support, the new medical paradigm became one that was heavily mechanistic, emphasizing disease as something to be attacked with drugs or surgery rather than prevented or treated holistically through lifestyle or behavior interventions. Rockefeller's Standard Oil empire was invested in petrochemicals, the base materials for many early synthetic drugs. Some historians argue that this created a symbiotic incentive to push pharmaceutical solutions derived from petroleum, rather than nutrient-based dietary therapies.

The newly reformed medical schools—modeled after Johns Hopkins and funded by Rockefeller—began training physicians to focus on diagnosing and prescribing, minimizing the role of nutrition, lifestyle, and the body's innate healing capacity. At the same time, Rockefeller poured money into public health initiatives and research institutions, further cementing the dominance of pharmaceutical science and biomedicine.

As allopathic medicine gained institutional legitimacy, traditional healers were delegitimized, ridiculed, or even criminalized. Herbalists, midwives, and natural medicine practitioners were pushed to the margins. Licensing laws were rewritten to exclude anyone not trained in the new paradigm. Medical journals, also funded through Rockefeller-aligned institutions, began promoting drug-based therapies and discrediting alternatives as unscientific.

This suppression wasn't merely academic—it was economic, legal, and cultural. The holistic health traditions that had thrived for centuries were now branded as quackery. And with the rise of the pharmaceutical industry—deeply intertwined with oil, chemistry, and capitalist structures—profit-driven medicine became the norm.

Rockefeller's vision reshaped the global health landscape. The biomedical model he helped establish has evolved into one that prioritizes treatment over prevention, pharmaceuticals over food, and specialization over systems thinking. While modern medicine has made extraordinary advancements in surgery and acute care, critics argue that it has failed spectacularly at addressing chronic disease, root causes, and whole-person wellness.

Today, echoes of that transformation remain. Most medical education requires no nutrition training whatsoever, while some programs devote less than 20 hours throughout the multiyear training to nutrition,[5] and pharmaceutical companies influence everything from research to prescribing patterns to policy. The dominance of this system is not accidental—it is the result of a century-old ideological and financial blueprint set in motion by one of the world's most powerful men.

Fast-forward to the present day. We are seeing the consequences of those decisions permeate Western medical orthodoxy. A recent example was the suppression of data on the effectiveness of vitamin D, an established intervention to protect immunity, during COVID-19. Indeed, an observational study conducted in Israel revealed that patients with higher vitamin D levels—particularly above 40 ng/mL[6]—experienced significantly better COVID symptoms and recovery time. In contrast, those with a deficiency were fourteen times more likely to develop severe or critical illness. Hazard a guess as to why this cheap, ubiquitous, and easy intervention was rejected by the medical establishment.

This elite bureaucracy of food, farming, and pharmaceuticals ensures that poor health isn't just common—it's great for bottom lines. Cheap, addictive foods make people sick. Industrial agriculture strips nutrition from our food and poisons our land. And when disease inevitably sets in, the pharmaceutical industry steps in as the savior—but rarely with a cure, only a lifetime prescription.

It's a highly coordinated, well-documented system designed to extract maximum profits from human illness.

MEDIA CONTROL

As legendary Soviet dictator Joseph Stalin apparently said, "Ideas are more powerful than guns. We would not let our enemies have guns, why should we let them have ideas?" The Toxic Triad appears to fully endorse this conclusion.

As though controlling our nation's food supply weren't enough, the consolidation of power within the food and agriculture industries is now having significant implications for the Fourth Estate.

Increasingly dependent on advertising revenue from large corporations, our once-independent media institutions are today merely mouthpieces for powerful interests. For instance, a study highlighted by the American Marketing Association found that media coverage of corporate misconduct is overwhelmingly muted or distorted when the offending companies are significant advertisers.[7] This financial dependency discourages negative reporting on these corporations, leading to a lack of critical (translation: real) journalism.

Investigative journalism is supposed to play a crucial role in holding powerful entities accountable. However, Big Food and Big Ag have employed tactics to undermine such efforts. Internal documents have revealed coordinated campaigns to discredit journalists and researchers who critique industrial agricultural practices—campaigns that often involve disseminating counternarratives and questioning the credibility of independent investigations.

The cumulative effect of these strategies is a media landscape where critical reporting on food and agriculture is often stifled and in some cases is explicitly prohibited. Recently, when I confronted a journalist friend about her parroting the phrase "the science is settled"—an oxymoron if there ever was one—she admitted, almost bluntly, that she knew it wasn't true... but the outlet required her to say it. That exact phrase was the approved talking point, handed down from editorial like gospel. Let that sink in. It is an absurd statement. Science is never settled. The whole point of science is to stay in the question. We used to think autism was caused by "refrigerator mothers"; ulcers were caused by stress, not bacteria; and aspirin was a miracle drug that all should take to prevent heart disease—until we recently discovered that it was more likely to kill you than prevent a heart attack if you were not a high-risk patient. The propaganda machine is well oiled. You may have heard or read the phrase in the media: "The link between autism and vaccines has been debunked." True or not, no theory in medicine is ever debunked. The very premise of science is to keep investigating, challenging our thinking and asking the questions. Not to stop questioning.

You might ask why someone with integrity would bend a knee to that kind of shameless bullying, but the sad reality is that, while we know the mainstream media is bought and paid for, even independent journalists who defect now face real repercussions—blacklisting, loss of access, and financial instability. For independent media outlets in particular, the threat of legal action, withdrawal of advertising revenue, and smear campaigns— and now, in the wake of the merciless assassination of legendary free thinker Charlie Kirk, murder—is existential, leading to self-censorship or biased reporting. Consequently, the public receives a skewed narrative that is rigged to reward compliance and punish truth telling.

THE CENSORSHIP INDUSTRIAL COMPLEX

The Toxic Triad doesn't just flood our supermarkets with unhealthy food—it shapes our perception of what's "healthy" through media manipulation, lobbying, and corporate-funded science. As we've seen, Big Food spends billions on advertising to manufacture demand for addictive, ultraprocessed products, while industry-funded research floods the scientific community with biased studies that downplay the harms of sugar, seed oils, and artificial additives.

Big Food companies have been accused of colluding with one another and with lobbying groups to influence public policy in their favor. They exert pressure on regulatory bodies to prevent the implementation of policies that could negatively impact their profits, and they often lobby against regulations that would limit the marketing of unhealthy foods, especially to vulnerable populations like children. They also fund research that supports the supposed health benefits of their products, creating a conflict of interest that can mislead consumers and policymakers. In one especially egregious example, it's no coincidence that the American Heart Association used to put its seal of approval on ultraprocessed cereals while demonizing natural saturated fats like butter and tallow that were dietary staples long before heart disease was the top killer in America.

Critics of Big Food and Pharma (well actually, most of Big Industry these days) often face coordinated smear campaigns designed to discredit them and undermine their influence. A notable example is the ongoing attacks on Dr. Casey Means as well as food activists like Vani Hari who have been vocal about the negative impacts of processed foods and our broader dietary practices, exposing the duplicity of large food corporations. Following her nomination for surgeon general, Means faced a barrage of criticism from various industry-backed groups and paid influencers alike, determined to tarnish her reputation, diminish her credibility as a critic of the food industry, and, presumably, prevent her confirmation.

Big Food companies also employ underhanded tactics to shift the narrative in their favor by funding front groups that appear to be independent but actually promote industry-friendly messages. For example, the Center for Consumer Freedom, funded by the food industry, has been known to attack public health advocates and promote messages that downplay the health risks associated with certain foods. And despite what we all witness with our own eyes, they claim that the obesity epidemic is a hoax.

Wrongspeak = Canceled

In recent years, a disturbing trend has emerged: If your opinions challenge the orthodoxy or inconvenience powerful industries, they don't just get debated—they get labeled as "misinformation," or a newer species, "malinformation." The difference? "Misinformation" means the information is supposedly false; "malinformation" means the information is *actually true*—but the deep state doesn't like it because it undermines the "right" narrative. Either way, it—and you—get canceled.

We saw this play out with the Biden administration's pressure on social media companies. The White House leaned on platforms like Facebook to remove posts they didn't like—even when the science was still evolving. Mark Zuckerberg (founder and CEO of Meta, which owns Facebook and Instagram) himself admitted that the government pushed Facebook to censor certain COVID-related content, including claims that later turned out to be accurate. So much for "trusting the science."

Big Food and Big Ag have mastered this game, slapping the "misinformation" label on anything that challenges their carefully controlled monopoly over what we eat. Exhibit A: raw milk.

Raw Milk: Public Enemy Number One or Threat to Big Dairy?

Few foods have been as aggressively demonized as raw milk, while pasteurized milk has been pushed as the only "safe" option. In the eyes of government regulators, Big Dairy, and the FDA, unpasteurized milk is practically a biological weapon, with officials warning of deadly bacteria, life-threatening infections, and imminent outbreaks if it's consumed.

Meanwhile, in Europe, raw milk is widely available, in some countries legally sold in vending machines, and even a dietary staple in countries like France, Italy, and Switzerland. So why was the FDA under Biden aggressively policing raw milk sales, making it illegal in many states?

Could it be because Big Dairy doesn't like competition, and because the government is in the pocket of Big Dairy? Meanwhile, the same regulatory agencies that treat raw milk like a Schedule I drug give a free pass to ultraprocessed, chemical-laden "dairy" products full of seed oils, synthetic additives, and hormone-disrupting preservatives. Because apparently, heavily processed cheese-like substances are fine, like Kraft Singles, which technically can't be called cheese because they are less than 50 percent cheese—but milk straight from the cow...dangerous.

The official narrative is simple: Raw milk is dangerous because it hasn't been pasteurized, meaning it could contain harmful bacteria like E. coli, listeria, and salmonella.[8] The CDC and FDA warn against it, citing potential outbreaks and cases of foodborne illness. And yes—if it is mishandled or if it comes from sick animals or from a contaminated farm, it can carry risk—like any raw food. And honestly, as a doctor, I don't recommend it (or really, most forms of dairy). Raw milk in America can come with serious risks, so I do get the caution. But it's the zeal and disingenuous motivations of the government in selectively targeting raw milk—while completely ignoring the health risks of the foods their biggest donors want them to actively promote—that irks me.

For example, here are a few things you might not know about raw milk and the milk industry:

- Raw vegetables are linked to far more foodborne illness outbreaks than raw milk—yet no one's calling for a ban on spinach.
- Industrial dairy operations—where cows are confined in horrific conditions and milk is mass-produced—are the primary reason pasteurization became necessary in the first place.
- Traditional small-scale farms with pastured cows have much lower contamination risks—but the same laws apply to them as to factory farms drowning in antibiotics and fecal contamination.

The safety concerns around raw milk conveniently ignore the actual source of most dairy contamination: industrialized, overcrowded factory farms that rely on pasteurization to "fix" their low-quality, bacteria-laden milk.

At its core, the raw milk crackdown isn't about public health—it's about protecting the dairy industry's monopoly. Big Dairy depends on centralized mass production, and it doesn't want small, independent farmers selling directly to consumers, because if more people bought raw milk from small farms, they wouldn't need to buy pasteurized, ultraprocessed milk from corporate giants like Dairy Farmers of America or Nestlé. And thus, Big Dairy lobbies aggressively to keep raw milk illegal or restricted, ensuring that the only "milk" widely available is the kind that has been stripped, fortified, homogenized, and processed beyond recognition.

Meanwhile, pasteurization allows Big Dairy to cut corners. Cows can be kept in confined, unsanitary conditions because any bacteria in the milk will be "killed off" later. Without pasteurization, Big Dairy would actually have to clean up its production methods—something it would rather avoid. If you just follow the money, it becomes clear which motives are being prioritized.

Despite the government's war on raw milk, grassroots rebellion has caused surging consumer demand. In many states, farmers and activists have fought back, leading to loosening restrictions and underground raw milk markets.

- In 2023, at least 30 US states allowed some form of raw milk sales, from farm-direct purchases to herd-share programs.[9]
- In states where raw milk is banned, farmers have resorted to creative loopholes—like selling "pet milk" labeled "Not for Human Consumption,"[10] which people buy for their own consumption anyway.
- Demand for raw dairy has surged[11] as consumers reject ultraprocessed foods and seek nutrient-dense, unaltered alternatives.

As I said, I am not an advocate of dairy milk, full stop. I don't really care where it comes from. Nutritionally speaking, it's not something we should be consuming in large quantities. But this point is purely illustrative: Raw milk bans are simply another example of Big Food and Big Ag controlling what we're allowed to eat. When corporate interests align with government regulations, consumer choice is restricted under the guise of "safety."

The same pattern repeats: If something threatens Big Food's profits—whether it's questioning the health effects of ultraprocessed food, advocating for regenerative farming, or challenging dietary guidelines—the response from Big food isn't open debate. It's de-platforming, suppression, and industry-funded hit pieces.

This isn't about "protecting the public"—it's about protecting corporate dominance. The minute you start asking inconvenient questions, you get thrown into the wrongspeak category. And once you're there? Big Tech, Big Food, and Big Government work together to silence, ridicule, and erase you.

The good news? Once you see the game for what it is, you can opt out. You can choose real, unprocessed foods. You can support regenerative agriculture. And you can take back control of your health—before Big Food, Big Ag, and Big Pharma do it for you.

CHAPTER 11

How the Food Industry Co-opts Public Health and Corrupts Nutrition Science

When Coca-Cola and Skittles first went on the market, we can give their manufacturers the benefit of the doubt that they didn't know just how much obesity and disease their products would cause. But this is no longer the case. Big Food companies are not innocent bystanders caught in the wake of their actions' unintended consequences. Big Food is now knowingly fueling the disability, disease, and premature death of billions—and trying to hide it. Rather than reformulating their products to reduce harm, these corporations have orchestrated a calculated, multibillion-dollar cover-up designed to silence critics, manipulate scientific research, distort the truth, and control the very institutions meant to protect public health. They have infiltrated media, politics, public health organizations, and consumer advocacy groups—ensuring that profits always come before people.

Wall Street isn't the only predator lurking in plain sight—Big Food is marching straight into your home, your schools, and your grocery stores, disguising itself as a friend. With deep pockets and ruthless tactics, they're not just selling food—they're engineering addiction, fueling chronic disease, and ensuring their grip on public health stays unchallenged. While Wall Street manipulates markets, Big Food manipulates your cravings, your health, and even the policies meant to protect you.

Let's see exactly how.

In the spring of 2012,[1] Coca-Cola was under attack. New York City mayor Michael R. Bloomberg had just announced a controversial new plan to ban local restaurants, movie theaters, and fast-food establishments from selling large cups of sugary beverages. Chicago, Philadelphia, and other cities were debating whether to institute sugary-drink taxes to drive down their obesity rates as well. And on social media, a video called "Sugar: The Bitter Truth"—which showed a charismatic endocrinologist named Robert Lustig explaining in gripping detail why sugar is so toxic to the liver and the body—was going viral, with millions of page views and more than 50,000 new viewers every month.

Sugar was suddenly under assault.

Americans were starting to look at their fizzy, sugar-laden beverages as the cause of their growing waistlines. Sales of full-calorie soft drinks across the United States were plummeting, reaching their lowest point in 20 years. Coca-Cola, the industry leader, was desperate to stop the bleeding.

The company deployed a powerful weapon: one of its top executives, Rhona Applebaum,[2] a tough corporate executive with a PhD in microbiology who was Coke's chief scientist. Just a few months later, Applebaum drew the battle lines. She warned the sugar executives at the International Sweetener Symposium that they needed to be more aggressive in defending their products from the public health onslaught. Applebaum put up a slide that showed a list of the food industry's biggest detractors. On the slide were photographs of Kelly Brownell—dean of the Sanford School of Public Policy at Duke University and an obesity expert and outspoken advocate of soda taxes—along with the logo of the Center for Science in the Public Interest, a consumer watchdog group and major critic of the junk-food industry.[3]

Applebaum outlined a cold-blooded strategy on how to weaponize science by funding "defensive and offensive science and research"[4] to promote industry-friendly studies. If you learned in school that the definition of science is "inquiry into truth," you might be reading this a bit cockeyed. *How can science be used as a munition for special interest groups?* you might be wondering. Well, sadly, what has come to light in the more than a decade since then reveals this as a common practice dating back to the turn of the twentieth century. "Science," rather than being an impartial tool for discovery, has often been leveraged as a strategic asset, shaped and manipulated to serve powerful agendas.

Back to Applebaum, though. She warned that the industry was under attack from "detractor activism."[5] She complained about Lustig's viral video on sugar, calling him a crusading "tube star" and pointing out that he and other public health critics were resonating with the public. These critics of the industry "basically go unchallenged," she told the crowd, lamenting that even Coke had sometimes been too complacent in the face of criticism.[6] Applebaum told the executives that Big Soda and the sugar industry were facing a do-or-die moment. To drive the point home, she put up a slide with a famous quote uttered by Benjamin Franklin during the Revolutionary War. "We must all hang together, or assuredly we shall all hang separately."[7]

At a closed-door meeting,[8] Applebaum made a direct plea on behalf of Coca-Cola: The industry needed to "work together and use science" to neutralize critics and sway public opinion. She unveiled a carefully crafted strategy to "balance the debate"—not through open dialogue, but by cultivating alliances, underwriting research, and positioning a narrative.[9] What I view as her most insidious tactic was embedding Coca-Cola within leading public health organizations, effectively turning watchdogs into allies.

Applebaum emphasized that the industry must take a proactive stance on the health effects of sugar. The key, she told the audience, was to "address the negatives—advance the positives."[10] In other words: acknowledge concerns, but spin them to serve corporate interests. The message was clear—if the public could be convinced that obesity was simply about caloric balance, Coca-Cola could remain a staple of the American diet.

Enjoy an ice cream cone shortly before lunch.

Sugar can be the willpower you need to undereat.

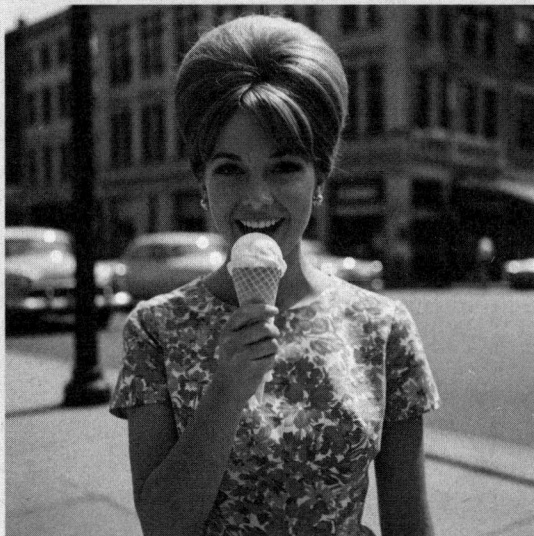

When you're hungry, it usually means your energy's down. By eating something with sugar in it, you can get your energy up fast. In fact, sugar is the fastest energy food around. And when your energy's up, there's a good chance you'll have the willpower to undereat at mealtime.

HOW'S THAT FOR A SWEET IDEA?
Sugar ... only 18 calories per teaspoon, and it's all energy.

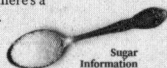

Sugar
Information

But Applebaum's efforts weren't just theoretical. Internal emails obtained from the Freedom of Information Act (FOIA) reveal a concerted effort to court influential scientists, inviting them to Coca-Cola's headquarters in Atlanta and discreetly funneling millions of dollars into their research (and personal bank accounts).[11] A steady stream of corporate-backed studies followed, reinforcing the myth of "energy balance"[12] — the idea that weight loss is just about calories in versus calories out, conveniently ignoring the metabolic impact of sugar-laden drinks.

To be clear, a thousand calories of Coke are *not* the same for the body as a thousand calories of broccoli. When burned in a closed-loop laboratory environment, yes, they both release the same amount of energy, but when you eat them, they have profoundly different and opposing effects on the body. But with enough money, influence, and strategic deception, Coca-Cola blurred that truth and made junk food part of the so-called balanced diet.

UNDER THE TABLE

In one case, Rhona Applebaum and Coca-Cola provided millions in funding to the Pennington Biomedical Research Center, where one of the country's leading obesity researchers, Peter T. Katzmarzyk, produced a study[13] of a dozen countries that pinned the blame for childhood obesity on sedentary behavior.

"Pennington Biomedical Research Study Shows Lack of Physical Activity Is a Major Predictor of Childhood Obesity," announced a news release published in August 2015. A footnote toward the end of the press release included an important disclaimer that few people reading it might have even noticed: "This research was funded by The Coca-Cola Company." Pennington's big study cited lack of sleep and "too much television" as additional factors that contribute to childhood obesity. But the study was perhaps most noticeable for what it did not say—it was strangely silent on the role of junk food and sugary drinks. For their services, Katzmarzyk and the other Pennington researchers received nearly $7 million in funding from Coca-Cola.[14]

Beginning in the year following that whiteboarding session, Coke provided more than $120 million to US universities, health organizations, and research institutions between 2010 and 2015.[15] From 2008 to 2016 Coke funded 389 articles in 169 journals concluding that physical activity was more important than diet and that soft drinks and sugar were essentially harmless.[16]

As a doctor, let me correct the facts for a second: On average, you have to walk 4 miles to burn off just *one* 20-ounce Coke. One slice of pepperoni pizza is equivalent to 30 minutes of jogging. And you'd need to run 5 miles to break even from a large order of fries. Has Coke ever told you that?

Any honest medical practitioner will tell you that you simply can't exercise your way out of a bad diet. But these companies continue to publish data that minimizes the effect of food and inaccurately pushes exercise as the solution to our obesity and disease epidemic.[17] Why? Because they manipulate, obscure, and selectively omit crucial data that doesn't align with their bottom line.

Furthermore, Applebaum and Coke's influence on researchers extended beyond money. One of the top scientists they courted was Jim Hill,[18] who was then a professor of medicine at the University of Colorado. Hill served on the National Institutes of Health (NIH) and Centers for Disease Control and Prevention (CDC) obesity panels. He cofounded the National Weight Control Registry, the most prominent, long-running weight-loss study in America. He was also a former president of the American Society for Nutrition, which once called him "a leader in the fight against the global obesity epidemic." It's no surprise that the society is heavily funded by the food industry.[19]

Beginning in about 2011, with cities and states increasingly proposing taxes on soda and other junk foods, Hill grew cozy with Coke. He published studies paid for by Coke[20] and the American Beverage Association (formerly known as the American Soda Pop Association) and traveled the country giving speeches and attending conferences on Coke's dime.

Some of his research findings were so baffling, they defied common sense.[21] One study,[22] published in the prestigious journal *Obesity,* claimed that obese individuals who drank diet soda lost more weight than those who drank only water—a conclusion that flew in the face of independent research consistently linking diet drinks to weight gain and type 2 diabetes. Behind the scenes, emails obtained through the FOIA revealed a different story. Coca-Cola executive Rhona Applebaum had been pressuring Hill to publish the study, eager to use it as ammunition against growing concerns about aspartame. In one particularly revealing exchange, Applebaum warned Hill that *The Dr. Oz Show* was about to air a critical segment on artificial sweeteners, making it clear that Coke was desperate for his research to hit the press. When Hill's paper finally appeared in May 2014, nutrition experts were stunned. The findings contradicted a mountain of independent research, and the timing reeked of corporate influence. The entire episode was a textbook case of industry-backed science being weaponized to mislead the public—another example of Big Food rewriting reality to protect its bottom line.

"How coincidental that right as diet soda sales take a significant tumble, the soda industry's main lobbying group helps fund a study that tries to claim diet sodas are superior to water," one skeptical nutritionist told a reporter at the time.[23]

Hill's deeds did not go unrewarded. Coke paid him $550,000 for "honoraria, travel, education activities, and research on weight management." The company paid for his travel to conferences and meetings in England, Mexico, and Grenada. It also picked up the tab for Hill and his wife to fly to Australia and New Zealand.[24] In 2014, the company gave Hill's university a check for $1 million to help him start an anti-obesity advocacy group called the Global Energy Balance Network (GEBN), which was Applebaum's brainchild. She not only conceived of the organization but also helped to recruit its 120 members, many of whom Coke had financially supported. Behind the scenes, emails show, Applebaum orchestrated the group's message, designed its website, and edited its mission statement.[25] Hill, with Applebaum's blessing, became the group's president.

THE PROBLEM WITH CALORIES

Science definitively proves that all calories are not the same: Sugar and starch calories act completely differently than calories from fat and protein inside your body. In a 2018 Harvard study, researchers fed two groups identical numbers of calories, but one group ate 60 percent of calories from fat with less than 20 percent from carbs while the other group had 60 percent from carbs and 10 percent from fat.[26] In the most overweight of the participants, the low-carb, high-fat group burned 400 more calories a day without any more exercise, and while eating the exact same number of calories. Sugar slows your metabolism. Fat, counterintuitively, speeds it up.

The reason is that our body is not a simple machine — it's more like a hybrid engine, designed to run on a combination of fuel sources including both carbs and fat, but they behave very differently inside your cells.

You see, calories are information, instructions that affect hormones, brain chemistry, the immune system, the microbiome, gene expression, and metabolism. They are not just fungible units of energy. Food sends biochemical instructions that tune up or down your cellular programming.

The outdated belief of the energy-balance hypothesis claims that weight gain or loss is simply about the number of calories consumed versus the number burned. But this model has been disproven by decades of science. It survives mostly only in the minds of those in the fast-food industry because they have a stake in pushing the idea that weight is all about calories in and calories out. But any third grader could tell you that 1,000 calories of soda and 1,000 calories of broccoli have profoundly different effects on the body.

In one internal memo that the nonprofit advocacy group US Right to Know obtained, Applebaum characterized the GEBN as "akin to a political campaign"[27] and said the goal was to "develop, deploy and evolve a powerful and multi-faceted strategy to counter radical organizations and their proponents." As Applebaum saw it, Big Food was at war with the public health community and science, and the GEBN would serve as the industry's war room. "There is a growing war between the public health community and private industry over how to reduce obesity. Sides are being chosen and battle lines are being drawn. The most extreme public health experts have gained traction with the media, with many policy makers, and with an increasing proportion of the general public."[28]

Unfortunately for Applebaum, the GEBN blew up in Coca-Cola's face. In 2015, the *New York Times*[29] and other news outlets exposed the organization as an industry-funded front group. When the news broke, Coke announced that Applebaum was suddenly "retiring" from the company and cut its financial ties to GEBN, which promptly announced it was ceasing operations because of "resource limitations."[30] Resource limitations? Really? Their "sponsor's" annual revenue in 2018 was more than $31 billion, for not much more than selling varieties of sugar water.

THE BIG FOOD PLAYBOOK

Coca-Cola's involvement in spreading disinformation is not unique. Its tactics exemplify a multipronged strategy that Big Food has been using to deceive the public for decades.

Junk-food companies don't just sell products—they manufacture science to protect the sales of their products. With marketing budgets that dwarf those of public health research, they recruit nutrition experts as hired guns, paying them hefty sums to endorse junk food and discredit inconvenient research. While the NIH scrapes together just $1 billion for nutrition studies, the food industry pours in more than $12 billion annually, flooding the scientific landscape with biased studies designed to confuse policymakers, mislead the public, and even deceive doctors and nutritionists.

And it works. Industry-funded studies are 8 to 50 times more likely[31] to produce favorable results for their products, not because the science holds up but because the food industry controls the design, the data, and the dollars behind it. Big Food buys influence in public health organizations, academic societies, and government agencies—tainting the very institutions meant to protect us.[32] The result is a food system built on corporate-funded propaganda masquerading as nutrition science— and a nation paying the price in skyrocketing rates of obesity, diabetes, and chronic disease.

Just looking at Coca-Cola as an example, researchers obtained 87,013 pages of documents through FOIA, including five agreements between Coke and public institutions in the United States and Canada.[33] The "research" contracts allow Coca-Cola to review research prior to publication and maintain control over study data, whether the study gets published, and any acknowledgment of Coca-Cola's funding of the study. If they don't like the results, Coke gets to bury the findings. And they support front groups that pose as independent organizations to mislead consumers. So much for the purity of science and independent researchers! No wonder the "clinical research" on nutrition begets such contradictory and confounding results.

Many ways in which Big Food is borrowing the tactics of Big Tobacco were documented in a landmark 2009 paper[34] written by Kelly Brownell and titled "The Perils of Ignoring History: Big Tobacco Played Dirty and Millions Died. How Similar Is Big Food?"[35] As Brownell noted, "Disputing science has been a key strategy of many industries, including tobacco. Beginning with denials that smoking causes lung cancer and progressing to attacks on studies of secondhand smoke, the industry instilled doubt. Likewise, groups and scientists funded by the food industry have disputed whether the prevalence figures for obesity are correct, whether obesity causes disease, and whether foods like soft drinks cause harm." Unbelievably, the food industry front group the Center for Consumer Freedom claims that the obesity epidemic is a hoax.[36] Guess they have never been to Disneyland or taken a walk down Main Street America.

If you were around in the 1980s and this all sounds uncannily familiar to you, your spidey senses are right on the money. Big Food's iron-clad plan to fool you with junk science and bogus claims is not just reminiscent of the tobacco industry's playbook to subvert the truth in past decades; it *is* Big Tobacco. The very corporations that spent decades denying the dangers of smoking, manipulating research, and marketing deadly products to children bought up and consolidated major food companies, applying the same deceptive tactics to ultraprocessed foods.

Tobacco behemoth Philip Morris acquired General Foods[37] in 1985 (which now includes Kraft and Oscar Mayer) creating one of the largest food conglomerates in the world before spinning it off as Mondelēz and

Kraft. RJ Reynolds, another tobacco giant, purchased Nabisco (which makes Oreo cookies, Ritz crackers, and Chips Ahoy!), among others. I would be shocked if these companies, famously steeped in the art of addiction, stumbled upon an opportunity in food—my guess is that they saw a new frontier for chemical dependency.

They perfected the science of craving, addiction, and deceptive marketing, ensuring that hyper-processed snacks and sugary beverages hook consumers just as effectively as nicotine. They learned to fund studies that downplay health risks, pressure regulators to look the other way, and market aggressively to vulnerable populations. The same playbook, just a different poison.

This coordinated industry-wide strategy aims to influence science, public health organizations, and professional societies and corrupt government policymakers and lawmakers. When one congressman gets $300,000 for his PAC to introduce the "cheeseburger bill," which will prohibit lawsuits against food companies for any injury caused by their food—and most of Congress votes for it—you don't have to wonder who is pulling the strings.

TAINTED SCIENCE

Dr. Jay Bhattacharya, a professor of medicine and health policy at Stanford University—now leading the NIH—has pulled back the curtain on the toxic role of sugar in America's chronic disease crisis. His 2014 study[38] exposed how sugar-sweetened beverages fuel obesity and type 2 diabetes in SNAP, making a clear case for policy interventions to curb their impact. His work is a direct challenge to the food industry's grip on public health, reinforcing the serious need to rethink our broken food system, overhaul outdated policies, and confront the root causes of chronic illness head-on.

As consumers, we depend on unbiased studies to shed light on the foods we should eat and the ones we should avoid. While some food companies do carry out legitimate and informative research, many fund their own studies for self-serving purposes. Why? One major reason is marketing—Big Food funds studies to prop up dubious health claims, using science as a sales tactic to push their products. But the other, more insidious reason is manufacturing doubt. When independent research exposes the dangers of their products, these companies retaliate with their own carefully orchestrated studies, designed not to uncover truth but to muddy the waters. It's the same strategy Big Tobacco used for decades—flooding the scientific landscape with research meant to confuse the public and stall regulation. And as we've seen with Coca-Cola, few industries have mastered this deception better than the soft drink giants.

In February 2001, *The Lancet* published a large independent study[39] ("independent" being the operative word) that was among the first to demonstrate the following links between sugar consumption and obesity:

- Sugar-sweetened beverages increase obesity rates in kids.
- A child's likelihood of being overweight increased in direct proportion to the number of soft drinks he or she consumed.

■ For every can of soda a child drank each day, their odds of becoming obese rose by 60 percent.[40]

The study was a bombshell. It garnered international headlines, and more than 1,000 other scientific articles would go on to cite it.[41] In the days and weeks that followed the study's publication, Coke's stock plummeted. Its share price declined 20 percent relative to the Dow Jones Industrial Average, a downswing that persisted for months. In total the drop represented a loss of $20 billion in the company's valuation. Can you imagine a bigger threat to their bottom line than if everyone found out that Coke is liquid diabetes? Obviously, they can't have that floating around.

So how did Coke and other soft drink makers respond? In the decade that followed, they funded a slew of studies that claimed that sugary drinks were innocent. Coke, Pepsi, the American Beverage Association, Tate & Lyle (a corn syrup producer), and other sugar and soda industry groups sponsored (funded) a half dozen systematic reviews that examined whether sugary drink consumption was linked to weight gain.[42] Every single one of these studies found *zero* association between sugary drinks and obesity.[43]

The scope of this problem is enormous. An analysis[44] published in *JAMA* in 2016 found that compared to independent research, industry-sponsored food studies are 30 percent more likely to produce conclusions that favor their corporate backers compared to independent research. This level of bias is on par with that of Big Pharma, an industry infamous for spinning data to make risky drugs appear safer and more effective than they actually are.

At the same time, independent researchers continued to conduct their own studies, publishing eleven extensive reviews that examined whether sugary-drink consumption was a strong determinant of weight gain and obesity. Of these eleven studies, nine of them found that the answer was a *resounding* yes. Many of the studies even noted that public health authorities had enough evidence to actively discourage people from drinking soda.

SCIENCE OR PROPAGANDA?

We Thank Our Sponsors

Platinum
Sponsors

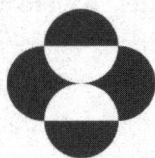

MERCK

Gold
Sponsors

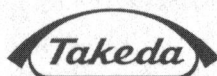 **GILEAD**　　*Takeda*

Silver
Sponsors

Genentech　*Lilly*　INTUÏTIVE　CERSI

In a report[45] entitled *Nutrition Scientists on the Take from Big Food,* Michele Simon details how the food industry has corrupted the nutrition science community. In a different review[16] of 206 studies, researchers found that not a *single* industry study published showed a negative outcome. Isn't that convenient?

Another review of 133 studies on sugar-sweetened beverages found that 82 percent of independently funded studies show harm from sugar-sweetened beverages, while 93 percent of industry-funded studies found that soda and sugar-sweetened beverages were not associated with any health problems.[47]

Coca-Cola and PepsiCo would have us believe they're acting as responsible corporate citizens by reducing calories in their drinks by switching to "zero calorie" artificial sweeteners. Because nothing says "good corporate actor" like decades of funding junk science to convince us that sugar water is part of a balanced diet. Don't fall for it. Despite the fact that industry-sponsored research miraculously detected zero harm from artificial sweeteners, independent studies uncovered significant risks. It's almost as if, when you fund the research, you get to write the ending.

For consumers, this means that you have to be hypervigilant. When you see a company touting the health benefits of their products on food labels, in an advertisement, or on a website or television show, there's a good chance that the claim came from a dubious study that was wholly bought and paid for by industry.[48] Equally, when you see studies casting doubt on the harmful effects of their products, don't believe those either. Take a look at the unbelievable studies that the food industry is feeding you...

Sweet Deception

In 2011 a study in the respectable *Food & Nutrition Research* journal looked at data on more than 7,000 kids and concluded that those who ate candy were up to 26 percent *less* likely to be overweight or obese than kids who didn't eat candy. The candy eaters did not have increased blood pressure, cholesterol, or other metabolic risk factors. In fact, they had *lower* inflammation than the non–candy eaters.[49] The findings were almost too good to be true. "This study suggests that candy consumption did not adversely affect health risk markers in children and adolescents," the authors wrote. Who knew candy was a health food? Well, probably anyone who checked the funding source.

The authors of this study received thousands of dollars[50] from the National Confectioners Association, a trade group that represents the makers of Skittles, Hershey's, and Butterfingers. This candy group not only paid for the study but was also involved in analyzing the data and writing the manuscript. Emails[51] show one of the authors, Victor Fulgoni, a former Kellogg's executive, acknowledging to his coauthors his incorporation of the candy industry's feedback in their study manuscript. "You'll note I took most but not (all) their comments."

As absurd as it was, the study nonetheless generated plenty of positive media play—precisely what the candy industry was looking for. "Does Candy Keep Kids from Getting Fat?" one CBS News headline declared.[52] No, it doesn't. But that hasn't stopped the candy industry from funding other studies that claim that candy consumption has no link to heart disease, obesity, or metabolic syndrome.[53]

If you think that top peer-reviewed scientific journals publish only objective research, think again. One of the most respected medical journals, the *Annals of Internal Medicine,* published a study in 2017 entitled "The Scientific Basis of Guideline Recommendations on Sugar Intake: A Systematic Review."[54] At first read I was taken aback. The conclusions contradicted almost all the science I had studied on sugar for 20 years. "Guidelines [to reduce] dietary sugar do not meet criteria for trustworthy recommendations and are based on low-quality evidence." Turns out the "study" was funded by the International Life Sciences Institute (ILSI), the food and agriculture industry front group founded by a Coca-Cola executive[55] and whose sponsors include, along with Coca-Cola, Bayer, Dow AgroSciences, DuPont, ExxonMobil, General Mills, Hershey Foods, Kellogg's, Kraft, McDonald's, Merck & Co., Monsanto, Nestlé, Novartis, PepsiCo, Pfizer, and Procter & Gamble. And the lead author was on the board of Tate & Lyle, one of the largest makers of high-fructose corn syrup.

This problem is global. In Australasia, Nestlé partnered with nutrition societies and funded dubious studies to promote its sugary powdered drink, called Milo, to millions of parents and children. Milo is a malted sugar beverage like Ovaltine with roughly the same glycemic index as Coca-Cola. With the backing of local nutrition experts, the company marketed the ultraprocessed concoction as a nutritious breakfast meal, running ads featuring cartoons, energized schoolchildren, and famous kid-friendly pop stars. They also promoted it as a health and sports drink targeted at kids who have an "energy gap," which they claimed four out of five kids suffer from. I must have missed the class in medical school where we learned about the dreaded energy gap that must be cured with a sugary drink. Nestlé enlisted Dr. E-Siong Tee to "prove" that Milo was a health drink.[56] He served as science director for more than 20 years for ILSI Southeast Asia. Is it any surprise that Malaysia is one of Asia's fattest countries?

Dr. David Ludwig, professor of nutrition at Harvard Medical School, reviewed Tee's study and found that its design was "wildly overstated."[57] The dietary analysis used was not validated and the Milo drinkers were more active and had far less screen time, which the analysis didn't account for. Oh, and Nestlé reviewed the manuscript.

Sugarcoated Research

While these examples are from recent years, the sugar industry has been duping Americans with deceptive research for more than a half century. Indeed, sugar executives acknowledged a link between sugar consumption and chronic disease back in the 1960s.[58] An industry trade group called the Sugar Research Foundation funded animal research as far back as the 1960s that looked at the relationship between sugar and heart disease. But documents show that when the research suggested that sugar might cause both heart problems *and* cancer—a result the researchers found terrifying—the industry buried the data and never published their results. Around the same time, the sugar trade group paid Harvard scientists the equivalent of $50,000 in today's dollars to publish an influential review[59] in the *New England Journal of Medicine* dismissing the idea that sugar caused heart disease.[60] The real culprit, they claimed, was saturated fat.[61]

In fact, the two authors of that review,[62] Fred Stare and Mark Hegsted, were the most prominent nutrition scientists at the time. Dr. Stare started the nutrition department at Harvard, the first in the country.[63] He and the school received $29 million over his career from the food industry, including sugar industry funding for thirty studies from 1952 to 1956, or about $305 million in 2025 dollars.[64] In 1976, Hegsted coauthored a report commissioned by the Sugar Association called *Sugar in the Diet of Man,* which downplayed the relationship between sugar and chronic disease. Need I say more? Hegsted later played a key role in shaping the first US Dietary Guidelines[65] under Senator George

McGovern, where he championed the now-infamous advice to cut fat while giving sugar and carbs a free pass—a decision that laid the groundwork for the greatest health crisis in human history. And let's not forget: In the 1960s, researchers weren't even required to disclose conflicts of interest, meaning the food industry's fingerprints were all over public health policy, unchecked and unchallenged.

Today a small handful of influential researchers are still deeply involved with the sugar and corn syrup industries. One of them is James Rippe, a scientist who runs an institute that specializes in churning out studies for the food industry. The lobbying group for the high-fructose corn syrup industry, the Corn Refiners Association, paid Rippe $10 million over a four-year period for his research and even kept him on a $41,000-a-month retainer to write editorials defending corn syrup from critics.[66] Rippe then produced a series of studies that reported the following:

- Guidelines on reducing added sugar intake are not warranted because "the scientific basis for restrictive guidelines is far from settled."[67]
- Eating added sugar doesn't promote insulin resistance[68] (which causes pre-diabetes and diabetes).
- Consuming even five times the upper limit of sugar recommended by the American Heart Association (AHA) doesn't increase blood pressure or screw up your cholesterol.[69]

With almost ten times as much of this "junk" research on junk food as of true independent science, the public, the media, and the policy-makers, sadly, remain confused.

Whole Grains: Not the Whole Truth

If you believe the federal government, whole grains are practically a superfood. But like most things in public health, the reality is far more nuanced. Ancient, heirloom, and unadulterated whole kernel grains definitely have their place in our diet. They've been a staple in human diets for millennia. But the refined, bleached, bastardized, mega-processed grains that dominate American grocery shelves? The ones soaked in cancer-causing glyphosate (Roundup) and stripped of all nutrients before being "fortified" back to life...not good for your health.

What most people don't realize is that when you grind the most commonly used "dwarf wheat"—the high-yield, increased-gluten-content variety developed during the Green Revolution—into flour, whole wheat or not, it is literally *worse* for your health than sugar. The glycemic index of sugar is 65 and that of American shelf-stable whole wheat bread is 74, which means that this type of bread raises your blood sugar more than table sugar. As I regularly tell my patients: Below the neck, there is basically no difference between a bowl of sugar and whole wheat bread. Well, actually, the bread is worse.

But what about my "heart-healthy" Cheerios? Or my Quaker Oats "high-fiber" healthy breakfast? you might be wondering. Well, let's start with the fact that Quaker Oats is currently facing a class-action lawsuit[70] over dangerously high levels of the pesticide chlormequat, a chemical linked to developmental and reproductive issues. And as for those glowing health claims plastered all over cereal boxes? They're nothing more than a slick marketing con designed to dupe consumers into thinking they're making smart choices.

Of course, it helps when you have the American Heart Association (AHA) on your payroll. Cereal makers pay hundreds of thousands of dollars to slap the AHA's seal of approval on their boxes, regardless of how much sugar is inside. Namely, Twix chocolate bars somehow made the AHA's list of "heart-healthy" foods—right alongside Froot Loops, Cocoa Puffs, and French Toast Crunch, all of which boast 7 teaspoons of sugar per serving. At this point, we should stop calling it breakfast and start calling it what it really is: dessert in disguise.

The scientifically independent group the Cochrane Database of Systematic Reviews concluded that the favorable studies on whole grains were so weak and mired in conflicts of interest that their results "should be interpreted cautiously."[71]

Alcohol Extends Your Life?

You might recall the trend a few years back alleging that red wine extends life. It was the golden age of "drink red wine, live forever"—a time when everyone gleefully believed their nightly glass of cabernet was basically a health tonic. The logic was simple: Red wine contains resveratrol, this magical compound that science suggested might improve heart health and reduce inflammation. So obviously, drinking wine = longer life.

Except for this minor detail: The amount of resveratrol in a single bottle of red wine is microscopic. On average, you get about 1.9 mg per liter[72]—which is great—until you realize that in clinical studies, researchers used doses of 250 mg to 1,000 mg per day to see benefits. To hit just 500 mg of resveratrol, you'd need to drink 263 liters of wine a day. That's 69 gallons—or, put another way, you'd have to turn into a human wine barrel and be permanently drunk until the end of time. If you try to get your daily dose through wine alone, your liver will file for early retirement long before your heart gets any benefit. This is textbook Big Business propaganda—take a tiny grain of truth, stretch it like taffy, and blast it into the public consciousness until people genuinely believe that red wine a health supplement. It's not nutrition science; it is marketing disguised as research, amplified by an industry that thrives on keeping the booze flowing. The result is a wildly misleading health claim that conveniently keeps their bottom line—and your wineglass—full.

Fortunately for public health, however, as recently as January 2025, an indictment of alcohol by the US Surgeon General Dr. Vivek Murthy highlighted the truths about alcohol: There is a direct link between alcohol consumption and increased cancer risk, represented as the third leading preventable cause of cancer in the United States.[73] Dr. Murthy's clarion call for updated warning labels on alcoholic beverages to inform consumers about these risks must have Big Alcohol shaking in its booties. It's only a matter of time before they start funding counter-research to downplay the risks. Or perhaps they'll throw in the towel and pivot to the booming cannabis market. After all, if you can't beat the health warnings, might as well join the green rush.

DOES THE STUDY PASS THE SNIFF TEST?

At the end of the day, much of the nutrition research published in major journals is legit. But the food industry is determined to keep you confused with bogus studies to promote their processed junk foods. Because industry studies tend to produce sensational findings, they are often picked up by blogs and news outlets, leading to eye-catching headlines. That's why you need to be skeptical when you see the latest nutrition science headline in the news. If it doesn't pass the smell test, then it's best to forget it. Don't share it on Facebook, don't send it to friends, and certainly don't take it as fact. You don't want to be part of the misinformation campaign that Big Food is implicitly recruiting you for.

So, before you buy into a headline (ranging from mainstream media to esteemed academic journals), take a moment to engage in a few self-education habits.

First, check who paid for the study. Does the story mention who funded it? If it's a study on breakfast cereal and weight gain, for example, did the NIH fund it or did Kellogg's sponsor it?

Second, you might need to dig a little deeper. If it says it is funded by the International Life Sciences Institute, you may feel relieved. Sounds legit. But do your own digging. Google the organization. See who is behind it. Be a sleuth.

Third, use your own common sense and don't believe everything you read. "To separate the truth from the bull," Hari says, "I have the

GET TO THE SOURCE

To find a funding source for a study, look up the study on the database PubMed (https://www.ncbi.nlm.nih.gov/pubmed/). Simply type in the name of the lead author and the subject of the study, click on the link to the study you're researching, and look for the part of the paper that mentions its funding source. If the funder sounds like a legitimate organization, don't trust it. Google it and see what you can find.

following suggestions: scrutinize the source of the information, the source's possible agenda, and the evidence provided in the message. If possible, ask: *Is the evidence science-based? Who funded the science? Does the evidence logically support the claims being made? Does it seem like relevant facts or context have been left out?* Remember that commercial pressures shape the form and content of research and news—and exert massive influence."

And lastly, remember that replication is the cornerstone of good science. One study that claims that soft drinks are not linked to weight gain should not distract you from the fact that dozens of independent studies have found otherwise. Instead of being led astray by one clickbait headline, think about the larger body of research. If one sensational new study contradicts a large body of research and sounds too good to be true, then it probably is.

FOOD FIX: BIG FOOD AND SCIENCE SHOULDN'T MIX

It is fairly innocuous for companies to carry out small studies looking at the potential benefits of their products. It makes sense for Pepsi to study whether the electrolytes in the Gatorade it sells can help athletes rehydrate more quickly, for example, or whether products like Quaker Oats might be more satiating than cornflakes. Food companies do research so they can use their findings to make marketing claims, and in some cases, spur innovation that genuinely benefits people.

But consumers should be aware that these claims are often exaggerated at best, and straight up health-crushing fake news at worst. Big Food is in the business of selling junk food. It should not be in the business of doing public health research. As outlined previously, there are ample reasons not to trust Big Food with this type of research. Its documented tactics include the promotion of harmful products, misleading marketing campaigns, targeting of children and other vulnerable groups, corporate lobbying, co-opting of organizations and social media with financial support, and attacks against science and scientists.

At the same time, we must also face the painful reality that government funding for scientific research is already scarce and continuing to dwindle year after year. Academic jobs and research positions at universities are becoming increasingly competitive, and these obstacles, combined with the outsized compensation packages the food industry offers, drive many well-intended scientists to work for industry.

If the food industry is going to be involved in funding studies, however, there must be transparent principles that they are obliged to follow to ensure that their research is untainted and public health remains protected. Any engagement with industry requires firm oversight and strict rules, like ensuring that researchers have full independence to report and publish their findings, and that the companies they partner with have commendable track records of environmental and social responsibility. More innovative ideas, like vetting companies that intend to fund studies, increasing funding for independent studies, or forming an oversight committee for all studies can reduce the problems that stem from food companies funding nutrition research. The companies should not, however, ever be involved in any way in study design, data analysis, authoring of the manuscript, or even review or comments on the manuscript. And obviously, they should not have final say on what gets published.

Another radical change would be to create a firewall between industry and science. This would allow the food industry to fund important studies without biasing the researchers and their results. To effectuate this, companies could pool their donations into a common research fund. This pool of money—perhaps called the Nutrition Fund—could be managed and distributed to scientists by the NIH. Companies could receive incentives to make donations to the fund through tax breaks and other benefits. This fund could then be used to support basic nutrition research on food, diet, and health, as well as food science research that could help companies develop products. A committee of independent scientific advisers could oversee the fund and review and approve research proposals. Ultimately, it could begin to restore the public's faith in industry-sponsored studies.

Such an idea would not be foolproof, of course. In fact, the USDA oversees a number of commodity checkoff programs, which are funded by mandatory fees levied on producers and food companies. While these programs are ostensibly to be used for research and to promote agricultural commodities, in practice they serve as powerful marketing programs for Big Food. Remember the campaigns "Got Milk?" or "The Other White Meat" or "Beef. It's What's for Dinner"? They were all paid for by your tax dollars, promoting agricultural products, regardless of their health benefits. What continues to blow my mind (as naïve as I may be) is that Congress actually introduced a bill to block FOIA requests from uncovering anything about the checkoff programs.[74] A taxpayer-funded program, supposedly designed to support farmers, is so secretive that lawmakers want to shield it from public scrutiny. What exactly are they hiding? And more importantly, why is the government acting as the marketing arm of Big Food?

FOOD FIX: FIXING BAD SCIENCE

Putting an end to Big Food's co-opting of scientists, academics, and health groups will only solve half the problem. The other problem is that nutrition science is in need of a major overhaul. Many of our dietary guidelines and health recommendations are based on what is known as "nutritional epidemiology," which relies on easily manipulated observational studies—types of research studies where scientists watch people's behaviors and health outcomes without interfering. Instead of running experiments, they look for patterns and connections. While useful for spotting trends, these studies can't prove cause and effect—just because two things happen together doesn't mean one causes the other.

This is why Big Soda can publish study after study claiming that children who drink soft drinks aren't on a fast track to becoming obese and diabetic—they use observational data that can easily be molded to get the outcomes they prefer. Large observational studies also gave us the disastrous advice to eat low-fat diets and six to eleven servings of bread, rice, cereal, and pasta every day! The conventional nutrition wisdom has changed again and again over the years depending on the direction in which the winds of the latest observational studies are blowing.

Large reviews of observational studies found that less than 20 percent were later confirmed in actual experimental trials.[75] Asking people what they ate once or twice in 20 years and correlating that to health outcomes or death is highly inaccurate and confounding.[76] For example, we often hear of large observational studies "proving" that eating meat increases the risk of heart disease, cancer, and death.[77] Sounds bad. But when you discount those studies based on the fact that the sample size eating meat also disregarded general health hygiene, it becomes clear that the outcome is biased.

To illustrate the shortcomings in observational studies, consider this example: If I ran a study of women over fifty-five years old (postmenopause) who had sex, I would conclude that sex never leads to pregnancy. It is 100 percent accurate but 0 percent valid. In the same vein, Bruce Ames, one of the world's leading scientists, once quipped that if you ask epidemiologists who did observational population studies about Miami, they would conclude that everyone is born Hispanic but dies Jewish.

So what is the purpose of observational studies? They are highly useful for generating hypotheses for future research and to assess whether correlations are real or just noise. Yet it's important to note that they *never* prove cause and effect. If the effect size is significant enough, then it can be convincing and worth acting on. For example, the increased risk of lung cancer in smokers was 20 to 1. You can take that to the bank. But when a new study, for example, showed that eggs caused a "17 percent" increased risk of heart disease and an "18 percent increased risk of death," that sounds scary, but for context, the trend was more like 1900 percent for smoking and lung cancer. If it is anything less than a 2-to-1 (or a 100 percent) increased risk, we typically aren't too concerned.

The problem with observational studies is that they are frequently subject to a phenomenon known as "data dredging"—scientists run repeated analyses on a dataset to extract insignificant findings that might otherwise be meaningless and then amplify them. That's why nutrition science headlines can cause whiplash, with studies telling us one week that butter, cheese, and chocolate are bad for us, and then the next week new studies telling us that these foods are the key to weight loss and a slim waistline. Nutrition epidemiologists (the ones for hire) are notorious for squeezing trivial findings out of observational datasets and then transforming them into splashy and sensational research papers that attract headlines. It's the very opposite of the scientific method. But sadly, both the food industry and nutrition policymakers use it to their advantage.

The studies worth placing faith in are called "large randomized controlled trials," which are experiments in their truest form. In a typical randomized trial, scientists manipulate one variable—sugar intake, for example—and then assign people to different groups where they are exposed to high levels of sugar or low levels of sugar. Then researchers follow them and measure things like changes in their body weight, cardiovascular biomarkers, appetite, and so on. This is how good science is done. A randomized controlled trial *can* prove cause and effect. An observational study cannot.

One great example was a study[78] by Dr. David Ludwig of Harvard, in which he tested the diet effects of a low-fat, high-carb diet, then switched to a high-fat, low-carb diet on 164 people. The study provided the food to participants and measured their metabolism and hormones. Ludwig and colleagues found that the low-carb, high-fat group burned 300 to 500 more calories a day even though they ate the exact same number of calories.[79] That is definitive. These results support the carbohydrate-insulin model, suggesting that reducing dietary carbohydrates can increase energy expenditure during weight-loss maintenance, potentially offering a strategy to address obesity.

Another interesting example is Dr. Kevin Hall of the NIH's 2019 study[80] examining the effects of ultraprocessed foods on calorie intake and weight gain. In this tightly controlled experiment, 20 adult participants were provided with either ultraprocessed or minimally processed diets for two weeks, followed by the alternate diet for another two weeks. Despite both diets being matched for calories, macronutrients, sugar, sodium, and fiber, participants consumed approximately 500 more calories per day and gained about 2 pounds during the ultraprocessed diet phase, while losing a similar amount during the minimally processed diet phase.

Building upon these findings, Dr. Hall's recent research has delved deeper into understanding why ultraprocessed foods lead to overeating. His studies suggest that factors such as faster eating rates, lower protein content, and the "hyperpalatable" nature of these foods — which combine high levels of fat, sugar, and salt to enhance taste — may contribute to increased calorie intake.[81] This ongoing research aims to inform dietary guidelines and public health strategies to address the obesity epidemic linked to the consumption of ultraprocessed foods. Admittedly, this was a small trial of short duration and there were some study challenges, so I wouldn't call this conclusive, but it's much closer to science than the observational studies.

Proposing a more reasonable set of guidelines to reform nutrition science (which are badly needed), we might consider the following:

- **Focus on large randomized controlled trials.** Instead of publishing a million more observational nutrition studies that give us contradictory findings, the nutrition community should do large and rigorous randomized trials that give us definitive answers. According to John Ioannidis, professor at Stanford University, the cost of randomized trials needed to answer critical questions in nutrition in definitive ways would add up to less than 1 percent of the NIH's budget.
- **Share raw data to increase transparency.** Journals should require that researchers share their raw data. This will increase transparency and reduce the likelihood of manipulation. All researchers should be able to access and analyze one another's data. Through Harvard, the NIH has funded some of the largest population studies, involving hundreds of thousands of people over decades. Many of our nutrition

beliefs are derived from these studies, including the Nurses' Health Study and the Physicians' Health Study. But even though taxpayers funded the studies, the researchers won't allow others to see or analyze their raw data. How does that make sense?

- **Enforce strict disclosure rules.** Every medical and nutrition journal should adopt strict conflict-of-interest disclosure rules, and they should impose penalties on researchers who violate the policies. First-time violations could result in a six-month to one-year suspension. Those who repeatedly violate the rules should face a lifetime ban from publishing in the journal. If all journals introduced a system of penalties for flagrant violations of disclosure rules, then researchers would take the policy more seriously. As Marion Nestle wrote in her book *Unsavory Truth: How Food Companies Skew the Science of What We Eat,* not everyone discloses, and many disclosures are incomplete. At the University of California, San Francisco, professor of clinical pharmacy Lisa Bero and her colleagues reported that one-third or more of authors in the studies they examined had undisclosed conflicts and that a similar percentage of published reviews omit statements of funding sources.

- **Media outlets should also be investigating conflicts of interest and should report transparently on the food industry.** They should have strict conflict-of-interest policies and disclosures for any articles published. For example, an article in *Forbes* that targeted me made no mention that Monsanto funnels money to the industry front group behind the article — the Genetic Literacy Project.[82] The author behind that paper, Kavin Senapathy, also declared that breastfeeding is not always the best choice because it could lead to starvation and malnutrition.[83] Sadly, most media advertising is from the food or pharmaceutical industry, making tough, critical reporting difficult for media outlets.

Now you know what's really behind all those confusing headlines and reports. The fine print reveals who is funding a study and how the data might be manipulated for profit rather than for your health. So next time you read a nutrition headline, be wary, be thoughtful, dig a little, and ask these important questions: (1) Who funded the study and what are the authors' conflicts of interest? (2) Is this a study that can prove cause and effect or just a correlation? If there is a correlation, is the increased risk or benefit over 100 percent? If not, move on.

One of my favorite quotes from Dr. Bhattacharya is that "the healing of the world starts by one person saying loudly, so the whole world can hear, an important true thing that he knows he's not supposed to say and that he knows will get him in trouble for saying it. Such courage is contagious." Let's be courageous together.

For a quick reference guide on the Food Fixes and resources to help you decipher real science from fake news, go to www.foodfixuncensored.com.

CHAPTER 12

FRONT GROUPS: HOW BIG FOOD BUYS FRIENDS AND INFLUENCES PEOPLE

The food industry strategy for controlling science, public health groups, professional health care societies, public opinion, schools, community organizations, the flow of information, political institutions, and policy is calculated, clear, and effective. And it is well hidden. On purpose.

When New York City mayor Michael Bloomberg introduced his controversial ban on large, sugary soft drinks back in 2012, the soda industry promptly sued.[1] The industry, led by the American Beverage Association, ultimately won that battle when a New York State judge struck down the ban in 2014.[2] But the industry did it with the help of some surprising allies: Dozens of minority groups came to Big Soda's aid, filing "friend of the court" briefs in support of the soda industry's lawsuit.[3] These advocacy groups represent the very communities that have been hardest hit by the diabesity epidemic (the continuum from obesity to pre-diabetes to type 2 diabetes).

The NAACP and the Hispanic Federation were among the groups that came to Big Soda's defense.[4] These groups are supposed to fight for the best interests of the communities they represent, which are plagued by chronic disease. Black American and Hispanic people have the highest rates of obesity and diabetes in America[5]—and it is precisely because the junk-food industry preys upon them. Fast-food restaurants are often concentrated in Black and Hispanic neighborhoods. Companies disproportionately target them with predatory advertising. And they are more likely to market their worst foods to minority children than to white children, plying them with ads for products laden with salt, sugar, and unhealthy fat.[6]

Researchers at the University of Connecticut[7] found that junk-food companies spend the most on ads that target Black American people and Spanish speakers. Guess which products were most heavily advertised toward minorities—Gatorade, Pop-Tarts, Twix, Cinnamon Toast Crunch, and Tyson Frozen Entrees. The worse the nutritional profile, the more heavily the products were promoted through advertising. Where are the veggie ads? These findings, the researchers noted, "highlight important disparities in the food and beverage industry's heavy marketing of unhealthy foods to Hispanic and Black youth, and the corresponding lack of promotion of healthier options."[8]

So why would groups like the Hispanic Federation and the NAACP support the soda industry in its battle against anti–obesity measures? Could it have something to do with the fact that Coca-Cola gave the NAACP more than $1 million in donations between 2010 and 2015?[9] Or that it gave the Hispanic Federation more than $600,000 in the same time period? In fact, many of the Black and Hispanic civil rights, business, and health advocacy groups that joined the beverage industry in opposing soda regulation in recent years have been the recipients of millions of dollars in gifts and funding from the soda industry. Soda companies sponsored NAACP scholarships,[10] financial literacy classes offered by the National Puerto Rican Coalition, and programs from the National Hispanic Medical Association.[11]

While these prominent groups and others cozied up to Coca-Cola, the soda industry has run roughshod over Black and Hispanic communities. Things came to a head when two prominent Black American pastors filed a lawsuit against Coke and the American Beverage Association in 2017, saying that the soda industry deliberately deceived Americans about the link between soft drinks, obesity, and diabetes—a practice that contributed to the devastating disease epidemic in minority communities. The pastors told the *Washington Post* that they filed their lawsuit because they were sick and tired of attending funerals for their parishioners whose junk-food diets gave them heart disease, diabetes, and strokes. One of the men, Delman Coates, the pastor at Mount Ennon Baptist Church in Maryland, told the *Post* that it was not uncommon for members of his church to give their babies bottles filled with sugary drinks.[12]

"It's become really clear to me that we're losing more people to the sweets than to the streets," he said. "There's a great deal of misinformation in our communities, and I think that's largely a function of these deceptive marketing campaigns." Pastor Coates pointed out that he was well aware that minority groups had been co-opted as well. "This campaign of deception has also been bestowed on the leadership of our major Latino and Black organizations," he told the paper.[13] This is a form of legal racism practiced by the food industry. And it is effective. The communities most affected are often completely unaware of this invisible, insidious form of oppression.

BIG FOOD'S MAFIA TACTICS: CORPORATE CO-OPTING AND MANIPULATION

While establishing links to minority groups is particularly insidious, the food industry uses corporate sponsorships and financial gifts to buy loyalty from a wide range of prominent organizations. In a report by the Center for Science in the Public Interest called "Selfish Giving: How the Soda Industry Uses Philanthropy to Sweeten Its Profits,"[14] these nefarious tactics are extensively documented. Here's their strategy:

- Link their brands to health and wellness rather than illness and obesity
- Create partnerships with respected health and minority groups to win allies, silence potential critics, and influence public health policy decisions
- Garner public trust and goodwill to increase brand awareness and brand loyalty
- Court growing minority populations to increase sales and profits

This strategy of investing in "corporate social responsibility" can make strange bedfellows, but that spending achieves two important objectives for the food industry: It can generate outspoken support, as we saw with the NAACP and the Hispanic Federation, and it can buy silence from groups that might otherwise criticize junk-food companies for their most shameful behaviors.

The seduction of soda money has created chilling conflicts for many influential organizations. We already saw in Chapter 4 how Big Food fights back against soda taxes; their tactics also include corrupting health groups. Save the Children, an international nonprofit that has long fought for children's rights, was once an outspoken proponent of soda taxes. The nonprofit group threw its endorsement behind soda tax campaigns in New Mexico, Philadelphia, Washington State, Mississippi, and Washington, DC. But in 2010, to the surprise of many in the public health world, Save the Children suddenly withdrew its support for soda taxes. It was perhaps no coincidence that around the same time the organization accepted a $5 million grant from Pepsi.[15]

Sadly, Save the Children was not alone. When Mayor Michael Nutter of Philadelphia proposed a soda tax in 2010, the soda industry offered to make a hefty donation to the city if it would agree to abandon the measure. Eager to receive a windfall, the city council voted down the tax, and the American Beverage Association followed through with a $10 million donation (aka bribe) to the Children's Hospital of Philadelphia for an obesity program.[16] Fortunately, years later, the tax passed on both diet and regular sugar-sweetened beverages. In Philadelphia, after the tax was implemented, daily consumption of regular soda dropped by 40 percent, energy drinks consumption was 64 percent lower, the thirty-day regular soda consumption frequency was 38 percent lower, and bottled water 58 percent higher.[17] In a follow-up study of the 1.5 cents-per-ounce tax there was a 51 percent reduction in sugar-sweetened-beverage consumption, or 1.3 billion ounces less, over two years.[18] However, the American Beverage Association has spent millions fighting back against this tax, trying to get it repealed, and has even taken the city to court. The judge ruled in favor of the city, upholding the tax, and the revenue from the soda tax went to creating 4,000 pre-K slots and twelve new community schools and to rebuilding crumbling parks and libraries.[19]

These tactics are used across the country. In 2012, the Chicago City Council proposed a soda tax to help reduce the city's growing obesity rates—and you'll never guess what happened next. Coca-Cola donated $3 million to launch fitness programs in Chicago community centers— and the soda tax that had been proposed magically disappeared.[20] In the 2016 election, three cities in California[21] had a soda tax on the ballot measure. In 2016, the American Beverage Association, along with major companies like Coca-Cola and PepsiCo, collectively spent more than $42 million[22] to defeat local soda tax initiatives across the United States. In response, public health advocates, supported by philanthropists such as former New York City Mayor Michael Bloomberg and Houston philanthropists John and Laura Arnold, contributed nearly $26 million to promote these measures.[23] They passed. But there are not that many billionaires who are willing to engage in heroic measures to defeat Big Food. We need to rely on better business practices, not just periodic billionaire philanthropy.

Nonetheless, as just outlined, studies show taxes work. If the United States passed a national penny-per-ounce tax it would save $23.6 billion[24] in health care costs and produce $12.5 billion in revenue for community-based programs or programs to address obesity.[25] The beverage industry has not taken this lightly and is fighting back. Taking a page from the tobacco industry's playbook, they have launched a stealth strategy of preempting taxes. When tobacco was under the gun it launched a campaign to create state laws that would prohibit cities or municipalities from creating their own taxes. In effect, the state laws could preempt any city from passing a law restricting tobacco use, for example, in public places. It worked for tobacco.

The beverage industry has taken the same tack, launching two ballots to preempt taxes in the 2018 election. The one in Oregon was called "Yes on Measure 103, Keep Our Groceries Tax Free," supported by the Parents Education Association PAC (an industry front group).[26]

The measure did not pass. However, in Washington State, "Initiative 1634, Prohibit Local Taxes on Groceries Measure" did pass.[27] Why? The beverage industry spent $21.8 million to pass the preemptive measure, preventing any future soda taxes, while opposition groups were able to spend only $100,000.

In the face of a growing soda tax movement, the soda industry is making states an "offer they can't refuse." In California, the most liberal state in the country, where four out of the seven cities with soda taxes are, Big Food played dirty. They spent $7 million pushing a ballot measure that has nothing to do with soda taxes. It would force local governments to require a two-thirds majority to pass any local taxes. This would have effectively paralyzed local governments and limited their ability to fund public services such as schools, fire and police departments, and public libraries. In five days, before anyone knew what was happening, behind closed doors, the beverage industry told Governor Jerry Brown (formerly known as Governor Moonbeam for his liberal views) that if he signed a law prohibiting soda taxes for 12 years, they would withdraw the ballot measure that would cripple local governments.[28] He buckled and signed it. They have done the same in Arizona, Michigan, and Washington.[29]

INFILTRATING PROFESSIONAL MEDICAL AND NUTRITION ASSOCIATIONS

It's gutting to watch nonprofits and lawmakers betray their principles — whether seduced by soda industry money or silenced by smear campaigns and takedown attempts. But what's even more infuriating is Big Food's hijacking of some of the most powerful health and nutrition organizations in the world. It's one thing for a politician to sell out to corporate donors — we almost expect that. But when public health institutions — the very groups meant to protect us — start doing the bidding of Big Food, it's a betrayal of the highest order.

If we can't trust leading health and nutrition experts to put public health first, who's left to fight for us? These organizations are supposed to be our last line of defense, offering impartial guidance based on science, not corporate influence. We count on their expertise. We expect them to stand up for families, children, and communities. And yet, time and again, they have allowed themselves to be co-opted. Take a look at the deception for yourself:

- **American Diabetes Association (ADA).** With diabetes debilitating or killing tens of millions of Americans every year, you would think that the ADA would take a hard stance against companies that peddle diabetes-inducing junk foods. And yet over the years the ADA has signed a number of major deals with more than a dozen companies, including General Mills, Coke, and Campbell's.[30] In one instance, the group signed a $1 million deal with Kraft Foods that allowed the company to slap the ADA logo on products like SnackWell's cookies, Post Raisin Bran cereal, Cream of Wheat, and sugar-free Jell-O. The diabetes group signed another mega sponsorship deal with Cadbury Schweppes, the world's largest candy maker, worth $1.5 million. In exchange, Cadbury was allowed to use the ADA logo on products that are abjectly terrible for people with diabetes, like Mott's applesauce, Snapple, and Diet Rite sodas. And yes, diet drinks have been linked to obesity and type 2 diabetes through their effects on appetite, hormones,[31] and the gut microbiome.[32]

    I once gave a talk at the ADA conference, and as I walked through the exhibit hall, a massive banner caught my eye: "Cure for Diabetes." Intrigued, I went closer—only to find it was an ad for gastric bypass surgery. That was their idea of a "cure." Meanwhile, the rest of the exhibit hall looked like a junk-food trade show—aisles packed with processed snacks, artificially sweetened products, and ultraprocessed garbage that I would never let my patients with diabetes touch. The irony was so thick you could spread it on a slice of white bread (which, of course, was probably being handed out at one of the booths).

- **American Academy of Pediatrics (AAP).** When it needed funding to create a website to promote children's health, the AAP turned to a company whose products have played a starring role in the childhood obesity epidemic: Coca-Cola. Between 2009 and 2015 the sugary-drink giant gave the academy roughly $3 million. The academy praised Coke for being a "gold" sponsor of its Healthy Children.org website, calling it a "distinguished" company for its commitment to "better the health of children worldwide." For a while parents and pediatricians who logged onto the academy's website were treated to a picture of the Coke logo—a major coup for the world's largest soft drink manufacturer.[33]

- **American College of Cardiology and the American Academy of Family Physicians (AAFP).** Both have received millions of dollars in junk-food funding.[34] The president of the American College of Cardiology carried the Olympic torch to help promote its CardioSmart initiative, which was funded by Coca-Cola.[35] In 2010 Coca-Cola spent $102 million to support charities, which sounds generous. But at the same time, it spent $2 billion marketing sugary drinks.[36] The good news is that many leading family doctors resigned from the academy in protest over the AAFP getting into bed with Coca-Cola.[37]

- **American Heart Association (AHA).** In 2017, the AHA received $182 million in funding from industry,[38] including PepsiCo, Kraft, Monsanto, Cargill, Unilever, Mars, Kellogg's, Domino's, Subway, General Mills, and Nestlé, to mention a few.[39] *They* are in charge of protecting our hearts? Trade groups and authors of guidelines that promote the use of more bean and seed oils, like soybean or canola oil, are consultants and receive funds from and sit on the boards of these groups or companies such as the Canola Council of Canada or Unilever. That is why the AHA came out hard against coconut oil despite the lack of evidence that saturated fat causes heart disease. One large review of seventy-six studies on 600,000 people in nineteen countries including randomized trials and observational studies found no basis for our current government recommendations to reduce saturated fat intake.[40] More than seventeen reviews of all the data on saturated fat and heart disease found no link.[41]

Promoters of High-Carb Diets Funded by Corporate Interests

*Denotes pharmaceutical company that manufactures cardiovascular and/or diabetes medications, medical devices, or diagnostic equipment.

It is offensively incongruent—like a magician's sleight of hand. The right hand puts on a show of doing good, while the left hand quietly undoes it all, wreaking havoc in plain sight.

NUTRITION ASSOCIATIONS OR PUPPETS OF THE FOOD INDUSTRY?

Our most revered and respected nutrition societies are often in bed with Big Food. A glaring example of how this undermines both consumers and the public health community is the Academy of Nutrition and Dietetics (AND)—the world's largest organization of registered dietitians. Founded in 1917, the academy is considered one of the nation's preeminent nutrition groups, with more than 100,000 registered dietitians who work in hospitals, schools, universities, the food industry, and private practice. Its initial stated purpose is "empowering members to be the nation's food and nutrition leaders." When it launched, it described its mission as "optimizing the nation's health through food and nutrition."

The academy has annual revenues exceeding $34 million, much of it from membership fees and sponsorships.[42] But it gets a healthy top-up from the food industry of roughly 40 percent of its total funding.

Public health expert Michele Simon published a fairly exhaustive and disturbing exposé on the academy entitled "And Now a Word from Our Sponsors: Are America's Nutrition Professionals in the Pocket of Big Food?" She found that in recent years the AND underwent a radical transformation. In 2001 it had just ten food industry sponsors. A decade later, that number had risen nearly fourfold to thirty-eight. Among its most generous sponsors was a cast of characters that included some familiar names: PepsiCo, Mars, Kellogg's, General Mills, Conagra, Unilever, the National Dairy Council, and Coca-Cola.[43]

So what perks do companies get in exchange for their generous academy sponsorships? Mostly they are after inroads to nutrition professionals so they can indoctrinate them on how to get people to purchase their products. As Simon explains in her report:

> For example, partners can co-sponsor "all Academy Premier Events," conduct a 90-minute educational presentation at the AND's annual meeting, and host either a culinary demo or media briefing also at the annual meeting. Partner status also confers this benefit: "The right to co-create, co-brand an Academy-themed informational consumer campaign." Examples include the Coca-Cola "Heart Truth Campaign," which involves fashion shows of women wearing red dresses and is also promoted by the federal government. Another instance of partner/sponsor co-branding is the National Dairy Council's "3-Every-Day of Dairy Campaign," which is a marketing vehicle for the dairy industry disguised as a nutrition program. The partnership consists of several fact sheets that bear the AND logo, demonstrating the value of the group's seal of approval. The National Dairy Council does not disclose that they paid for the right to use the AND logo.[44]

The thing is that the AND's and the government's nutrition advice is, at best, questionable science and, at worst, entirely backward. Remember the skim milk ads? They billed skim milk as the "healthy" choice, but it turns out it's actually more likely to cause weight gain.[45] And milk itself, the holy grail of calcium? Studies[46] now link it to osteoporosis, cancer, allergies, digestive problems, and autoimmune disease. The single ingredient we were told would strengthen our bones might actually be breaking them. Oops.

The AND literally lets food corporations teach dietitians. That's right—the same companies pushing ultraprocessed junk get a front-row seat in shaping the nutrition advice we're supposed to trust. The academy oversees the credentialing process for registered dietitians and requires them to complete continuing education credits—which sounds great, until you realize those courses are often sponsored by Big Food itself. Imagine if Marlboro were in charge of medical school lectures on lung health. You can't make this shit up.

A 2022 study published in *Public Health Nutrition* exposed a symbiotic relationship between the academy and multinational food, pharmaceutical, and agribusiness corporations, revealing that the AND often acts as a pro-industry voice even when the industry's policy positions contradict the AND's mission to promote health.[47] Between 2011 and 2017, the AND accepted more than $15 million from corporate sponsors, including Conagra, PepsiCo, Coca-Cola, Hershey, Kellogg's, General Mills, and Abbott Nutrition.[48] Internal documents obtained through public records requests show that the AND has invested in ultraprocessed food and pharmaceutical companies, consulted for industry giants, and shaped policies to align with its sponsors' interests. This isn't just about funding...it's surreptitiously about influence. These companies don't just write checks; they get a front-row seat in shaping the nutrition advice we're supposed to trust.

The "education" sessions they provide to dietitians, for example, teach them that obesity is all about calories; that artificial sweeteners are safe for small children; and that health concerns about sugar are an "urban myth" and "a misconception."[49] The "calories in, calories out" myth is one of Big Food's greatest marketing triumphs—a neat, science-y sound bite that conveniently lets them off the hook for pushing ultraprocessed junk. They love to cite the first law of thermodynamics—energy in equals energy out—but this logic falls apart for two big reasons: First, your body isn't a vacuum (a necessary condition for the first law to apply); it's a biochemical factory with a lot of leaky energy systems. Second, as outlined above, not all calories are created equal—your body processes energy differently depending on where it comes from, whether it's sugar, protein, or fat. But acknowledging that would mean admitting that 100 calories from soda doesn't have the same effect as 100 calories from salmon—and that's a truth Big Food can't afford for you to believe. Much of it is unscientific nonsense and food-industry propaganda that is passed off as fact.

The companies are also granted prime real estate at the academy's annual food and nutrition trade show. At one recent expo, the Sugar Association sponsored a booth where its representatives handed out flyers stating that mothers could placate kids who are picky eaters by sprinkling sugar on their vegetables. In her report, Michele Simon found that at one of these annual expos, many of the largest booths were occupied by processed-food companies. Among the largest expo vendors were:

Organization	Booth Fee
Nestlé	$47,200
Abbott Nutrition	$47,200
PepsiCo	$38,000
Unilever	$28,800
General Mills	$21,900
Cargill	$19,600
Kraft Foods	$19,600
Campbell Soup	$15,800
Coca-Cola	$15,800
Conagra	$15,800

These industry partnerships and financial arrangements tarnish the academy's credibility and ultimately influence its policies. In 2015, the

AND gave Kraft Foods the green light to plaster its "Kids Eat Right" logo on Kraft Singles[50]—a product so aggressively engineered that Kraft legally isn't allowed to call it cheese. Why? Because less than 50 percent of it is actually cheese.[51] So what's the rest of it? Well, according to the label, it's a "pasteurized prepared cheese product"[52]—which sounds less like something you'd eat and more like something you'd use to insulate a house. But sure, let's slap a nutrition endorsement on it and call it a day.

Getting the academy to provide its seal of approval was a major coup for Kraft, which boasted to news outlets that the arrangement marked the first time the academy had ever endorsed a product. Health advocates across the country were understandably in disbelief. After a fierce public backlash, Kraft and the academy rightfully decided to terminate the logo deal.[53]

The academy's behavior even drew the attention of comedian Jon Stewart, who lambasted the organization on *The Daily Show*[54] for selling out to a food company that "wants the positive PR of going healthy but doesn't want the hassle of actually improving their product. And here's how you know Kraft has not changed their ingredients: Kraft is still not legally allowed to call their product cheese," Stewart scoffed. "It turns out the Academy of Nutrition and Dietetics is an academy in the same way that Kraft Singles is cheese."

If Kraft were to brand its Singles accurately, it might look a bit more like this:

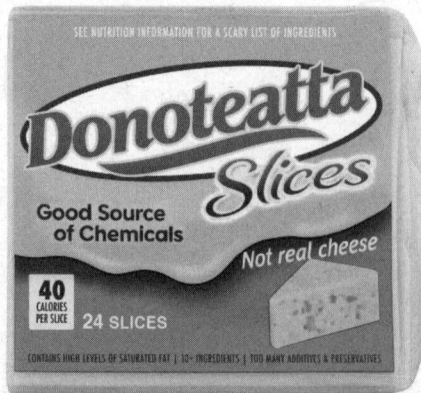

Over the years, the AND and the soda industry became so entwined that it was hard to tell them apart. Coke and the American Beverage Association recruited some of the academy's most high-profile dietitians to act essentially as their public relations machine. The company paid them to:

▪ Promote mini-cans of Coca-Cola as a healthy snack.[55]
▪ Write articles disputing the notion that sugary drinks play a role in the obesity epidemic.[56]
▪ Criticize soda taxes on social media. They paid more than $2.1 million to "independent nutritionists" to oppose soda taxes on social media.[57]

In 2017, the soda industry almost pulled off a hostile takeover of the academy, staging what can only be described as an aggressively shameless coup attempt. Here's how it went down: That year, the academy held an election to select its next president. Two prominent dietitians ran for the position, but one of the two candidates, Neva Cochran, left some critical details out of her official bio[58] that was circulated to voters: She failed to disclose that she had spent 27 years working as a consultant for Coke, McDonald's, Monsanto, the Corn Refiners of America, the Calorie Control Council[59] (which promotes artificial sweeteners), and the American Beverage Association. She was also one of the registered dietitians whom the soda industry had paid to write social media posts opposing soda taxes and promoting beverage industry products. "Plain water isn't that appealing," she wrote in one social media post. In another, she encouraged parents to give their "active teens" soft drinks, lemonade, sweet tea, and chocolate milk and accompanied her recommendation with a vintage advertisement of a young cheerleader with the caption "Jenny needs a sugarless energyless soft drink like a Beatle needs a hairpiece. Two-four-six-eight, what does she appreciate? Sugar."

Jenny has been in orbit since breakfast time. From school she rushed off to a Girl Scout meeting, a trampoline class, and then the pep rally. Jenny needs a sugarless, energyless soft drink like a Beatle needs a hairpiece.

Two-four-six-eight, what does she appreciate?
Sugar.
It quenches fatigue.

NOTE TO MOTHERS
How much energy does your child get from the synthetic sweetner in a bottle of diet soft drink? Exactly none. And how much energy does she need? You tell us—and ask yourself if you're doing her a favor when you stock the refrigerator with no-sugar soft drinks. She'll drink them—her thirst craves anything that's cold and wet. But if you want her to have the energy she needs, you'll bring home the kind with sugar.

SUGAR'S GOT WHAT IT TAKES
... 18 calories per teaspoon—and it's all energy
Sugar Information, Inc.

As Kyle Pfister, the founder of Ninjas for Health, a public health advocacy group, explained it: "Never before has an Academy's presidential candidate been so compromised by corporate conflicts of interest."[60] Cochran could have very easily won the election and been installed as the academy's new president, had it not been for Pfister and several courageous dietitians, who called attention to Cochran's deep industry ties. They sounded the alarm on social media, igniting a firestorm of criticism that embarrassed the academy leadership. Many dietitians who were already uncomfortable with the academy's sugarcoated allegiance to Big Food said that allowing an industry consultant to head the organization was simply beyond the pale. Cochran's opponent, Mary Russell, ultimately won the election, and a crisis was narrowly averted. As one nutritionist and academy member explained it, the election outcome showed that dietitians "want change and professional integrity, not more food-industry insiders."[61]

AMERICAN SOCIETY FOR NUTRITION: WHO PULLS THE STRINGS?

The other main nutrition association in the US is the American Society for Nutrition (ASN), which publishes the world's premier nutrition journal, *The American Journal of Clinical Nutrition,* a journal that deserves the subtitle "where peer-reviewed studies meet corporate sponsorships." This "respected" organization has actively fought against sugar taxes, which isn't exactly shocking when you realize it's been bankrolled by Coca-Cola, PepsiCo, Kellogg's, McDonald's, and Monsanto. But I'm sure that had *nothing* to do with their publishing a "scientific" paper[62] titled "Processed Foods: Contribution to Nutrition," which somehow concluded that there's no difference between processing food at home and processing it in a factory. It's not even common sense, let alone trusted science.

Yes, technically cooking is processing—baking, broiling, sautéing. But does making a home-cooked meal even remotely resemble the industrial chemistry required to produce a Pop-Tart with forty-seven ingredients, half of which most adults cannot even pronounce? According to these guys? Apparently, yes.

They also launched a Smart Choices Program to place their seal of approval on "healthy food," like Froot Loops.[63] When questioned about this endorsement, their response was, "Well,...Froot Loops are better than doughnuts." (Fortunately, the program didn't last; it shut down in 2010.) But is that really the advice we expect from one of the country's leading nutrition societies? They have a long and sullied history of being in bed with the food industry, compromising science, and placing the welfare of their sponsors above public health.[64]

ASTROTURFING, FRONT GROUPS, AND OTHER TOOLS OF INDUSTRY DECEPTION

Not only does the food industry infiltrate and influence existing groups; it also creates "grassroots" groups that are largely, or even entirely, funded by them to manipulate public opinion. One of the most insidious ways that Big Food controls public opinion is through innocuously named front groups like the "Alliance for Safe and Affordable Food" (originally funded by the Grocery Manufacturers Association and Monsanto) that pretend to promote the interests of citizens and the science. Among their core objectives is a fight against GMO labeling along with the disparagement of organic food.

Another is the Center for Food Integrity, also funded by Monsanto,[65] as well as the National Restaurant Association[66] and the United Soybean Board. All of these organizations discredit organic food production, defend pesticides and antibiotics in animal production, and promote the benefits of artificial sweeteners, trans fats, and GMO foods. Some of the worst groups funded by Big Food, Big Ag, and Big Pharma are documented in a report[67] by Friends of the Earth entitled *Spinning Food: How Food Industry Front Groups and Covert Communications Are Shaping the Story of Food.*

These groups have spent hundreds of millions of dollars to manipulate public opinion, discredit legitimate science, and influence policymakers. In just four years, from 2009 to 2013, four of the biggest trade groups spent more than $600 million to promote the "benefits" of pesticide use, GMOs,[68] and the interests of Big Food, conveniently omitting the literally lethal "side effects." Fourteen front groups spent $126 million using stealth tactics to corrupt the truth. Their efforts are focused: discredit organic food production, defend pesticides and antibiotics in animal production, and promote the benefits of artificial sweeteners, trans fats, and GMO foods. They attack investigative journalists as "uncredentialed" and health influencers as "ideological conspiracy theorists," and undermine the credibility of independent scientists by funding seemingly neutral platforms (like the old *SciMoms* blog[69] on "evidence-based parenting") and pressuring them to instead publish industry-aligned content disguised as independent analysis. These efforts are amplified through covert social media campaigns and astroturfing tactics that simulate grassroots consensus. It's seriously so dark that it if it were a prime-time drama, critics would call it too unrealistic to be believable.

There are many of these groups. The American Council on Science and Health (ACSH) might just have the most deceptively legitimate name of any industry front group. It sounds trustworthy, authoritative, and science-y—which is exactly the point. But make no mistake: The ACSH is a mouthpiece for some of the world's largest corporate interests. Over the years the ACSH has received millions in funding from the likes of Big Food, Big Pharma, Big Oil, Big Tobacco, and other industries. According to the Center for Media and Democracy, their donor list has included names like Monsanto, McDonald's, Pfizer, Coke, Pepsi, ExxonMobil, and Dr Pepper Snapple.[70]

The ACSH portrays itself as an important defender of science. But it has a history of proclaiming that smoking, pesticides,[71] and sugar are "not harmful."[72] It dismisses the benefits of organic produce and dietary supplements as "unproven science,"[73] emphasizing the lack of large randomized controlled trials, branding them as dangerous quackery. All the while, it defends things like GMO crops, high-fructose corn syrup, e-cigarettes, and artificial colors and sweeteners. It also routinely attacks people who raise concerns about drug side effects and toxic chemicals in food, labeling them pseudoscientists, alarmists, or fearmongers (all in an effort to smear or deflect). They accuse whistle-blowers of "spreading misinformation" and "contributing to the erosion of public trust in scientific expertise." This playbook is frustratingly effective, as we have seen in the rise of cancel culture, where dissenting voices are swiftly silenced. The famous quip often attributed to Vladimir Lenin—"a lie told often enough becomes the truth"—isn't just a saying to them; it's practically their mission statement.

In 2015 a group from the ACSH wrote a letter requesting that Columbia University remove Dr. Mehmet Oz[74] from the faculty after his show raised questions about GMOs. Dr. Gilbert Ross, one of the signatories on the letter, is the acting president and executive director of the ACSH. He is also an ex-convict who was sentenced to forty-six months in prison for defrauding Medicaid of $8 million and at one time had his medical license revoked for professional misconduct.[75] Getting the memo yet?

There are literally dozens of similar groups. The benevolent-sounding names mask their true intentions. Their aggressive tactics, blatant lies, and half-truths are an attempt to dupe the public. While food industry corporations incubate and underwrite these front groups, they try to conceal information to protect the public images of their funders. They do the bidding of the food industry so that food companies can keep their hands clean. But don't be deceived by their propaganda. When you're tempted to believe the latest campaign ads or sensational headline, I urge you to dig a layer deeper to uncover the sponsor. Disturbingly often, you'll discover that a front group or astroturfing efforts are behind it.

Industry watchdogs are bad for business, and for Big Food, they must be squashed.

FOOD FIX: ETHICAL SPONSORSHIP OF PROFESSIONAL SOCIETIES AND ASSOCIATIONS

Professional medical and nutrition associations like the ADA, the AHA, the ASN, and the AND should, under no circumstances, accept money from junk-food companies. John Ioannidis of Stanford University wrote an important review of corruption in these professional associations and recommended that they abstain from authorship of guidelines and disease definition statements.[76] In other words, they should not be in the business of giving "objective" advice or recommendations. Professional health organizations must face the reality that Big Food has a long history of lobbying against public health, influencing public policy to the detriment of society, and manipulating scientific research.

But as is often the case with researchers, it is unrealistic to expect health organizations to sever all ties with the food industry. Plenty of food companies have missions that align with professional health organizations. You don't have to look too far to see that in many cities a growing number of restaurant chains, grocery stores, health start-ups, and other food establishments are providing healthy, sustainable, and delicious options to consumers. Relatively new and popular farm-to-table food chains such as Sweetgreen and True Food Kitchen are competing with McDonald's and Burger King. There are plant-based chains such as Veggie Grill, Freshii, and Salad and Go (the drive-through salad chain). And stores like Whole Foods and Thrive Market make it easy to find wild, organic, and sustainable foods. Professional health organizations should be looking to promote, commend, and form partnerships with these food companies—not the ones that make all their profits from junk food.

To objectively determine what food companies are ethical to work with, there needs to be a set of guidelines that will help sort out worthy food companies from junk-food peddlers. In 2013, a group of registered dietitians who were frustrated with the AND and its ties to Big Food formed a splinter group called Dietitians for Professional Integrity (DFPI). DFPI has been speaking out against Big Food's infiltration of the academy and demanding change. The splinter group actively petitioned the AND to sever ties with sponsors like Coca-Cola, PepsiCo, and Kraft, collecting more than 24,000 signatures and meeting academy leadership in October 2013. As a result, the AND terminated Coca-Cola's sponsorship in 2015, ending a multimillion-dollar relationship.[77] DFPI has also devised a set of guidelines to help ensure ethical and responsible industry sponsorships. The recommendations are so simple and sensible that there's no reason all professional health organizations shouldn't abide by them. Companies that sell alcohol, soft drinks, and confectionery are automatically disqualified from consideration, but beyond that, the guidelines work in part through a scoring system. Companies are awarded points based on how they do on the following criteria:

- The extent to which they market their products to children
- Whether their products contain artificial colors and sweeteners
- How they rank on animal welfare and the use of hormones
- Their use of fair-trade ingredients
- Their organic production practices
- Whether they use trans fats

- Whether their meat and dairy products are grass-fed, organic, or conventionally raised
- Their fishing and aquaculture practices
- LEED certification (a green building rating system)

Companies are scored in all applicable categories. A company that attains a final average score of 1.5 or higher out of 2 is considered an ethical and responsible sponsor. In the event that a larger company owns a prospective sponsor, the parent company should be scored as well— which is important because most smaller good-for-you brands are now owned by about nine Big Food companies.

FOOD FIX: ETHICAL POLICIES IN MEDICINE

One of the reasons major conflicts of interest are so rife in the public health world is that many universities and medical centers do not have rigorous conflict-of-interest policies, nor do they impress upon future doctors and health professionals the importance of navigating potential conflicts. This is such a critical issue that the prestigious Pew Charitable Trusts convened an expert task force and published a report on conflicts-of-interest policies for academic medical centers.[78] If you work in a university or medical center, take these recommendations to your leadership team:

- Faculty members, staff, students, residents, trainees, and fellows should not accept any gifts or meals from industry.
- Faculty should be required to disclose to their institutions any industry relationships.
- Faculty should not accept industry funding for speaking engagements.
- Continuing medical education courses should be stewarded and funded by scientists and domain experts, not be supported by industry.
- Faculty, students, and trainees should not participate in promotional or educational events that are paid for by an industry.

- Pharmaceutical sales representatives should be prohibited from liaising with faculty, students, or trainees in academic medical centers or affiliated entities.
- Conflict-of-interest education should be required for all medical students, residents, clinical fellows, and teaching faculty.

It is a bit harder to ferret out the truth from fiction when professional associations, public health groups, and top scientists are co-opted by Big Food, Big Ag, and Big Pharma. I encourage you to be a healthy skeptic. Get your information from independent nonprofits, independent journalists, and public advocacy groups such as the Union of Concerned Scientists, the Environmental Working Group, and the Sustainable Food Trust, as well as academic institutions. Remember to follow the money and ask yourself when something fishy appears in the marketplace or media: Does it pass the sniff test? Is Froot Loops really a "Smart Choice" as our esteemed nutrition experts advise?

For a quick reference guide on the Food Fixes and resources to expose food industry partnerships and a deeper dive into front groups, go to www.foodfixuncensored.com.

PART IV

FOOD AND SOCIETY: THE DESTRUCTION OF OUR HUMAN AND INTELLECTUAL CAPITAL

"Structural violence is one way of describing social arrangements that put individuals and populations in harm's way," said Paul Farmer of Partners in Health. "The arrangements are structural because they are embedded in the political and economic organization of our social world; they are violent because they cause injury to people....Neither culture nor pure individual will is at fault; rather, historically given (and often economically driven) processes and forces conspire to constrain individual agency. Structural violence is visited upon all those whose social status denies them access to the fruits of scientific and social progress."

The food industry is part of the story of structural violence that hurts minorities, the underserved, and the food insecure. Those who consume our industrial diet suffer from cognitive and behavioral problems, violence, suicide, homicide, and more chronic disease and premature death and mental health problems. Many of these crises stem from a toxic flood of ultraprocessed junk and a tragic lack of real nutrition. Even the US military—literally at the forefront of our nation's strength and resilience—can't find enough healthy recruits. The food system also harms the very workers who farm and harvest our food. It's an injustice that we can no longer ignore.

In this section, we take a deeper look at the role food injustice plays in our current crises of obesity and chronic disease, our poor national academic performance, the perpetuation of poverty, the challenges facing food workers and farmworkers, violence, mental health, behavioral problems, and even national security. Spoiler alert: They are not separate problems.

Chapter 13

The Hidden Oppression and Social Injustice of Big Food

A few years ago, I had the opportunity to go on a whitewater rafting trip with Robert F. Kennedy Jr. in Utah led by Waterkeeper Alliance, a non-profit dedicated to protecting our waterways. The trip was designed to bring awareness to the tar sands mining of the Tavaputs Plateau at the head-waters of the Colorado River.[1] Tar sands mining for fossil fuels will pollute the waterways critical for local and Indigenous populations and the long-term health of the Colorado River. On the trip was a Hopi chief and his wife, both severely obese and diabetic. While rafting, I observed that they mostly drank Coca-Cola. The chief got sick from his diabetes on the walk down to the river, vomiting and becoming weak. After a few days' floating down the Green River on a raft together, I suggested to him that he could reverse his diabetes if he wanted. I told him he'd need to eliminate refined carbs, starches, and sugars. He paused for a minute and said that it would be very difficult to do this, because it would be impossible to do the traditional Hopi ceremonies without their traditional ceremonial foods.

"What foods?" I asked.

He replied, "Cake, cookies, and pies."

How did this man come to believe that his traditional ceremonial foods were processed flour and sugar and refined oils that didn't even exist 100 years ago? The story of the chief's answer is the story of sickness, poverty, social disenfranchisement, loss of food sovereignty, and internalized racism. It's what Paul Farmer calls *structural violence*[2]—the social, economic, political, and cultural factors that determine disease.

The chief's ancestors had almost no obesity, type 2 diabetes, or alcoholism. Now 80 percent of his people get diabetes by the age of thirty and life expectancy is fifty-three.[3] So, what happened? First, the Hopi were moved to reservations, where their access to many resources is extremely constrained. Second, the water they depended on for drinking and to grow their own traditional foods was usurped by the damming and diverting of the Colorado River to supply California and desert cities such as Phoenix. This pattern was repeated throughout Native American communities. Nearly 60 million bison were slaughtered by the US government to cut off the food supply of tribes on the plains. Buffalo Bill Cody once said, "Kill every buffalo you can! Every buffalo dead is an Indian gone."[4]

Unable to continue their traditional food systems, the Hopi received government-supplied commodities—white flour, white sugar, and shortening. They created new foods like "Indian fry bread." Let me tell you, though, there is nothing in the Native American heritage that includes deep-fried flour, sugar, and shortening. Their Hopi genetics were adapted to scarcity and a high-fiber, plant-rich diet. This is often referred to as the thrifty gene (or genes)[5] because throughout history they were more threatened with starvation than with abundance and thus became efficient at storing excess calories. The recent flooding of their bodies with starch and sugar has made them unusually obese and diabetic. The tribes even have a word for the type of obesity caused by these highly refined processed commodities provided by the government to "help" their people. They call it "commod-bod."[6]

This is a form of internalized racism. It is definitely not as obvious as limiting voters' rights and employment opportunities, the bombing of churches, or hate speech and hate crimes, but in a way it is perhaps more pernicious and destructive, in part because most of the victims have not identified it as a problem in need of fixing.

To put this in perspective: Of all deaths in America, 1.5 percent are caused by gun violence.[7] Roughly 80,000 people die every year from the opioid epidemic. Of course, these problems are real and tragic and we need to help them end. But roughly 75 percent of total deaths, or more than 2 million per year, are caused by chronic disease such as heart disease, diabetes, cancer, high blood pressure, and stroke—mostly the result of our toxic food system.[8] As a consequence, it can be reasonably concluded that more Black Americans, Hispanic people, Native Americans, and people with low incomes are killed by bad food than by anything else. The silent crisis is that drive-through fast food kills far more people than drive-by shootings. Yet we remain in the dark about the role of the food system in killing millions of Americans. Shouldn't we be litigating this with at *least* the same rigor as gun violence and opioid addictions?

RETHINKING THE CAUSES OF DISEASE AND SOCIAL INEQUITIES

Clearly, what we are doing is not working. More and more people are chronically ill, as costs and suffering escalate dramatically. I first began to think deeply about this issue in 2010 when I had the opportunity to be one of the first doctors on the ground in Haiti after the earthquake. In Haiti, I met Paul Farmer, who cofounded Partners in Health. Partners in Health created a powerful and successful model for treating drug-resistant tuberculosis and AIDS in the most impoverished nations in the world during a time when most public health officials had dismissed these nations and diseases as too tough to address.

The brilliance of Paul Farmer's vision wasn't coming up with a new drug regimen or building big medical centers but a very simple idea: The missing ingredient in curing these patients was not a new drug, but addressing the socially driven structural violence that perpetuates disease.[9]

Recruiting and training more than 11,000 community health workers across the world, Farmer proved that the sickest, lowest-income patients with the most difficult to treat diseases in the world could be successfully treated. The *community* was the treatment. It was about providing clean water, access to food, and support from community members. The model is called "accompaniment" because the idea is that neighbors accompany one another to health.

I realized that this model was important not just for infectious disease but for chronic "lifestyle" diseases as well. What determines your lifestyle? The community in which you live, your access to healthy food, the safety of your environment, your education, your family and your friends, and your level of income and employment.[10]

In Chapter 2, we discussed how "noncommunicable" diseases are strongly correlated with community and lifestyle. Only 10 percent of our health is determined by direct medical care. More than 60 percent is related to the social determinants of health.[11] In other words, your zip code is a greater determinant of your health outcomes than your genetic code. Speaking of zip codes, here's a scary stat: For every subway stop heading north from Midtown Manhattan to the Bronx, life expectancy drops by six months, or about 10 years in total.[12] But in health care we focus on the wrong end of the problem. Even though it is clear that the social determinants of health drive most disease, we continue to focus on the molecular pathways of disease, drug targets, and surgical innovation. We are promoting gastric bypass as the cure for diabetes even though it fails 25 to 50 percent of the time,[13] because people go back to the same environment and culture without the health system addressing the real cause of their obesity or diabetes.[14] Shouldn't we be asking why so many need a gastric bypass to begin with?

Shifting our perspective from "blame the victim" to "change the system" is essential for addressing the social injustice that drives our chronic disease epidemic, obesity, poverty, food insecurity, and toxic nutritional landscape, where making good choices is nearly impossible for many. Food is a social justice issue and our industrial food system is an invisible form of oppression.

FOOD APARTHEID: POVERTY, DISEASE, AND FOOD INJUSTICE

A 2016 *JAMA* landmark study compared the difference in life expectancy between the highest-income and lowest-income 1 percent of the population. The difference between those two groups was 15 years for men and 10 years for women. That is equivalent to the loss of life expectancy that results from a lifetime of smoking.[15] More than 38 million Americans live in poverty and almost 100 million live in near poverty.[16]

Life on the other end of the spectrum is also shortened. The United States has the worst infant mortality rate of the top twelve richest industrialized countries.[17] But infant mortality among Black Americans is two and a half times that among white people![18]

Over the past two decades, type 2 diabetes rates have surged among youth, with the highest increases seen in Black, Native American, and Hispanic children. From 2001 to 2017, the prevalence has nearly doubled in Black youth and increased by approximately 80 percent in Hispanic youth.[19] Native American youth also face disproportionately high rates, with a 68 percent increase in diagnoses observed between 1994 and 2004.[20] Additionally, the Native American, Native Hawaiian, Pacific Islander, and Asian communities remain twice as likely as the white community to develop diabetes.[21] And if you are a Black American person you are more than four times as likely to have kidney failure and three and a half times as likely to suffer amputations as a white person.[22]

Is this just bad luck or bad genetic lottery, or could it be something else? The easy cop-out is to blame genetics. But a more intellectually honest truth is that our food system predates a whole class of unwitting casualties.

When we talk about racism, we often picture white supremacists, police brutality, job discrimination, systemic poverty, or hate speech. But rarely do we consider what may be one of the most insidious and overlooked forms of institutionalized racism: food.

You've probably heard of "food deserts"—neighborhoods where fresh fruits, vegetables, and whole foods are nearly impossible to find. Instead, what's available is mostly ultraprocessed junk from gas stations, corner stores, and fast-food chains. For 23 million Americans, the nearest grocery store is more than a mile away, and they often are without access to transportation.[23] But the issue goes deeper than food deserts.

Enter the "food swamp"—communities oversaturated with fast-food outlets, convenience stores, and bodegas, aggressively pushing hyperpalatable, addictive, and nutrient-poor foods. In these areas, it's easier to find a 64-ounce soda than a single piece of fresh produce. Burgers, fries, and fried chicken are on every corner, while anything remotely nourishing is scarce or unaffordable. No real food in sight. This maze of fast-food chains and convenience stores is a leading culprit behind disease, disability, and suffering. These swamps are one of the strongest predictors of obesity, diabetes, and chronic illness, disproportionately impacting low-income communities and communities of color.[24]

In the 40 years since obesity and diabetes exploded in America, the fast-food market has grown seventy times.[25] One in three Americans visits a fast-food restaurant *every single day*.[26] Americans spend more money on fast food than on movies, books, magazines, newspapers, videos, and music *combined*.[27]

The USDA found that only 5 percent of Black Americans follow a healthy diet today.[28] That's a staggering drop from the 1960s, when Black American diets were apparently twice as healthy as the national average — rich in fruits, vegetables, fiber, and healthy fats.

So what happened?

This isn't just about personal choice — it's about systemic sabotage. Today, Black communities are flooded with nearly twice as many fast-food restaurants as white neighborhoods. When every corner is packed with ultraprocessed, high-sugar, high-salt foods — and fresh, affordable, nourishing options are nearly impossible to find — it's not a mystery why health outcomes have deteriorated. It's a direct result of how the food system has been weaponized against communities of color.[29]

Though we often hear about food deserts and food swamps, a more accurate term might be "food apartheid" — a deliberate, systemic form of discrimination that dictates who gets access to real food and who is flooded with ultraprocessed, disease-causing junk. Unlike a desert, this isn't a natural phenomenon — it's the result of policy, economics, and industry influence. Communities most affected by food disparity are increasingly adopting this term to expose the reality: Food access isn't just an issue of geography; it's an issue of power.

Speaking of power, I bet you didn't know that the history of sugar is closely linked to slavery. The slave trade served the growth of sugar production. Legal American slavery is thankfully over (although forms of slavery certainly still occur), but today sugar, especially in its new form, high-fructose corn syrup, is connected to a new kind of oppression—food oppression, which makes people of color sick, fat, and disabled.[30] It is a form of apartheid in which the underserved and minorities live in areas that lack healthy food and have an overabundance of fast-food outlets and convenience stores. Compounding this is the targeted marketing of the worst food to low-income communities and people of color. Children are the biggest targets. Not only are they more susceptible to manipulation but they also represent long-term investments for Big Food.

STEALING LAND, SLAVERY, AND BROKEN PROMISES

Our country has a history of racism in agriculture and landownership. We displaced Native Americans through Manifest Destiny and stole their lands. Our farming system and our nation's early prosperity were built in large part on the backs of enslaved people. After the Civil War, formerly enslaved people were promised forty acres and a mule by President Lincoln to start a self-sufficient life, but his promise was revoked by President Andrew Johnson, so formerly enslaved people were never allowed to establish a foothold in the economy and self-determination. If formerly enslaved people had actually been given that land, today it would be worth roughly $6.4 trillion.[31]

Not surprisingly, at the turn of the twentieth century, Black people owned 14 percent of farms. This was a threat to white people, who stole Black land via raids on Black farmers, lynchings, and murders. Now there are few Black farmers, and fewer who own their land. Moreover, because many in the Black community have forgotten—or were never told—that their ancestors were brought to the United States (as enslaved people) to bring their agricultural wisdom and crops to the New World, now many in the Black community equate farming with slavery.

As of 2022, less than 2 percent of farmers are Black and less than 2 percent are Native American, according to the USDA Census of Agriculture.

FOOD INSECURITY

Even when food is available to disadvantaged communities, fresh whole foods can be expensive, which leads to the purchase of cheap, unhealthy junk food. When the decision is between facing hunger and eating cheap processed food, the choice is inevitable.

Food insecurity can also have incredibly detrimental effects on pregnant mothers. A colleague grew up in East Cleveland, a place with no job opportunities and even less real food. Until recently, they didn't even have a McDonald's. They have Rally's, a fast-food chain that makes McDonald's look like a gourmet restaurant. You can get two burgers for $3. Who knows if it is even meat? Through hard work she pulled herself out of her environment, something rarely seen in that neighborhood. She had a role model, her mother, who was a police officer. She recounted the story of one young woman of fifteen who begged my colleague to help the young woman find a way to get out of that neighborhood. The young woman knew she would end up like her mother, on welfare with multiple children, living in the projects with no way out. Yet getting pregnant made her eligible for $20-a-month subsidized housing in the projects, food stamps, health care, and social services. It was her only way to survive. How is this a just society?

Data shows that preterm labor and infant mortality decrease if we provide housing and food to pregnant mothers, and this reduces overall health care costs.[32] The same goes for people living unhoused. Provide housing and food, and health care costs plummet.[33] But the perverse financial systems in health care and social programs don't encourage us to do the right thing—the thing that will reduce costs, save lives, and protect our citizens.

The Food Research and Action Center produced a white paper in 2017 called *The Impact of Poverty, Food Insecurity, and Poor Nutrition on Health and Well-Being*.[34] The consequences of our current food system on malnourished mothers are staggering. When children are born to malnourished mothers and grow up on a diet of artificially cheap sugar and processed and fast foods, they are stunted, developmentally delayed, and cognitively impaired, they suffer from learning disabilities, and they have behavioral and emotional challenges and increased rates of violence, obesity, and chronic diseases. The "food" they eat as children doesn't change when they grow older, and the malnutrition continues, perpetuating mental health issues and increased rates of obesity, type 2 diabetes, heart disease, depression, disability, and premature death, with a loss of an average of 10 to 15 years of life.

Living in poverty drives food insecurity, overconsumption of cheap processed foods, higher rates of obesity and diabetes, and a whole host of other chronic diet-related diseases. The risk of diabetes for any ethnic group is twice as high (100 percent increase) for those with less than an eighth-grade education. If you are food insecure, you are also twice as likely to be diabetic.[35] Diabetes rates are lowest in white people, at 8 percent; they are 16 percent among Black people and 22 percent among Hispanic people, and much worse in people with low incomes of all ethnicities.[36] Education is also a huge determinant of health status, regardless of income.

It is both the overconsumption of bad food and the underconsumption of real food that drive this problem. Not surprisingly, the research shows that those who are the most food insecure use more health care services and have the highest health care costs. Junk food is a devil's bargain: you may pay less now, but you'll pay much more later.

JUNK-FOOD PUSHERS: HOW BIG FOOD SELECTIVELY TARGETS LOW-INCOME COMMUNITIES AND MINORITIES

Of course, the food industry welcomes those suffering from food insecurity with open arms, aggressively advertising unhealthy foods to them. One day I was working in an urgent care center as a medical resident and a Hispanic woman came in for back pain with her seven-month-old baby in tow. The baby was sucking a bottle of brown liquid.

"What is that?" I asked. "Coke," she replied, as if it was the most normal thing in the world. I asked her why she would give her baby Coke, and she said, "Because he likes it."

Earlier you read about Big Food's marketing ploys to reach children. That trend is amplified even more for minority children. In 2019, the Rudd Center for Food Policy and Obesity published the damning report *Increasing Disparities in Unhealthy Food Advertising Targeted to Hispanic and Black Youth,*[37] showing that Big Food companies actively target Black and Hispanic youth with their least nutritious products, including fast food, candy, sugary drinks, and snacks. From 2013 to 2017, food advertising on Black-targeted TV increased by 50 percent. Black teens viewed 119 percent more junk-food–related ads—mostly for soda and candy—than white teens. The average teen saw more than 6,000 junk-food ads a year just on television. Even if you talk to your kid about healthy eating three times a day, there is just no way to compete with the subliminal messaging their subconscious is assaulted with on a daily basis.

You see, food companies know to use cultural icons to influence minorities. LeBron James promoting Sprite.[38] McDonald's using Serena and Venus Williams and Enrique Iglesias in their TV ads to attract Black and Hispanic consumers. Do you think a Big Mac, fries, and a Coke were really Serena's pre-match meal? No matter, their dollars are well spent. Race-based advertising works.[39]

Our government is complicit in the perpetuation of these behaviors and the support of the production and sale of the very foods it tells Americans not to eat in its dietary guidelines. What may shock some is that government-guaranteed loan programs support fast-food outlets, which are far more prevalent in underserved communities of color.[40] Why should government loans pay for the expansion of food that kills Americans?

CORPORATE SOCIAL RESPONSIBILITY OR CORPORATE SOCIAL EXPLOITATION?

A while ago I was part of a documentary called *Fed Up*—a movie about how our food system makes us sick and fat with addictive sugary, starchy products. While on the road promoting the movie, I met with Bernice King, Martin Luther King Jr.'s daughter, and she explained to me that nonviolence also includes nonviolence to ourselves; thus, she was excited about showing *Fed Up* at the King Center in Atlanta. Then, unexpectedly, a few days later I got a call from her, sounding defeated as she announced that we couldn't show the film. Turns out that Coca-Cola funds the King Center.[41] And that story got a hard no from Coke execs.

I was so shocked I decided to double-click on this behavior. I met with the dean of Spelman College in Atlanta, who confided to me that half the incoming class of Black American freshman women were already battling a chronic disease—whether it was type 2 diabetes, hypertension, or obesity. I asked her the obvious question: Then why are there Coke machines and soda fountains everywhere on campus? The answer was just as obvious. Coca-Cola is one of Spelman's biggest donors.[42] In fact, Helen Smith, Coca-Cola's vice president of global community affairs and president of the Coca-Cola Foundation, sits on the college's board of trustees.[43] You don't need a degree in public health to see the problem here.

FOOD FIX: FOOD JUSTICE, FOOD SOVEREIGNTY, AND EMPOWERMENT

Often the people living in these circumstances are not aware that they are victims of food oppression, food apartheid, and internalized food racism. The work of transforming this system of oppression must come from multiple sectors, like changes in government policies at the local, state, and federal levels, regulation, litigation, health care reimbursement for food as medicine, nonprofits creating local programs to educate and empower people, and grassroots efforts of citizens working to change their communities and regain food sovereignty. Illustratively, in Atlanta, the Ebenezer Baptist Church—Martin Luther King Jr.'s church—started a 2-acre urban garden where parishioners participate in growing food for the local community. There are hundreds if not thousands of these stories of hope and empowerment.

One of the leaders working to transform their ravaged neighborhoods is Ron Finley (who goes by the endearing pseudonym "Gangsta Gardener"). From South Central Los Angeles, a place of gangs, drugs, violence, and desperate poverty, he grew up in a food prison where he had to drive forty-five minutes to buy a tomato. Through a simple act of turning the dirt by the curb in front of his house into a garden, he started a small "horticultural revolution." That patch of dirt technically belonged to the city, and he was slapped with a citation for gardening without a permit. But he didn't back down. Instead, he kept going— until he had a warrant out for his arrest for the crime of growing carrots[44] and 12-foot sunflowers by the curb. Rather than give up, he fought back, got the laws changed, and transformed the urban landscape. He pioneered curbside gardens, turned lawns into food forests, and built raised-bed gardens in abandoned lots—giving gang members, ex-convicts, and former drug dealers a new way forward, one seed at a time. Finley now wants to transform the food desert into a food forest and is leading a movement to bring the education and skills needed to the youth in his community and beyond.

Strange Bedfellows: Faith and Food Justice

Increasingly Black American pastors see the link between the plight of their congregations and food apartheid. Some have taken it upon themselves to help their congregations link food and theology and are improving their congregations' lives through food.

Methodist pastor Christopher Carter, who's also an assistant professor of theology and religious studies at the University of San Diego, focuses his work on helping link the health of humans, the treatment of animals, and the destruction of the environment to the food we eat and how it all connects to racial equity and Christian theology. He invites his congregants to ask: How was this food raised? Were the animals treated humanely? Were the farmworkers subject to harsh working conditions, underpaid, or abused? What is the impact of industrial food on the health of individuals and communities? He believes this is central to shifting deeply held notions that allow Black American communities to be held hostage by the food they consume. He seeks to do what he describes as an effort to "decolonialize the plate" and reclaim old traditions.

Reverend Dr. Heber Brown III, the senior pastor of Pleasant Hope Baptist Church in Baltimore, Maryland, founded the Black Church Food Security Network. He recognized that in most food deserts (or areas of food apartheid), there was an abundance of churches, and he created a movement, not from farm to table but from "soil to sanctuary." His network empowers Black churches to grow their own food and partner with Black farmers and urban growers to bring fresh produce to churches. They create pop-up farm stands at churches, start gardens on church-owned land, and lead lectures and small group meetings that focus on food justice and food sovereignty.

Imagine if Black church leaders (or any affected minority group) collectively joined in a campaign to link the struggles of minority communities to food, food apartheid, and racial targeting by the food industry. They could strike back at the invisible form of oppression that keeps communities down, a form of racism that is internalized and insidious, that disables and kills more people of color than anything else, and create a call to action to change all that. Black lives matter. But Black health matters too. What if Black American churches boycotted soda or junk food, echoing Martin Luther King Jr.'s Montgomery bus boycott in the 1950s challenging segregation on buses? I see a truly powerful untapped movement that could shift culture, shift the physical and economic health of communities of color across the country.

Art, Social Justice, and Food

Understanding the link between social justice, food, and disease, the University of California, San Francisco Center for Vulnerable Populations and a youth development and arts education program called Youth Speaks partnered to create "The Bigger Picture," a public health campaign through spoken-word poetry and hip-hop music videos to call out the connection between the social injustice of stress, poverty, and violence, and food insecurity, lack of access to whole foods, and a plethora of ultraprocessed and fast food in their communities.[45] The value teens place on social justice, their anger at manipulation by the food industry, and their witness to the death and destruction in their families and communities empowered them to create art that inspires awareness, agency, and change. It takes the blame away from individual choices and places it on the structural systemic problems that drive disease, disability, and poverty.

In his piece for the Bigger Picture, "Empty Plate," Anthony Orosco, age twenty, addresses the legacy of poverty of those who pick and pack the produce that we buy at Whole Foods but don't make enough money to buy the very food they pick.

> *Abuelas y abuelos, tías, tíos, primos y carnales*
> *Who picked processed and packed produce*
> *Their pockets couldn't afford to begin with.*
> *Backs breaking, bones aching*
> *Harvesting healthy fruits and veggies*
> *Acre by acre,*
> *The bounty of California's breadbasket*
> *That almost never blessed the tables of farmero families*

In her piece "The Longest Mile," Tassiana Willis, age twenty-four, an obese Black American woman, highlights the toxic food environment that drives disease.

> *This about how I starve myself before blood work*
> *Praying it doesn't pick up the candy from my last time of the month*
> *This is me praying I don't forget diabetes knocked*
> *2 uncles off their feet*
> *And one is barely standing*
> *This is my battle between diet and dialysis*
> *About being stuck between two Burger Kings*
> *And never having it your way...*

Whether through church leaders, activist farmworkers or farmers, or artists calling out social injustice, a growing awareness of food injustice attempts to correct the systemic conditions that fuel it. These are just a few examples of the movements happening across the country and the world, directed by local leaders and community organizers to reclaim the food system. It is a long road, with many obstacles, but we can drive change slowly from the margins. This is how all movements start. The abolitionists weren't deterred that it might take 100 years to pass civil rights legislation or 150 years to have a Black American president.

Admittedly, many other systemic problems perpetuate the food system crisis of injustice; we need bigger, policy-wide reform (many of those ideas are discussed in Parts 3 and 4). These reforms are very difficult to employ given our current political environment and campaign finance laws that make corporations able to contribute literally billions of dollars to influence policy and elections. The First Amendment protects speech, including apparently the right of corporations to target children and minorities with advertising. The most important reforms would be those akin to what we implemented for smoking and those that have been effectively implemented in other countries such as Chile (see Chapter 3).

It is important to transition from a business model where corporate interests privatize the profits but socialize the costs of their products and where the harmful consequences of their products are not taken into account. If these costs are not accounted for, we the taxpayers, our citizens, and our environment all pay the price.

FOOD FIX: SPREAD THE WORD

1. **Start a faith-based wellness program in your place of worship.** In 2011, Pastor Rick Warren, Dr. Daniel Amen, Dr. Mehmet Oz, and I launched the Daniel Plan, a faith-based wellness program in Warren's church. In the first week 15,000 people signed up; they lost a quarter of a million pounds in the first year by supporting one another in small groups to live healthier lives. Now the program is in more than one hundred countries and thousands of churches around the world. You can learn more at www.danielplan.com.

2. **Be an agent of change in your community or workplace.** Start a lunch group, rotating who brings healthy lunches for your group. Start a wellness group for walking or being active together. Get rid of the candy, doughnuts, and sodas. They are bad for absolutely *everyone,* increasing sickness, disability, and costs.

For a quick reference guide on the Food Fixes and resources on combating structural violence and social injustice, go to www.foodfixuncensored.com.

CHAPTER 14

COULD FOOD CAUSE OUR MENTAL HEALTH EPIDEMIC?

In 2009 I wrote *The UltraMind Solution,* linking diet, nutritional deficiencies, and lifestyle to mental illness, memory, and attention issues. These ideas were not widely understood at the time but my learnings were born out by my empirical experience. As I treated my patients for a multitude of physical conditions, I saw how changes in their diet resolved their behavioral, mood, memory, or attention problems.

One twelve-year-old boy, a patient of mine with severe ADHD, completely reversed his attention and behavioral problems after he got off processed and junk foods, ate a real-food diet, and added supplements to fix his deficiencies of omega-3 fats, magnesium, zinc, and B vitamins. Look on the next page at his handwriting before and after just two months of improved nutrition and supplementation. What might be the implications for all our brains if we could treat the root of the problem?

Since then, mounting science has connected the links between diet, mood, behavior, and violence. As a nod to my unexpected prescience, entire departments at leading academic and medical institutions including Harvard and Stanford have been set up to study "metabolic psychiatry and nutritional psychiatry" focusing on the intersection of diet, metabolism, and mental health. This approach posits that metabolic dysfunction (issues like insulin resistance, obesity, and inflammation) plays a significant role in the development and progression of psychiatric disorders. It's actually quite logical if you really think about it: The brain, being highly energy dependent, is particularly sensitive to metabolic changes. It requires a

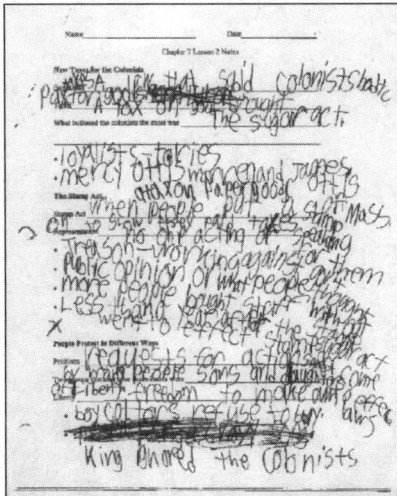

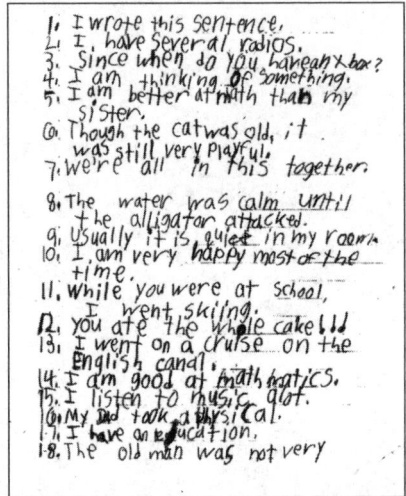

certain cocktail of micronutrients, which are primarily accessible through diet, to perform its essential functions, like producing the happy hormones and neurotransmitters we rely on for emotional stability.

HOW FOOD CHANGES MENTAL HEALTH AND BEHAVIOR

By now, major medical journals have shown the link between nutrition and mental health. *The Lancet Psychiatry*—a top medical journal—maps out just how nutritional medicine is a key to mental health and psychiatry.[1] Studies increasingly show that adults suffering from a variety of mental health symptoms and conditions, and children with ADHD, often have very low levels of antioxidants[2] (which come from fruits and vegetables).[3] Nutritional deficiencies, particularly in essential nutrients like omega-3 fatty acids,[4] B vitamins,[5] and magnesium,[6] can impair mitochondrial function (energy) and therefore brain health. And chronic inflammation, often resulting from a toxic diet like the industrial Frankenfoods described earlier in this book, can dramatically negatively impact brain health.[7] We have discussed the costs of obesity and chronic disease, which I think are becoming increasingly self-evident, but the connection of mental illness to the costs of chronic disease is not as easily identifiable. It's been posited that the economic burden of mental illness may even be greater than the costs of heart disease, diabetes, and cancer.

Mental health issues may not lead to the same death rates as diabetes or heart disease, but they lead to more years of disability and lost productivity. And their prevalence is growing astronomically. Years of life lost to disability and loss of productivity from mental illness are more than eight times those of heart disease, in part because mental health affects younger people with potentially decades of life ahead of them.[8] Population studies have found that diets rich in fruits and vegetables and low in French fries, fast food, and sugar are associated with a lower prevalence of mental illness,[9] and that junk food creates moderate to severe psychological distress.[10] The encouraging news is that interventional studies[11] have demonstrated that improving diet can be an effective treatment for mental health conditions (an especially important finding given that mood-altering drugs are the fastest-growing segment of the pharmaceutical market and as a group constitute the second-biggest class of medication in total sales and prescriptions).[12] Changes in diet have even been proven to reverse bipolar disorder and schizophrenia, conditions that often respond poorly to medication.

EDUCATIONAL INEQUITIES: THE ACHIEVEMENT GAP

Disturbingly, mental health and psychiatric issues are starting to develop earlier and earlier. I suppose it is no surprise knowing the state of nutrition in most schools. But what else does this affect? Juvenile academic performance and hence future potentials are being squandered as a direct consequence.

It's not uncommon to hear Americans lament our low global standing in academic performance. Unbelievably, we, the great American superpower, currently stand at thirty-seventh in the world in math (we dropped six points since the publication of the first edition of this book). To put that in perspective, the emerging economy of Vietnam, a nation we waged war on not too long ago, is fifteen points ahead at twenty-second.[13] One in six US children has a neurodevelopmental disorder.[14] More than one in ten children have ADHD.[15] Depression, learning disabilities, and behavioral problems are rampant in schools. School nurses have to contend with boxes of prescription medications they dole out to kids during the school day. Academic performance is the worst in low-income neighborhoods but also declining in more affluent areas. Brain development is the worst in the least-advantaged kids (who also have the worst diets), with brain sizes roughly 10 percent smaller and IQs an average of 7 points lower than developmental norms.[16] Why are so many children not graduating from high school? Why are kids in the most disadvantaged neighborhoods more likely to go to jail than college? There are many reasons for this including social determinants like poverty, crime, parenting, culture, and failure of government policies, but one of the biggest unspoken factors in cognitive development and behavior is most certainly nutrition.

To paraphrase President Clinton: It's the food, stupid.

This phenomenon of poor school performance in kids who face health issues, who consume poor diets, who are obese and often diabetic, is called the achievement gap.[17] A 2014 review of the science by the CDC entitled "Health and Academic Achievement" documents the clear link between poor nutrition and academic performance, including lower test scores, lower grades, poor cognitive function with less alertness, attention, memory, processing of visual information, and problem solving, and increased absenteeism.[18] Lack of fresh fruits and vegetables and vitamin and mineral deficiencies lead to the same problems. How can you expect kids to learn and function when their brains are starving for essential nutrients? The result is that kids are inattentive, disruptive, late, absent, or worse.[19]

Food is driving many of these problems.[20]

The average kid in America consumes 34 teaspoons of sugar a day![21] Even in spite of the fact that the cognitive and behavioral effects of sugar for children are well documented,[22] kids literally bounce off the walls. Ever been to a birthday party where chaos ensues in the aftermath of a cake binge? We are literally destroying the intellectual capital of our youth, with broad consequences for our whole society: less productive citizens who are more likely to earn less, suffer more, get sick early in life, and be incarcerated.

We are raising the first generation of Americans who will live sicker and die younger than their parents.

Not only that, but special education costs are skyrocketing across the country. In San Diego Unified School District, special education enrollment has surged, reaching 20,423 students in 2023–24, an increase of nearly 10 percent in *just one year*.[23] Meanwhile, overall school enrollment has declined by more than 10 percent since 2015, exacerbating financial pressures. While the district's total 2024–25 budget is $1.1 billion,[24] rising special education costs continue to strain resources. There are multiple causes for this, but the majority of cognitive dysfunction in kids can be linked to poor nutrition. As just described, healthy brain chemistry depends on nutrients to function properly. Neurotransmitters like serotonin and dopamine, responsible for mood stability, focus, and motivation, require key vitamins, minerals, and healthy fats to be produced. These are not "nice to haves." They are absolute biological imperatives. Your brain *cannot* function properly without them. Illustratively, insufficient iron (a common deficiency) leads to lower dopamine function and impaired concentration.[25] Vitamin and mineral deficiencies including B vitamins, iodine, zinc, and vitamin E are linked to diminished cognitive abilities and poor concentration.[26] And as a double whammy, when a child's diet is filled with ultraprocessed foods—first, devoid of these essential nutrients, and second, fueling brain inflammation—their brain is trapped in a cycle of emotional instability, brain fog, and poor impulse control.

COULD OUR DIET BE THE CAUSE OF OUR OVERFLOWING PRISONS, BULLYING, AND CONFLICT?

Another culprit behind mental hijacking is chronic brain inflammation—the silent saboteur fueled by poor diet, stress, and environmental toxins, quietly rewiring your brain from the inside out.

When the brain is inflamed, it doesn't just make you feel foggy or tired—it completely rewires how you think and behave. The prefrontal cortex—the brain's "adult in the room," responsible for reasoning, impulse control, and decision-making—stops working properly. Without it keeping things in check, the amygdala, the brain's emotional command center (fight or flight), takes over, making you more reactive, impulsive, and emotionally volatile.

Think of it like this: An inflamed brain essentially regresses to a childlike state. Just as young kids struggle with emotional control and long-term planning because their prefrontal cortex isn't fully developed (which takes until about age 25 for full maturity), adults with an inflamed brain lose those same executive functions. The result? Knee-jerk reactions, poor judgment, and acting on emotion instead of logic.

The food we eat modulates all our biology, including all our brain functions. Food affects our hormones, brain chemistry, nutrient status, and essential chemical and biological functions. There is nothing that you do to your body that you don't also do to your brain, which is why it's ignorant to abstract our diet from our mental health outcomes. Clearly, they are coupled.

Consider the following research:

- Data shows that junk food makes kids act violently—bullying, fighting—and suffer more psychiatric distress, including worry, depression, confusion, insomnia, anxiety, aggression, and feelings of worthlessness.[27]
- In an article entitled "Impact of Nutrition on Social Decision Making," scientists fed two groups different breakfasts.[28] One group got a high-carb breakfast, the other a high-protein, low-carb breakfast. The high-carb group was more likely to engage in "social punishment" behavior such as negative comments and actions toward others in structured behavioral experiments. Now consider that most Americans eat dessert for breakfast, full of sugar and carbs—cereal, muffins, bagels, sugared coffees, pancakes, French toast, oatmeal. This does not make for a very nice society.

■ Those who consume high levels of refined oils (currently more than 10 percent of our diet and found in all ultraprocessed foods) and low levels of omega-3 fats from fish have higher rates of depression, suicide, and homicide.[29] Our consumption of these refined oils (mostly soybean oil) went up 248 percent from 1970 to 2014.[30]

Think about this: We incarcerate Black Americans at six times the rate of white Americans.[31] Thirty-seven percent of inmates are Black, but Black Americans make up only 13 percent of the population.[32] That is the result of multiple complex factors. But I would hazard a guess that a significant portion of violent crime is also the result of a diet that robs people of their minds, impeding their thinking, judgment, and ability to make good choices. Naturally, the communities with the highest rates of food insecurity and the worst food apartheid also have the highest rates of incarceration.

One day I walked into my office and found a handwritten letter from a violent criminal still in prison. He said he read one of my books, changed his diet, and realized that much of his life of violence was driven by his diet. Changing his diet in prison transformed him. Studies have shown similar results.[33]

In one double-blind randomized controlled trial, researchers found a 37 percent reduction in violent crime in those taking omega-3 fats and vitamin and mineral supplements.[34] The author of the study said, "Having a bad diet is now a better predictor of future violence than past violent behavior....Likewise, a diagnosis of psychopathy, generally perceived as being a better predictor than a criminal past, is still miles behind what you can predict just from looking at what a person eats."

One study of violent juveniles found that among those given a vitamin and mineral supplement violent acts dropped by 91 percent compared to a control group.[35] These kids were deficient in iron, magnesium, B_{12}, folate—all nonnegotiable for proper brain function. Researchers wired these kids up to EEG machines to look at their brain waves and found a major decrease in abnormal brain function after just thirteen weeks of supplementation. They also advised kids to improve their diets. The ones who didn't showed no reduction in violent behavior. The kids who improved their diets showed an 80 percent reduction in violent crime.

Another experimental study of 3,000 incarcerated youth replaced snack foods with healthier options and dramatically reduced refined and sugary foods. Over the twelve-month follow-up there was a 21 percent reduction in antisocial behavior, a 25 percent reduction in assaults, and a 75 percent reduction in the use of restraints. There was also a 100 percent reduction in suicides. This is stunning. As the world struggles to deal with the exploding rates of teenage suicide—suicide is the third leading cause of death in children ages ten to fifteen, and rates of suicide increased 33 percent[36] between 1999 and 2014, with an increase of 57 percent for those age fifteen to nineteen[37]—a simple diet change could be a key to dramatic improvements.[38]

Yet another study[39] showed the same pattern. Violent behavior for incarcerated juveniles dropped by 47 percent once they were placed on nutritional supplements.[40] They showed lower rates of antisocial behavior in nine types of recorded infractions: threats/fighting, vandalism, being disrespectful, disorderly conduct, defiance, obscenities, refusal to work or serve, endangering others, and non-specified offenses. Depression, suicide, ADHD, and violent behavior are all, in one way or another, linked to food.[41] The low-income communities who live in food swamps and consume the most processed food and the fewest nutrients are often the ones who suffer from mental illness and violence and higher rates of incarceration.[42]

This is true not just in adolescent prison populations but also among adults. A rigorous randomized controlled trial of nutritional supplements in 231 adult prisoners found a 37 percent reduction in violent offenses. A Dutch study of 221 prisoners found a 47 percent reduction in violent crime with nutritional supplementation, and when drug offenders were removed from the analysis there was a 61 percent reduction in violent crime, comparable to a California study of 402 adult inmates.[43]

Clearly crime and antisocial behavior arise from a complex set of social, economic, and environmental factors. But what if a big part of the solution to our increasing social strife, exploding rates of depression, mental illness, ADHD, bullying, violence, and crime, and over-flowing criminal justice system is fixing our food system? What if we could fix the epidemic of broken brains by fixing the nutrition of those most at risk (and ideally all of us)?[44]

Our kids' brains are inflamed, and they're developmentally compromised because of it. I feel like I need to shout this from the rooftops: WHY AREN'T WE TALKING ABOUT THIS?!

UNFIT TO FIGHT: FOOD AND THE THREAT TO NATIONAL SECURITY

In a time of increasing global political instability, America is unable to find enough healthy recruits for military service with more than 77 percent of recruits being rejected as unfit to fight![45] In 2018, a group of retired admirals and generals from the organization Mission: Readiness published a report entitled *Unhealthy and Unprepared*,[46] showing that today, the military cannot meet its recruitment goals. Plenty of people try to enlist, but most get rejected, mostly due to health or weight issues. Not only are recruits overweight and sick, but also active-duty soldiers are 73 percent more likely to be overweight than in 2011. Overweight soldiers are 33 percent more likely to suffer from musculoskeletal injuries. In fact, there were 72 percent more medical evacuations from Iraq and Afghanistan for injuries related to obesity and poor fitness than for combat wounds.

One in four teenage boys is currently pre-diabetic or diabetic, meaning that solving health and food problems is crucial for military readiness.

The Department of Defense can transform food procurement for active duty soldiers who are currently overweight. It can focus on food for performance enhancement, health, and fitness. These are all essential in order to create and maintain a healthy military and save billions in taxpayers' money required to address the high cost of taking care of overweight soldiers and veterans.

Our nation's future—our global standing, economic power, and very survival—hinges on the intellectual strength of the next generation. Yet, we're raising children who are less capable of learning, less equipped to succeed, and less able to contribute to society than those before them. This isn't just a health crisis; it's a national security and economic disaster in the making.

What's the price of an entire generation handicapped by poor diet and malnutrition? How much innovation, productivity, and global influence are we sacrificing because we've allowed our food system to prioritize profits over people? If we don't address this now, we're not just failing our kids—we're surrendering our future.

FOOD FIX: HEAL MENTAL ILLNESS WITH NUTRITION

While it goes without saying that not all mental illness is caused by food, poor nutrition can worsen mental health conditions. Solving the problem of mental ill-health is complex and requires addressing poverty, inequities, trauma, violence, and more. But a few simple things can help integrate our nutritional knowledge into society and science.

First, if you suffer from a mental health issue, as much as possible, try to seek help from a functional medicine practitioner or functional dietician to help you address the dietary needs that will improve the health of your brain. The eating guidelines in the Chapter 2 Action Guide will be a key component. You can also refer to my book *The UltraMind Solution* or my upcoming course focused on metabolic psychiatry at www .hyman-health.com for a detailed plan on how to fix your brain.

The National Institutes of Health must also prioritize funding research on the link between food and mental illness, with a strong focus on clinical trials that establish cause and effect. Key areas of study should include depression, anxiety, ADHD, autism, and bipolar disorder—conditions that already have a growing body of research in nutritional psychiatry but require more robust evidence to shift mainstream medical treatment toward root-cause solutions rather than symptom management.

Additionally, health care reimbursement policies must evolve to cover food-as-medicine programs for treating mental illness. Health systems should integrate nutrition-based interventions, ensuring that patients receive dietary treatment and therapeutic supplementation alongside conventional therapies. Finally, medical education must be reformed so that doctors are trained in nutritional and metabolic psychiatry, equipping them to apply dietary interventions in clinical practice—a crucial shift that could transform mental health care as we know it.

FOOD FIX: GOOD SCHOOL NUTRITION MAKES KIDS SMARTER (AND BETTER BEHAVED)

Innovators and parents around the country are trying to create new ways to feed hungry kids in schools. In the lowest-income part of Washington, DC, a local philanthropist started a charter school and provided three meals a day of healthy whole foods to children. These children lived in extreme poverty with food insecurity and unsafe environments. Children from this neighborhood rarely went to college and few graduated high school. They were destined to repeat the vicious cycle of poverty and disease from which they came. Yet simply feeding these children real food and providing a safe and supportive environment changed the trajectory of these children's lives. Most went to college instead of jail. The program became so successful that even affluent families wanted to send their kids to this school because the academic performance on standardized tests was higher. But it wasn't the school or the children that drove these incredible results; it was access to real food essential for brain development, cognitive function, and emotional health.

The same experiment played out in the Academy for Global Citizenship on the South Side of Chicago, whose student body is mostly low-income, minority, or immigrant children. At twenty-three years old, teacher Sarah Elizabeth Ippel started this charter school and figured out how to get the Chicago Public Schools food service program to provide real whole foods to her students at the same cost as the processed foods served in most other schools. On the concrete playground were raised-bed gardens. I visited the school and saw the children ravenously eating all the vegetables and whole foods.

Check out the Food Fix Action Guide (accessed by scanning the QR code at the end of each chapter) for more examples of parents, chefs, and community leaders who are chipping away at the horrible school lunch landscape. Here are just a few notable ones:

1. **Brigaid,** started by top chef Daniel Giusti, aims to reform school meals through building real kitchens, creating delicious recipes, and training food workers who are used to microwaves and deep fryers to cook real food from fresh whole ingredients.[47] He started in the Bronx, New York, and Connecticut and continues to expand.

2. **Common Threads** is a nonprofit that teaches low-income children and families in schools and the community how to cook real food on a budget as a way to lift themselves up from food scarcity, poverty, and social injustice. They view cooking as the key tool to fix the obesity and chronic disease epidemic. And it's true. We have raised generations of Americans who don't know how to cook.

3. **Conscious Kitchen** is a California nonprofit that partners with schools to address food equity, nutrition education, and access by changing school food service, linking local sustainable farm systems to the schools, and cultivating nutrition literacy in the schools. They created a model for zero-waste kitchens and serve food that is local, organic, seasonal, and non-GMO, and once these conscious kitchens are built, the schools and students take over. The kids in the program are happier and healthier and have fewer academic and behavioral problems. Even better, Conscious Kitchen does this within the federal school lunch budget and nutritional guidelines. For those who say this can't be done, this model proves otherwise.

4. **Big Green** is a program started by my friend Kimbal Musk to bring learning gardens to nutrition education in schools across the country at scale and has expanded to support other nutrition and farming efforts throughout the country. Teaching the basics of farming and healthy eating, these outdoor classrooms aim to improve community

access to healthy produce through practical, garden-based education opportunities.

5. **Eat Real** is a nonprofit organization dedicated to transforming food in K–12 schools across the United States, aiming to create a healthier next generation. The organization collaborates with school district food service leaders to enhance the nutritional quality and sustainability of school meals. Eat Real's award-winning certification program currently supports over 600 schools, impacting more than 360,000 students and improving the quality of up to 129 million meals annually.

These programs need to be expanded and taken up as standard for all public and private school systems and local and federal policy. Real whole food should not be the privilege of a few schools and students. Real whole food that supports children's development and learning must be a right for all children. The tax of not doing this for all children is a lifetime of struggle with obesity, disease, poverty, impaired cognitive development, and learning and mood disorders.

FOOD FIX: CHANGE THE FOOD IN PRISONS AND REDUCE VIOLENCE

Some aspects of the food system are going to be hard to fix, but prison food and its link to behavior, mood, and violence should be an easy target. The federal government, states, and cities all maintain jails or prisons and engage in food procurement and meal service. They have sole power to contract only with food service providers that have health in mind and on their menu. They have the power to mandate that private prisons provide healthy food.

Some prisons have already started programs that teach inmates about healthy eating, growing food, preparing food, and other food education. How cool would it be for us to totally reform our—frankly tragic—prison system to one where we rehabilitate our disenfranchised, rather than just continue to impose suffering? Here are a few examples of successful stories:

- **Bastøy Prison** in Norway provides monthly stipends for prisoners to buy and cook their own meals and provides education about sustainable farming.
- **Harvest Now** in Connecticut, a nonprofit active in more than eighty-five prisons, links underserved food-insecure communities with prisons. They provide prisoners with seeds and the education to farm. Most of the produce is then donated to local food banks, up to 24,000 pounds a year in some counties.
- **Michigan Department of Corrections** stopped buying food from Big Food service vendors and started buying from local farms and improved the nutritional quality of the food for 43,000 prisoners.
- **The Richard J. Donovan Correctional Facility** in San Diego has a Farm and Rehabilitation Meals program to address the link between prison violence and a poor prison diet. The prison buys farmland and hires inmates to grow and harvest the food, which is then fed to the prisoners.

Not only is our food system causing an economic crisis by spreading chronic disease across the globe, it is also damaging the intellectual capital of our children, driving crime and violence and mental illness, and threatening our national security. These are not all separate problems. They are one big, interconnected problem that can only be solved by multiple solutions across the entire food chain, from seed to fork and beyond.

For a quick reference guide on the Food Fixes and resources to help you understand the impact of ultraprocessed foods on your mental health, go to www.foodfixuncensored.com.

CHAPTER 15

FARMWORKERS AND FOOD WORKERS: THE NEGLECTED VICTIMS OF OUR FOOD SYSTEM

Most of us don't give much thought to the people behind our food—the farmworkers, packers, truckers, cooks, and servers who make it all possible. Cheap food magically appears in grocery stores and restaurants, and while we may obsess over whether it's organic, grass-fed, or "clean," we rarely ask who grew it, harvested it, or prepared it. The human cost of our food system is invisible to most consumers, yet every bite we take is shaped by the labor of countless individuals whose struggles and working conditions remain largely unseen.

Farmworkers and food workers combined are one of the largest sectors of workers in America, numbering more than 20 million. Without farmworkers and food workers we wouldn't be able to eat. They rarely make a living wage and are subjected to harsh working and living conditions, including modern forms of slavery, sexual harassment, abuse, lack of health care, and exposure to toxic agricultural chemicals that leave them sick at our expense. And most of them are people of color. Three-quarters of those living below the poverty line and the 50 million food-insecure people in America are mostly Black, Latino, or Native American.[1] And, as we demonstrated above, people of color suffer disproportionately from diet-related diseases, labor abuses, lack of access to resources, and the environmental consequences of our food system.

THE COSTS WE PAY FOR FARMWORKERS AND FOOD WORKERS

Farmworkers face high risk of injury and harm from agricultural chemicals—many of which trace their origins to World War II, when chemicals like ammonium nitrate, originally used as explosives, and organophosphates, developed as nerve agents, were repurposed after the war for fertilizers and pesticides in agriculture. This wartime innovation laid the foundation for the modern chemical-intensive farming industry, with lasting consequences for human health and ecosystems. For those who work on a farm—there are 1 million farmworkers in our country—they have one of the most dangerous jobs in America.[2] They die at seven times the rate of other workers.[3] The Environmental Protection Agency (EPA) estimates that 10,000 to 20,000 farmworkers are harmed by *acute* pesticide poisoning every year,[4] which doesn't even account for the long-term effects of being exposed to toxins day after day, year after year.[5]

The herbicides and pesticides that farmers use on their crops are known neurotoxins, carcinogens, and hormone disruptors, demonstrated by the fact that many of these chemicals used in the United States are banned in countries abroad. The government agencies (the FDA and the EPA) that should be regulating these chemicals for human safety are asleep at the wheel.

Furthermore, the population of farmworkers is notoriously underpaid and increasingly exploited. They aren't protected by minimum wage or overtime pay requirements. Many of them live below the poverty line and have no health care, instead depending on emergency rooms and Medicaid to treat the diseases that our highly toxic agricultural chemical infrastructure forces upon them. The ugly truth is that the food system disproportionately affects low-income communities, immigrants, and people of color who actually work in the food system.

Farther down the food value chain, the average restaurant worker earns only about $11 an hour.[6] That's why we offset their salary through billions in tips and, by my math, another $16.5 billion in food stamps.

But their dependence on food stamps limits their food choices at the checkout aisle, and healthy options are often not affordable enough or government approved. The people feeding us are suffering from our food system the most.

FOOD SERVICE WORKERS AND THE OTHER NRA

According to the Labor Department, seven out of the ten lowest-paying jobs are in the food industry, all paying less than $20,000 a year.[7] The very people who grow and serve our food are often not able to feed their own families on the wages they receive. These workers have been left out of the protections afforded most other workers in our economy. In 1935, the National Labor Relations Act passed and a few years later the Fair Labor Standards Act, which established the minimum wage, protecting many workers. But it explicitly excluded farmworkers and domestic workers from these basic worker rights[8] (rooted in a racial compromise by President Franklin Roosevelt with the Southern Dixie Democrats to protect the interests of white landowners).

These antiquated labor laws don't provide the protections afforded to most other workers. Restaurant and other tipped workers' minimum wage is $2.13 an hour, unless state laws provide higher wages. Fifty-two percent of fast-food workers require food stamps and other government assistance, costing taxpayers $153 billion a year. More than 50 percent of workers reported illness or injury on the job, and the majority didn't have health insurance. This means that they rely on emergency rooms or urgent care centers, offloading the cost of underpaying workers to the taxpayers. Workers of color make an average of $5,600 a year less than white workers in the food sector.[9]

The powerful trade lobby the National Restaurant Association (the other NRA), is one of the most influential lobbying groups in the country. It vigorously opposes minimum wages[10] and has been able to keep the minimum wage for food service workers at $2.13 an hour.[11] After the Civil War, the restaurant industry lobbied to hire formerly enslaved people, pay them nothing, and have them work for tips alone. Today, on average, workers of color get paid $4 less an hour than white workers, and immigrant workers are subject to exploitation and fear of their employer's control over their visa status. Female workers often have to accept sexual harassment so they can feed their families on tips. Yet the reality of a dignified working wage is that if food workers received a minimum wage of $12 an hour, it would only increase the average household's food cost by 10 cents *a day*. Think we can all eat that tax.

In 2013 One Fair Wage launched a campaign to raise the minimum wage for food workers to $12 an hour; they have seen success in eight states and two municipalities and continue to raise awareness and advocate for change. These and other grassroots efforts can help raise awareness and create local change but must be scaled to become national policy. We need to be honest about the true cost of our food; the price we pay at the checkout counter or the restaurant is not reflective of the cost of our food or of the effects it has on humans, nature, and our economy.

THREATS AND VIOLENCE

Pay and working conditions aren't the only problems. Often through threats of violence and intimidation, workers are forced to work against their will, perpetuating harsh, unfair, and often illegal working conditions. More than 80 percent of female farmworkers in California's Central Valley have reported sexual abuse or harassment.[12] Much of our produce comes from Mexico and Central American countries, where workers suffer even worse abuses. The average farmworker in Mexico makes just $8 to $12 a day, and farming in Mexico "employs" nearly 600,000 children.[13] They are routinely subject to slavery and violence. A tragic example was when, after protesting and reporting their employers' illegal wage deductions for food and housing, eighty Mexican farmworkers just..."disappeared."[14] In Mexico — our biggest source of avocados for our smoothies, guacamole, and avocado toast—many of the farmers are extorted and even murdered by the drug cartels who sell their "blood avocados" to Americans.[15] Local farmers in Mexico have fought back against the cartels, but it is often not enough.

These stories are pervasive in our food system, affecting the poor and disenfranchised who are just trying to make a living. Chicken processing workers at industrial farms are a gruesome case study in how far corporations will go to keep food cheap—at someone else's expense. Americans are projected to consume a staggering 104 pounds of chicken per person per year in 2025,[16] and to keep up with demand, poultry production lines have doubled[17] their speed over the last 30 years. Workers now process 35 to 45 chickens per minute,[18] repeating the same exact motion every two seconds for eight hours straight, with just one 30-minute break. This causes carpal tunnel syndrome and other repetitive stress injuries to run rampant, with poultry workers suffering illness at a rate of five times higher than the average worker. All this for just $11 an hour, often in jobs filled by immigrant workers terrified of being fired, deported, or harassed. Even basic human dignity is sacrificed—bathroom breaks are often denied, forcing workers to wear diapers on the line just to keep the operation running.

So, next time you bite into your pre-breaded, pre-fried, pre-seasoned chicken nugget, remember this: Ninety percent of American chicken has been processed into these "chicken-like substances," and behind every bite is a worker enduring brutal conditions, stripped of rights, and sometimes forced to relieve themselves in a diaper—all so your McChicken stays cheap.

HEALTH RISKS

As mentioned earlier in this chapter, being a farmworker is one of the most dangerous jobs in America. The official numbers of those being poisoned would be even higher if we account for the long-term effects of chronic toxin exposure, including cancer, type 2 diabetes, neurodegenerative diseases, and developmental disorders, among others.[19] Farmers' risk of Parkinson's disease is 70 percent higher than that of the average population because of pesticide exposure.[20] Vandana Shiva, an environmental activist, doesn't pull punches when it comes to characterizing the harm Big Ag causes—she calls them the "poison cartel."

And yes, disturbingly, the United States has one of the laxest regulatory systems in the world on environmental poisons that saturate our food. Despite many other countries banning chemicals, we in the United States continue to use the following ubiquitously:[21]

- Atrazine, which disrupts hormones, damages the immune system, and is linked to birth defects
- Paraquat, which is linked to Parkinson's disease
- Neonicotinoids, which are linked to the disappearance of honeybees (which are essential for pollination)
- Glyphosate, which we have discussed at length, and which is linked to cancer[22]
- 1,3-dichloropropene, which is linked to cancer and is one of the most widely used pesticides in California

These chemicals are also known as *obesogens* and can cause obesity and type 2 diabetes.[23] It's all starting to make sense, right?

The risks of injury and harm from agricultural chemicals are also borne by taxpayers. These workers, often living below the poverty line, have no health care and depend on emergency rooms and Medicaid, both of which we all pay for through our taxes.

A study[24] of Hispanic agricultural workers in Salinas, California, found that these workers were 59 percent more likely to get leukemia, 70 percent more likely to get stomach cancer, and 63 percent more likely to get cervical cancer than the average population. They also have about 40 percent more organophosphate pesticides in their urine, including pregnant and breastfeeding women. Babies exposed to these chemicals have lower IQ and cognitive function, and higher rates of behavioral issues and attention deficit disorder. It is estimated that children younger than age five have lost 41 million IQ points because of exposure to environmental chemicals including pesticides, mercury, and lead.[25] What is the cost of that to future generations' happiness and productivity? *These kids are born pre-polluted.* Unlike medications regulated by the FDA for human safety, these chemicals are (poorly) regulated by the EPA, also asleep at the wheel. They operate from a model that could be described as: Approve first, ask questions later (or not at all).

And it is not just farmworkers who are at risk. It's also the food workers involved in the production, processing, distribution, and retail sectors of our food system. They are exposed to repetitive stress injury, physical risk, cleaning chemicals, biological hazards (from bacteria), and carcinogenic compounds.[26] Food workers have a 60 percent higher risk of occupational injury and illness than nonfood workers, and their risk of death is nine and a half times higher.[27]

FOOD FIX: THE VICTORY OF TOMATO FARMWORKERS

The story of the tomato farmworkers in Florida is one of tragedy as well as hope, possibility, and the power of grassroots efforts to transform communities and find a path to justice and fair food. Just outside Fort Lauderdale, Florida, in the small town of Immokalee, immigrant farmworkers grow and harvest 80 percent of America's tomatoes. The average backbreaking day of labor would yield the farmworkers $62 if they could pick 4,000 pounds, or 125 buckets, of tomatoes. That leads to an average income of less than $10,000 a year with no benefits and few rights. These workers are also subjected to abuse including beatings, sexual harassment, child labor, forced labor, and lack of shade, water, and breaks.

A disparate group of farmworkers from Mexico, Guatemala, and Haiti banded together in 1993 to create the Coalition of Immokalee Workers to fight for better wages and working conditions. Appealing to the growers failed, so they went to the big purchasers of tomatoes like Yum! Brands, including Taco Bell, Burger King, and KFC, and asked them to pay an extra penny a pound for their tomatoes. At first, they refused, but after the coalition launched campaigns like "Boycott the Bell" in 2004, they agreed, and other big companies followed suit, including McDonald's, Walmart, Whole Foods, Trader Joe's, Chipotle, Subway, and the big food service providers including Aramark, Sysco, Compass, and Sodexo (notably, Wendy's and Publix supermarket chain refused to participate). These companies have agreed not to increase the price of tomatoes in stores or restaurants and to sign on to the Fair Food Program, which mandates that growers provide basic protections for their workers.

"The Coalition of Immokalee Workers created a student/farmworker alliance. And now their model is being replicated by folks in the dairy industry, and it might get translated soon to folks in the poultry industry," says Navina Khanna, director of the HEAL Food Alliance. "They have set up a fair food standards council where they're the ones holding the corporations or the farms accountable and doing third-party verification."

The documentary *Food Chains* exposes the abuses of farmworkers and provides hope with the story of the Immokalee farmworkers. There is still much to be done across other farm systems and products, but this is a start.

FOOD FIX: EMPOWERING FARMERS AND FOOD WORKERS

That American workers should have basic rights would seem to be a given. But for farmworkers and many food workers it is not. Here's how we can change that.

1. **Restaurant and food retailers must agree to the Fair Food Program**[28] and pressure growers to adhere to its basic tenets for workers' rights:

- No forced labor, child labor, or violence
- At least minimum wage for all employees
- Pay workers for all their work
- No sexual harassment or verbal abuse
- Freedom to report mistreatment or unsafe working conditions without the fear of losing their job—or worse
- Access to shade, clean drinking water, and bathrooms while working
- Time to rest to prevent exhaustion and heat stroke
- Permission to leave the fields when there is lightning, pesticide spraying, or other dangerous conditions
- Transportation to work in safe vehicles

These rights are enforced through worker-to-worker education, audits, transparency, complaint resolution, and market-based enforcement. If restaurants and food retailers want to be part of the Fair Food Program, they must ensure growers abide by those rights, or stop buying from them.

2. **Support Fairtrade products.** Fairtrade International is an organization that supports farmers and farmworkers in dozens of low-income countries while also working to protect the environment. Part of its mission is to promote fairness and justice in trade. Low-income farmers in developing countries are frequently exploited. Fairtrade ensures that any product that carries its certified logo meets strong standards. The organization requires that products be sustainably sourced, that they be made in a way that doesn't pollute the land or waterways, and that farmers and workers receive fair prices. It's comforting to know this when you buy a Fairtrade certified product. Look for their logo and support the important work they do.

3. **Support advocacy groups ensuring safe and fair working conditions.** A growing movement, exemplified by the Coalition of Immokalee Workers, is ensuring safe and fair working conditions for

our food workers and farmworkers. The two groups most active in organizing and advocating around these issues are the Food Chain Workers Alliance and the HEAL Food Alliance.

For a quick reference guide on the Food Fixes and resources to help you support food workers and farmworkers, go to www.foodfixuncensored.com.

PART V

THE ENVIRONMENTAL IMPACT OF OUR FOOD SYSTEM

Our food system isn't just wrecking public health—it's quietly sabotaging our future. When we grab a burger, fries, and a soda—or even a so-called healthy green smoothie—we're not exactly thinking about where it came from, who grew it, or whether the soil was depleted to the point of producing nutrient-bankrupt food. If we're honest, we mostly just care if it tastes good and keeps us out of that hangry-sugar-crash mania.

But here's the problem: The way we grow and produce food today is directly tied to whether we'll be paying skyrocketing health care bills, dealing with food shortages, or watching our cost of living explode in the future. Most people don't connect their dinner plate to things like rising food prices, economic instability, or even national security—but we should. Industrial farming practices aren't just an "environmental issue"—they determine the quality of our food, the stability of supply chains, and how much of our paycheck goes to medical bills because we've been fed nutritionally bankrupt garbage instead of real nutrition. We've been lulled into complacency by the convenience and anonymity of our food, but that ignorance is going to cost us—not just in some abstract way, but in our wallets, health, and survival.

Learning what we have done to create these problems and what we have to do to solve them is essential to our collective future. I wish this were just hyperbole, but sadly it is not. This is not so much about saving the planet as about saving humanity.

Chapter 16

Why Agriculture Matters: Not Charity, But Survival

Since the dawn of agriculture in Mesopotamia 10,000 to 12,000 years ago, we have been growing food, which has enabled the rise of civilization. However, the history of agriculture is littered with our destructive habits born of a lack of knowledge of natural systems, resulting in vast ecological damage. The Roman Empire fell in part because of the demise of its agriculture, the result of destructive practices that depleted the soil.[1] Many other civilizations have suffered the same fate.[2] In *Sapiens: A Brief History of Humankind,* Yuval Noah Harari disabuses us of any notions of an idyllic past when humans lived sustainably on the Earth. In previous eras, however, the scale of our destruction was smaller, and there was more unspoiled territory, which meant new lands to farm.

At the turn of the twentieth century, half of all Americans were farmers; now it's only 1 to 2 percent, thanks in large part to the industrial economy that spurred massive technological efficiencies. Though while these innovations in agriculture enabled us to produce food in abundance, they came at some serious costs. The methods we use to grow food today are contributing to our future inability to grow food by depleting soil to the point where current cropland will become unfarmable. Not to mention the extractive methods of farming, which deplete soil and water and create chemical pollution (from nitrogen fertilizers, pesticides, and herbicides), destroying species including pollinators, rivers, lakes, and oceans in the process. Back in 2014, the UN

Food and Agriculture Organization report determined that we may have only sixty harvests left before we run out of soil.[3] While projections like these are notoriously murky and the exact number of harvests remaining is uncertain, the consensus is clear: Soil degradation is a pressing global issue that requires immediate attention.

If we don't stop erosion and soil loss, by 2050 we will lose 1.5 million square kilometers of farmland—equivalent to all the farmable land in India.[4] Water scarcity is also a huge issue; at a World Economic Forum meeting, I recall hearing Jim Kim, the former head of the World Bank, say, "The wars of the future will be fought over water, not oil."

The good news is that the science of how to grow food that properly feeds humans, regenerates land, conserves water, and reverses climate change provides a path to fix it all. Whether we take that path remains to be seen given the powerful economic incentives to continue in our current ways—incentives present only because the true costs of farming and food are not paid by those perpetuating the destruction.

TRAPPED IN THE SYSTEM: HOW BIG AG KEEPS FARMERS DEPENDENT

When we think of farmers, we imagine fiercely self-sufficient folk doing the hard work of feeding the population. In reality, farmers are no longer independent—they've been forced into a system where they answer to big dogs of Big Ag, Big Food—really the whole global industrial food machine. Instead of growing food that nourishes people and the planet, they're trapped in a cycle of producing crops that fuel disease, degrade ecosystems, and accelerate climate change.

The real power lies with seed and agrochemical giants and corporate food conglomerates, which dictate what gets planted, how it's grown, who buys it, and at what price. This stranglehold leaves farmers with fewer choices, shrinking profits, and mounting environmental damage.

Recent megamergers have consolidated control of agriculture; just a very few CEOs control most of our global food system, and their decisions impact every person on the planet:

- Four companies (Syngenta, Bayer, Corteva, and BASF) now control 70 percent of agrochemicals.[5]
- Large seed companies have bought up more than 100 seed companies since the 1990s, and now just four companies (Bayer [which now owns Monsanto], ChemChina, BASF, and Corteva) control more than 60 percent of the seeds sold to farmers (see figure following).[6]
- Ninety percent of the global grain trade is controlled by just four multinational corporations.[7]
- Nine big food companies control what is sold and bought in retail outlets, including most health foods and organic brands.[8]
- Seventy-five percent of our food comes from just twelve plants (all controlled by Big Ag and chemical companies) and 60 percent comes from only rice, corn, and wheat.[9]
- Fertilizer giants (Yara, Mosaic, and Koch Fertilizer) control most of the world's fertilizer market.

THE BIG 4: COMPANIES THAT CONTROL MORE THAN 60 PERCENT OF GLOBAL SEED SALES

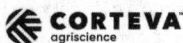

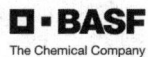

BAYER MONSANTO • CORTEVA agriscience • CHEMCHINA • BASF The Chemical Company

These corporations' singular focus—and frankly, their legal fiduciary duty—is the economic bottom line. Ignoring the impact on human, social, and natural capital provides short-term profits, but it also threatens our collective well-being. Their decisions impact everyone along the food chain: producing poor-quality calories for the junk-food industry, driving down food prices, affecting the working conditions of migrant workers and food service workers, and increasing the cost of inputs for farmers for their proprietary chemical-resistant seeds (soybean costs had risen 325 percent by 2012; by 2023 they had escalated even further—rising over 260 percent since 1997, with 2023 costs reaching $71 per acre, compared to just $19.72 per acre in 1997 — raising the economic pressure on farmers worldwide), pesticides, herbicides, and fertilizers, threatening the viability of farms across the world.[10]

Current large-scale agribusiness and the policies that support it are slowly harming farmers and the land on which they and we depend. As I write this, close to 60 percent of our 880 million acres of farmland is unplantable, the result of extreme weather, tornadoes, flooding, and the inability of degraded land to hold enough water. In testimony submitted to the House Committee on Agriculture in May 2019, farmer Mike Peterson of Twin Oak Farms and the Minnesota Farmers Union spoke about farmers' dire financial conditions: "The last five years have been incredibly challenging on my farm and on farms across Minnesota," Peterson said. "Market consolidation and the increase of monopoly power has caused our input costs to rise dramatically. Overproduction has driven commodity prices low — a situation that is further exacerbated by the impacts of ongoing trade disputes. Our current environment is unsustainable."[11]

Victims of a broken system, the farmers and ranchers aren't calling the shots. Rather, a small number of corporate executives control the majority of agriculture and the food system. "The American food supply chain — from the seeds we plant to the peanut butter in our neighborhood grocery stores — is concentrated in the hands of a few multinational corporations," agricultural economist Austin Frerick points out. "Because the supply, processing, distribution, and retail networks are concentrated in only a handful of firms, farmers face higher costs for their inputs and lower prices for their goods. In the 1980s, 37 cents out of every dollar went back to the farmer.[12] Today, farmers take home less than 15 cents on every dollar.[13] This new economic reality forces farmers to survive on volume, creating a system where only the largest farms can make a living."[14]

Ranchers face the same economics. "The nation's meatpacking industry is now more concentrated than when Upton Sinclair wrote *The Jungle* more than a century ago," Frerick says. "Four companies, two of which are foreign-owned, now slaughter 52 percent of all meat consumed in the United States,[15] more than twice the market share that the four largest companies held in 2002."[16]

It gets worse. In 2018 Monsanto's GMO seeds accounted for 90 percent of US corn, 91 percent of cotton, and 94 percent of soybeans grown.[17] It is probably even more now. Monsanto, the company that brought you dioxin, Agent Orange, PCBs (industrial chemicals), and glyphosate (Roundup), was acquired by Bayer a few years back. Strikingly, the Monsanto brand quietly disappeared—or rather, when it was absorbed by Bayer, it conveniently dropped the tainted name. My guess is that it's a classic case of corporate rebranding to erase a guilty past. As of April 2019, Bayer stock lost $34 billion in market value[18] because of successful lawsuits compensating cancer victims exposed to glyphosate. In 2018 and 2019 three large lawsuits against Bayer-Monsanto were successful, with one judgment of $2 billion for cancer victims.[19] There are approximately 67,000 of these lawsuits pending[20] against the makers of the herbicide glyphosate, which have cost the company so much it has recently asked the Supreme Court to indemnify it against future lawsuits.[21] They didn't just ask; they threatened to stop making the herbicide, which would force the US farmers to buy it from China (the only other producer of glyphosate), now subject to increasing tariffs, raising the price of growing crops and potentially putting US farmers out of business. That's just downright nefarious.

The results are easy to see in economic data. The USDA Economic Research Service report *Three Decades of Consolidation in U.S. Agriculture* illustrates that over the past 30 years, the number of farms with less than 1,000 acres has fallen from more than half of American farms to roughly a third. The number of farms with at least 2,000 acres has more than doubled over that same time frame.[22]

HOW FARMS WENT DOWNHILL

How did agriculture get to this point? Here is the CliffsNotes version: government farm policy, changes in technology, and the unchecked power of corporate agribusiness.[23] The mainstream ideology was well summarized by Earl Butz, President Nixon's secretary of agriculture, in his infamous advice to farmers in the 1970s: "Get big or get out."[24] And that's exactly what happened.

Over the past century, as small farms gave way to larger farms, agriculture faced major environmental crises. In the 1930s, the introduction of mechanized farm equipment used without ecological knowledge of soil and erosion, combined with eight years of drought, created the Dust Bowl[25] (one of the worst environmental crises in our country's history, during which dark clouds of wind-blown soil covered the sky and forced thousands to migrate, leaving farmland abandoned). While some environmental programs like soil conservation districts—sustainable practices to help farmers manage erosion—came out of that experience, the dominant trend leaned heavily on synthetic inputs, such as pesticides and fertilizers, mechanization, and corporate consolidation to drive productivity and harvest. Seemed like a good idea at the time, but that was before Rachel Carson's *Silent Spring* sounded the alarm over pesticides like DDT, before we sufficiently grasped the risks of soil erosion and the value of organic matter in soil, before we faced water shortages, and before we knew the danger of ultraprocessed food to human health.

It's important to know that consolidation didn't happen purely for profit. Economic, political, and technological factors started the trend toward large-scale agribusiness. Changing agricultural technology—including machinery, fertilizers, and pesticides—made it possible to produce more food. Who would have thought that was a bad idea at the time?

Today, fewer farmers produce more food than ever—but with a catch. As productivity increases, prices drop, forcing farmers to grow even more just to survive in a vicious, never-ending cycle. The result is a food system flooded with cheap grain and meat, produced with less labor, lower wages for farmers, and more environmental destruction than ever before.

It's relatively easy for a small number of people to run a pesticide-drenched and synthetically fertilized crop field or operate a confined animal feeding operation—the factory farms with nightmarish conditions you see on environmental activists' sites. But the real cost of this system isn't reflected in your grocery receipt. We all end up paying for it through contaminated water, drained aquifers threatening our water supplies, dead zones in rivers, lakes, and the oceans from the harmful effects of fertilizer runoff, depleted soil, climate disasters, and a public health crisis fueled by nutrient-depleted foods. What looks like cheap food today is a massive bill we'll be paying for generations.

What corporate consolidation did was accelerate the practice of extractive agriculture—using up our natural resources to get as much profit as we could out of the ground. In other words, abusing the land with intensive mechanical plowing, diesel-powered irrigation, and other petrochemical-based inputs. Artificial nitrogen, pesticides, and herbicides dramatically increased after World War II as bomb factories and biological weapons like nerve gas were retooled into agricultural products (if a biological weapon could kill an enemy, it could certainly kill a few insects, right?). The motivation was to improve yields and increase production. Yet those grand promises have failed to deliver. Chemical inputs keep getting higher, yet yields are no better, and costs are higher than those for agricultural systems using regenerative practices or even conventional agriculture in Europe that prohibits GMO crops and produces higher or equivalent yields with less fertilizer, pesticides, and herbicides. As farmers increase production, they may see initial gains, but over time, yields stagnate, costs rise, and environmental damage escalates—while profits shrink. It's a classic race to the bottom.

In fact, according to a 1992 agricultural census report, small diversified farms produce *twice as much food* per acre as large conventional farms. On degraded soils, higher chemical inputs may produce higher yields, but not on healthy soils. What has happened has led us to an agricultural and food crisis. Remember, we are projected to have only sixty harvests left from our soil if we continue farming as usual.

Unfortunately, our government policies aren't helping. You read about the issues with subsidies and the latest Farm Bill in Chapter 7, so it won't surprise you that the political power of the food system owners has greased the wheels of consolidation as well as changed the laws to benefit agribusiness (fertilizer, pesticide, seed, and machinery companies) and hurt independent small farms. The Farm Bill subsidizes monoculture crops like corn, wheat, and soy, and meat from confined animal feeding operations, which deplete the land, making it harder and harder to produce crops and meat without chemicals, antibiotics, and genetic engineering.[26] At the same time, these foods that produce disease and obesity are cheap and are in the highest demand. Our government policies are not only promoting disease-causing foods but also supporting agricultural practices that hurt the climate and the land.

"Despite the rhetoric of 'preserving the family farm,' the vast majority of farmers do not benefit from federal farm subsidy programs and most of the subsidies go to the largest and most financially secure farm operations," the Environmental Working Group reports. "Small commodity farmers qualify for a mere pittance, while producers of meat, fruits, and vegetables are almost completely left out of the subsidy game (i.e. they can sign up for subsidized crop insurance and often receive federal disaster payments)."[27]

Farms that continue to produce food in ways that are unsustainable in the long run—requiring large inputs of fossil fuels and water—are now known to drive soil erosion, climate change, and loss of biodiversity, and are also far less resilient than well-managed regenerative, organic, and sustainable farms (which now account for only 1 percent of agriculture). What these farmers need is a clear path to break free from industrial farming's treadmill and transition to regenerative agriculture, where both the land and their livelihoods can thrive.

THE GREEN REVOLUTION: SUCCESSES AND UNINTENDED CONSEQUENCES

You might be wondering—how did we get here?

Not too long ago, in the mid-twentieth century, the Green Revolution promised to solve world hunger by supercharging agriculture with high-yield hybrid crops, synthetic fertilizers, pesticides, irrigation, and mechanization. The idea was simple: grow more food on less land and feed the world. Small farmers would thrive; food insecurity would shrink—it seemed like a win for everyone.

And to some extent, it worked. The Green Revolution dramatically increased food production and helped reduce hunger.

Agronomic scientists like Norman Borlaug made huge advances in plant breeding to take advantage of artificial fertilizer and irrigation. In places like Mexico, where Borlaug did his graduate research, the history of yield results is remarkable.[28]

In many developing countries, more people had access to food because of Borlaug and his peers. Since World War II, Americans haven't faced significant crop shortages resulting in hunger (although poverty still perpetuates food insecurity). When asked about the criticism from environmentalists, Borlaug replied, "Some of the environmental lobbyists of the Western nations are the salt of the earth, but many of them are elitists. They've never experienced the physical sensation of hunger. They do their lobbying from comfortable office suites in Washington or Brussels. If they lived just one month amid the misery of the developing world, as I have for fifty years, they'd be crying out for tractors and fertilizer and irrigation canals and be outraged that fashionable elitists back home were trying to deny them these things."[29]

It's hard to argue against something that helped so many hungry people. While addressing hunger and food insecurity were crucial to the Green Revolution, the downsides are clear. Its unintended consequences now define our modern food crisis: an overabundance of cheap raw materials for ultraprocessed foods, excess calories with fewer nutrients, and massive environmental destruction, including polluted water from fertilizer and pesticide runoff, depleted soils, and loss of biodiversity. It also contributed to about one-third to one-half of the global environmental degradation that we've seen in the past half century, and to the consolidation of corporate power at the expense of small farmers and human health.[30] In the end, the Green Revolution didn't fulfill its promise of ending world hunger; 800 million people still go to bed hungry every night.

AN ALTRUISTIC WRAPPING: THE MYTH OF FEEDING THE WORLD

Fast-forward to today: Big Food and Big Ag push the myth that only they and their products can feed a growing world. The truth is we already produce enough food to feed the world, but that doesn't mean the hungry get access to that food.

The world has long produced enough calories. There are hungry people not because food is lacking, but because a third of calories produced go to feed animals, nearly 5 percent are used to produce biofuels, and more than a third is wasted downstream, all along the food chain.

The real problem is actually overproduction. "Though hunger and malnutrition are actually getting worse, we've been producing one and a half times more than enough food to feed everyone on the planet for half a century," says Eric Holt-Giménez of Food First, an institute for food and development policy.

> The glut of food keeps prices low for grain traders and processors of animal feed and junk food. Competition drives these companies to out-produce each other, each coming out with cheaper and cheaper processed food products. We end up with lousier food than the market can absorb and with meat fattened on grain in feedlots that hungry people can't afford. Prices drop and margins shrink, but "cheap food" hasn't ended hunger, and it comes at a tremendous social and environmental cost.... Overproduction results in monopolization up and down the food chain, giving agri-food corporations tremendous economic and political power to continue doing business as usual. These unregulated firms pay for none of the "externalities" they produce—we do.[31]

The truth is that the Green Revolution model didn't solve hunger through better seeds or increased chemical inputs or the increasing problems with corporate agriculture. And the Green Revolution also led to a more than 200 percent increase in the need for irrigation.[32] Even Dr. M. S. Swaminathan, the "Father of the Green Revolution in India," has since written scientific papers questioning the safety and sustainability of that very model. His main observation was that despite increasing yield, the quality of life for farmers was actually decreasing along with the health of the land.

"There is no doubt that genetically engineered Bt-cotton has failed in India: it has failed as a sustainable agriculture technology and has therefore also failed to provide livelihood security of cotton farmers who are mainly resource-poor, small and marginal farmers," he says.[33] Dr. Swaminathan and his colleague Dr. P. C. Kesavan also cited scientific evidence that the glyphosate-based herbicides, used on most genetically modified crops, have been found to cause birth defects, cancer, and genetic mutations.[34]

This recognition comes after years of warnings from social movements and scientists like Dr. Vandana Shiva, who have documented the human and ecological impacts of the Green Revolution including a wave of suicides by Indian farmers who become indebted because of the high costs of fertilizers, seeds, and pesticides. Their method of suicide — drinking pesticide — is a tragically ironic reminder of the human consequences of the extractive model of agriculture.[35]

GMOS: HELPFUL OR HARMFUL?

GMOs came out of the Green Revolution. However, genetic engineering wasn't new even then. Humans have modified the genetics of plants and animals for thousands of years. Remember high school biology where we learned about Gregor Mendel breeding different pea varieties in the 1800s?

What is new is both the scale of genetic engineering technology and the proprietary profit logic that underlies it. For example, in April 2019, PepsiCo filed lawsuits against nine farmers in Gujarat, India, alleging they were cultivating its patented FC5 potato variety, used exclusively for Lay's chips.[36] The company sought damages of approximately $142,840 from each farmer, which would bankrupt every farmer (for context, the average farmer in India earns US$1,440 per year). Local activists contended that these small-scale farmers were unaware of the patent and accused PepsiCo of employing private investigators who posed as buyers to gather evidence. Following significant public backlash and protests from farmers' organizations, PepsiCo withdrew the lawsuits in May 2019.[37]

If corporations control the seeds and plants that make our food, we disenfranchise the small farmers who feed most of the world's population, shift the profits to the top of the food chain, and perpetuate destructive agricultural practices, all of which ultimately threaten the stability of our food supply.

The promise of GMO crops requiring fewer chemicals to grow and resulting in higher yields has also failed, as demonstrated by comparative studies of agriculture in Europe (which prohibited the use of GMO seeds) and the United States.[38] In fact, GMO seeds have, in part, driven the rampant use of herbicides and pesticides, as pests and weeds have mutated to become more resistant. Ironically, agriculture is now locked in a hubristic arms race against superbugs and superweeds, which have evolved to resist the very chemicals that are supposed to kill them.

As for the health effects of eating GMO foods, in an interview with Steven Druker[39] from the Alliance for Bio-Integrity, he pointed out that while certain scientists have long rushed to declare GMOs safe, there has always been substantial disagreement among scientists about the health risks of genetically engineered (GE) foods. "Eminent scientific organizations have not only critiqued the safety claims about GE foods but have also cautioned about the risks and called for stricter regulation," Druker says.

The National Academy of Sciences, our nation's "independent" scientific advisers to the government, issued a report on GMOs and biotechnology, determining that they posed no risk. But in a damning investigative report by the *New York Times,* conflicts of interest on the expert panel were significant.[40] Seven of the thirteen members had clear ties to the GMO and biotech industry, calling into question their findings. And a few had conflicts that violated the National Academy of Sciences' own conflict-of-interest policies yet were allowed to remain on the panel. Just as food companies infiltrate scientific bodies and taint research, so do Big Ag and biotech companies.

Although proponents of GE foods also routinely claim that these products are harmless, a substantial body of research in peer-reviewed journals[41] has demonstrated adverse effects[42] on laboratory animals that were fed GE food, some of which have been in the human food supply for years. The Public Health Association of Australia has repeatedly issued warnings about GMOs[43] and called for an "indefinite freeze" on the commercial cultivation and the importation of these crops until long-term testing can prove their safety. In the European Union, the regulatory approach to GMOs is notably stringent. Employing their precautionary principle, they require comprehensive pre-market authorization and post-market environmental monitoring for any GMO intended for release.[44]

Relying on industry data for a product's safety, whether it's tobacco "science" proving cigarettes don't cause cancer or aren't addictive, or the soda industry data showing that sugar doesn't cause obesity or artificial sweeteners are safe, is just foolish. History has been full of "advances" like DDT and trans fats that turned out to be deadly after 50 or 100 years of use.

ROUNDUP OR COVER-UP?

Even if it turns out that consuming GMO products is not so bad, their use is currently a large uncontrolled experiment on humans, and there is no doubt about the toxic health impact of pesticides and herbicides.

Take glyphosate (or Roundup), for example. Before they're picked and fed to animals or sold to humans, GMO crops are routinely sprayed with toxic herbicides, the most famous of which is glyphosate, sold under the brand name Roundup. In the four decades since Monsanto released its blockbuster weed killer, the amount of it sprayed on the nation's crops has risen more than a hundredfold. According to the EPA, some 220 million pounds of Roundup's active ingredient were used in the United States in 2015. In California alone, more than 10 million pounds of glyphosate are applied to crops every year. Glyphosate now is the world's most commonly used herbicide and accounts for almost 72 percent of all herbicides used around the world, and since 1974, 1.6 billion kilograms (more than 3.5 billion pounds) have been used on crops in the United States.[45]

The EPA openly admits that glyphosate—the active ingredient in Roundup—is sprayed on more than seventy different food crops. It's not just on corn and soy; it's drenched into the very foundation of the American diet—wheat, oats, canola, you name it. So, if you're eating a slice of bread, a bowl of cornflakes, a sushi roll, a plate of pasta, a slice of pizza, or even a chicken nugget, you're most likely ingesting a nice helping of herbicide. Cheerios might be the grossest distortion of health claims. Proudly stamped with the "heart-healthy" label, Cheerios have tested off the charts for glyphosate residue. Glyphosate defoliates the plants, making the wheat easier to harvest. That's why Honey Nut Cheerios have more glyphosate per serving than vitamin D and vitamin B$_{12}$, which have to be added to enrich the cereal. Maybe instead of a cute little heart, the box should come with a skull and crossbones—or at the very least, a big "Doused in Weedkiller" warning.

Glyphosate is increasing our cancer risk,[46] according to a report by a working group of seventeen experts from eleven countries published by the International Agency for Research on Cancer.[47] Glyphosate also harms our microbiome, causes negative behavior changes in animal models, and causes epigenetic changes that lead to disease.[48] Studies clearly show harm in animal models, including birth defects, low sperm counts, low testosterone, ovarian and uterine abnormalities, and liver damage, among other harmful effects.[49] It also damages the microbiology of the soil on which we all depend.[50]

Even more concerning was a 2019 study that glyphosate can have transgenerational effects.[51] When you eat your GMO soy burger, or your Cheerios effectively laced with glyphosate, it may not just be affecting your health; it may also be putting your grandchildren and great-grandchildren at risk. In this study[52] of mice, direct exposure to glyphosate had negligible effects on the mothers and their offspring, but significant effects on little grand- and great-grand-mice that were never directly exposed to glyphosate. This effect is presumably driven by changes in epigenetics, tags on our genes that are carried forward to our offspring. The unexposed little grand- and great-grand-mice suffered from prostate disease, obesity, kidney disease, ovarian disease, and birth defects.

More recent studies have revealed alarming levels of glyphosate in *human* biological samples. A 2024 French study[53] found glyphosate in 57 percent of semen samples from infertile men, with concentrations four times higher in seminal plasma than in blood. This raises concerns about potential impacts on male fertility. And research in Thailand[54] detected glyphosate in 85 percent of maternal serum samples and 44 percent of umbilical cord blood samples, indicating that this herbicide can cross the placental barrier and expose developing fetuses. David Bellinger of the Harvard School of Public Health has shown that American children under the age of five have lost 17 million IQ points because of the harmful effects of pesticides.[55]

All in all, there's nothing healthful about a side of glyphosate on your breakfast cereal.

THE NEXT GENERATION OF AGRICULTURE

Jennifer Dempsey, director of American Farmland Trust's Farmland Information Center, projects that ownership of 40 percent of the forty-eight states' 991 million farm and ranch acres will change hands from 2015 to about 2035.[56] The question remains: Who will be the farmers of the future? How will the land be farmed? What policies are needed to encourage a new generation of farmers who can solve the challenges of our current agricultural system?

Young people who want to become farmers, or even people in inner cities and in suburbs becoming urban farmers, immediately run up against the problem of land access. Land is too expensive and is often worth more for its financial value than its agricultural value. The corporate profits from overproduction have gone into buying up land. Millions and millions of acres, an area about the size of France, have been bought up as a repository for excess capital because there's been no regulation on land purchases. The result is inflated land values around the world that prevent people from being able to go into agriculture as a livelihood. We need to change the incentive structures across the scale from federal to state to local initiatives that support young farmers and ranchers. We should also consider creating a federal program, a "Farmer Corps," to support a new generation of regenerative farmers.

HISTORY AND CO-OPTION OF LAND-GRANT COLLEGES BY BIG AG

Land-grant colleges were established under the Morrill Act of 1862, signed by President Abraham Lincoln, to democratize higher education and promote practical studies like agriculture, engineering, and military science. The act granted federally controlled land to states to fund the creation of public universities aimed at supporting farmers, rural communities, and the broader public good. A second Morrill Act in 1890 extended this model to include historically Black colleges and universities (HBCUs).

Initially rooted in service to small-scale farmers and public welfare, many land-grant institutions gradually shifted toward serving the interests of industrial agriculture. Starting in the mid-twentieth century, increased funding from corporate agribusiness, chemical, seed, and biotech companies—coupled with declining public investment—fueled a transformation. Agricultural research and extension services increasingly prioritized high-yield commodity crops, synthetic fertilizers, pesticides, and genetically modified organisms, often to the detriment of ecological practices, small farmers, and public health.

Today, critics argue that many land-grant universities function more as research arms of Big Ag than as public institutions serving community needs. Their ties to industry influence academic agendas, undermine independent research, and limit innovation in regenerative, organic, and sustainable farming systems. This co-option has helped entrench a food system that favors scale, monocultures, and corporate consolidation over resilience, diversity, and equity.

What was designed by Abraham Lincoln to support American farmers has become fully co-opted by Big Ag. Rather than train farmers how to farm in ways that regenerate soil, increase production, restore the environment, increase biodiversity, preserve our water resources, and create more economic abundance for farmers, the land-grant colleges have become nothing more than a training ground for industrial agriculture that encourages and teaches farmers to use more and more fertilizers, pesticides, herbicides, and proprietary seeds, harming farmers, the environment, and the consumer.

FOOD FIX: CONNECTING THE DOTS

The unintended consequences that emerged from our agricultural industrial revolution and the policies that supported it and the food system it created were hard to foresee. But now that we know, we can't unknow it.

Changes across the board from farmers, corporations, and government policies can help shift the entire system. We must move away from an extractive, destructive, fossil-fuel, chemical-dependent model to one that understands and restores natural systems and employs agroecological and regenerative practices.

In Chapter 7, we talked about the importance of implementing a national food policy. Instead of working within dysfunctional silos, the solutions need to integrate all aspects of the food system and build policies and initiatives based on solving the big problems of healthy nutrition, sustainability, social equity, and economic benefit. In fact, these are not separate problems; they are one problem. Thankfully many groups of very smart people are tackling this complexity and mapping out a new vision for our food and agricultural system. Here are just a few examples:

1. Among the most coherent comprehensive attempts to connect the dots for a common policy is the report[57] from iPES Food (International Panel of Experts on Sustainable Food Systems) entitled "Towards a Common Food Policy for the European Union." The iPES report has key objectives that require coordinated effort across all sectors of policy agencies, businesses, and farmers, including shifting to regenerative agriculture, shortening supply chains (i.e., emphasizing local food), and fixing trade policies to support local agriculture. Read the executive summary or full report at www.ipes-food.org under "Our Reports." If its principles were implemented at scale, we could solve many of our food, climate, and health crises.

2. In 2018, the UN Environment Program hosted an initiative called TEEB, or TEEBAgriFood,[58] that brought together more than 150 scholars from thirty-three countries to assess the impact of and solutions for our food and agricultural systems. According to the TEEB-AgriFood report, our food system accounts for 44 to 57 percent of human-created greenhouse gas emissions when you include soil loss, factory farms, deforestation, food waste, food transportation, refrigeration and freezing, and processing and packaging.[59] Their Scientific and Economic Foundations report mapped out a very different future that addresses some of the biggest global challenges today linked to food and agriculture—climate change, environmental damage, and loss of biodiversity, among others. No small task.

3. Another important report, *Fixing Food 2016: Towards a More Sustainable Food System,*[60] focused on how to address sustainable agriculture and food loss and waste. The authors created a Food Sustainability Index that ranks twenty-five countries on fifty-eight indicators: environmental, societal, and economic. Sustainability is defined as the ability of our food system to not deplete or exhaust natural resources or compromise health. The United States was ranked eleventh, followed closely by Ethiopia and China. Not the best company in terms of sustainability. France, Japan, and Canada topped the list. This tool can help countries assess their progress in meeting benchmarks for building a sustainable food system.

4. In the United States, there are voices of change in Congress. For example, Earl Blumenauer, a former Oregon congressman, has laid out a road map called *Growing Opportunities: Reforming the Farm Bill for Every American* to address the problems of our current agricultural system through Farm Bill reforms.[61] Incremental changes won't be sufficient to address the magnitude of the problems in our current food system. The current bill undermines human health, carbon reduction, economic development, land conservation, and animal welfare. More than 88 percent of our agricultural production comes from only 12 percent of farms.[62] Eighty-five percent of subsidies go to the biggest 15 percent of farms,[63] while those wanting to shift to regenerative agriculture don't get much support.

The road map for a new Farm Bill would focus on reforms to crop insurance, incentives and support for regenerative agriculture including more research, and investment in local food systems and urban farming, and would address food waste. Imagine if farmers were incentivized by the amount of soil organic matter on their farms. If they didn't create more good soil, then they would have to pay higher insurance rates. Good soil helps reverse climate change, reduce water use, build resistance against droughts and floods, and increase ecosystem biodiversity.

For a quick reference guide on the Food Fixes and resources to help you support regenerative agriculture, go to www.foodfixuncensored.com.

Chapter 17

Soil, Water, Biodiversity: Why Should We Care?

Our food doesn't magically appear on grocery store shelves—it comes from a delicate natural system that we've been recklessly depleting. But instead of respecting these cycles, we've spent the last century waging war on nature, convinced we can outsmart it. We bulldoze the land with machines, pump synthetic fertilizers into the soil, drench crops in chemical pesticides, and rely on fossil fuels to supercharge industrial farming. And for a while, it worked—sort of. But in the process, we've burned through millions of years' worth of natural resources, gutting the very ecosystems that make food production possible.

We are now running on borrowed time and borrowed resources. Much like an overdrawn bank account, this continued depletion of a fixed amount of our natural capital—soil, water, pollinators, microbes—is driving us toward bankruptcy. Every five seconds, we lose a soccer field's worth of soil due to destructive land management practices. According to the UN's FAO report, at the current rate of degradation, we have only sixty harvests left before our soil is too depleted to grow food. While this may be an oversimplification, it's definitely true that we're crushing our precious soil reserves. Seventy percent of the world's fresh water is used for industrial crop and livestock production, draining aquifers faster than they can be replenished. Even industrial organic farming is part of the problem, pulling water from deep aquifers, which brings up salt and selenium—one destroys soil, the other kills birds. The soil is so degraded that most of this water never even reaches the roots of plants, instead running off and contributing to sea-level rise.

And then there are the pollinators—responsible for 75 percent of our food production[1]—disappearing at alarming rates. The very pesticides designed to kill crop pests are also wiping out the bees, butterflies, and other species essential to agriculture. No pollinators, no food. No food, no humans.

IT'S THE SOIL, STUPID!

We must treat the whole problem of health in soil, plant, animal and man as one great subject.

—SIR ALBERT HOWARD, *THE SOIL AND HEALTH,* 1947

Why do I keep talking about soil, and why should you care?

There is a big difference between soil and dirt. Healthy soil is alive, teeming with microbes that contribute to the thriving ecosystem beneath our feet. Healthy soils extract nutrients from the earth, making them available to plants and to humans; just a single gram of soil contains billions of microbial cells.[2] Soil feeds plants by making the micronutrients and macronutrients available to the plants (and then to you, when you eat them). Soil can hold hundreds of thousands of gallons of water per acre,[3] absorbing the water for later use, which naturally protects against droughts and floods. Soil is also the biggest carbon sink on the planet. Think of soil as the rain forest of the prairies;[4] in fact, it can sequester more carbon and reverse climate change more than all the rain forests in the world.[5]

Dirt, on the other hand, is lifeless. Dirt contains very few microorganisms, fungi, or worms, all of which are needed to produce healthy plants. Dirt requires chemical inputs to grow plants; lacking the living organisms to metabolize requisite nutrients, dirt cannot on its own generate produce, which means it also fails to nourish the plants that we then consume. Dirt cannot hold water, nor sequester carbon. A dead mass, it is unable to feed plant growth unassisted, so it requires massive inputs of fertilizer, pesticides, herbicides (all of which are synthesized from fossil fuels!), and extensive amounts of water to generate even a single crop. These synthetic chemicals only further ruin the soil. This has caused the depletion of naturally occurring essential minerals in our food supply, all of which our human health is entirely reliant upon.[6]

Soil is a renewable resource we have squandered. We have lost 430 million hectares of arable land to soil erosion, which is one-third of the world's available farmland.[7] We have mined the land, turned it to dust, and lost the 60 to 80 feet of topsoil that existed in some areas of the Midwest. Through tillage and erosion, soils have lost 133 billion tons of carbon[8] into the atmosphere since we started farming, which many scientists believe contributes to global warming.[9]

Research shows that by 2050, increasing CO_2 levels and poor soil quality will worsen the nutrient composition of the food we grow, which could result in zinc deficiency for 175 million people, protein deficiency for 122 million, and iron deficiency in 1 billion.[10] There is less calcium, magnesium, iron, and other minerals[11] in food today compared to 100 years ago. Just as you can't get blood from a stone, you can't get nutrients from dirt.

Across the globe, farmland is becoming desert (or dirt) at alarming rates. The UN's Food and Agriculture Organization (FAO) says 12 million hectares of arable land (or about 23 hectares a minute), enough to grow 20 tons of grain, are lost to drought and desertification annually, which affects 1.5 billion people in more than one hundred countries.[12] According to President Obama's 2016 initiative *The State and Future of U.S. Soils: Framework for a Federal Strategic Plan for Soil Science,* soil erosion is a profound risk to future food production, and in another report, by the Union of Concerned Scientists,[13] it is estimated that we will lose 300 years' worth of soil by 2100 at current trends. That's a terrifying projection for a nation that is such an important exporter of grain and soybeans.

Experts say we have globally lost 50 percent of our topsoil.[14] This is caused primarily by:

- Livestock overgrazing (poor livestock management)
- Industrialized agriculture
- Deforestation
- Urban industrialization
- Overfertilizing
- Monocrop agriculture
- Tilling
- Bad crop rotation
- Bare fallows (leaving bare ground) and not using cover crops

In other words, our modern form of industrial agriculture has strip-mined our soil rich in organic matter. We ran mechanized plows through the soil for years, rupturing normal biological and chemical cycles. Then we added chemicals and started killing off organisms. Big fertilizer conglomerates such as Yara, Mosaic, and Koch Fertilizer (the infamous Koch brothers) produce 25 million metric tons of fertilizer a year using fossil-fuel-intensive processes.[15] When that fertilizer is applied to farms, the damage is wrought on the soil, weakening the plants, polluting water systems, and driving huge external costs. The bacteria in the soil convert the nitrogen fertilizer into huge amounts of nitrous oxide, which is released into the air as a greenhouse gas that has 300 times[16] the heat-trapping potential of carbon dioxide.[17] Adding nitrogen fertilizer to soil paradoxically makes the soil less fertile because it depletes the soil organic matter, which then results in the need for more fertilizer.[18] Good for big fertilizer companies, bad for the soil, for us, and for the climate.

Halting land degradation has become an urgent global imperative.

THE LOSS OF BIODIVERSITY: WHY IT MATTERS

You've probably heard climate activists, academics, and systems thinkers alerting us to the public health emergency that is the loss of biodiversity and destruction of natural ecosystems due to our chemical runoffs, but you may not quite connect the dots between your health and that of the planet. While it may seem like a simple altruistic preference for protecting our environment, it is actually a profound recognition that we are intimately connected to our ecosystems, and the degradation of these systems *directly* risks our future stability.

The chemical inputs (which are routinely mandated in America) used to cultivate industrial crops not only damage human health but also disrupt natural ecosystems, deplete the diversity of life in the soil, threaten the loss of most of the plant and animal species we have consumed for millennia, and severely affect pollinators like honeybees and butterflies, which we depend on for agricultural crops.[19] (Chapter 15 explains these consequences in depth.) The predictable loss of biodiversity due to industrial agriculture—quaintly referred to as "externalities" by economists—is a much bigger problem that threatens global food security and, by definition, our future survival as a species.

According the FAO, more than 90 percent of plant varieties and half of livestock varieties have been lost to farmers (and the world).[20] Thirty percent of livestock breeds are facing extinction, with approximately six breeds becoming extinct each month.[21] Most of our modern industrial food comes from just twelve plant varieties and five animal species,[22] threatening our food security. As shared above, just three crops (wheat, corn, rice) account for 60 percent of our food in America. But why does this matter to you? Well, in all ecosystems, complexity can be considered a staple of health and resilience; whereas simplicity tends to make systems more vulnerable. Think of monocrop corn (meaning it's the only crop grown on a farm) compared to a rain forest. One plant dies in a rain forest, no problem; there are many remaining to compensate. One plant dies on a monocrop corn or soy megafarm—no food. Aside from the fact that the most resilient species are those that benefit from diversity, if a natural disaster or drought were to wipe out even one of these, it leaves us irreparably exposed to food insecurity worldwide.

Today, as a result of the consolidation of major agricultural conglomerates, farmers cannot even collect, store, or breed their own seeds and plants. Most farmers no longer grow local, resilient, genetically diverse and nutrient-dense varieties. They only use genetically uniform (or GMO) high-yield varieties that require intensive use of fertilizers, pesticides, and herbicides—further destroying the organic matter and biodiversity of the soil, which results in less nutrient-dense plants and increased need for irrigation. Big Agriculture lobbyists architected regulations designed specifically to trap farmers in a vicious cycle requiring them to sacrifice their future yields to generate higher profits today.

How do we measure the costs to human health and the threats to our pollinators and the loss of biodiversity? The calculus is actually fairly straightforward: No more bees, no more pollination, no more plants, no more animals—no more humans.

THE DESTRUCTION OF SOIL AND RAIN FORESTS: CLIMATE CHANGE AND DESERTS

As mentioned previously, only 1 percent of corn grown in America is sweet corn actually consumed by humans. The rest is *dent* corn, used for food oils, animal feed (for cattle), ethanol, biodiesel, high-fructose corn syrup (for your sugary soda), biodegradable plastic, alcohol, food starch, and food additives (for your hamburger bun). Soy and corn monocrops account for 74 percent of all farmland.[23] Much of that food goes to feed animals on confined animal feeding operations (CAFOs), or factory farms, which in many places in the developed world are now the main way we produce animals for human consumption. It varies globally, but in the United States, only 27 percent of cropland is used to grow food for humans, while 67 percent is used to grow food for factory-farmed animals.[24]

The problem is not only that portions of the crops are grown for feedlot animals (including the cattle for your burger and high-fructose corn syrup for your soda). How those crops are grown also creates massive destruction. The crops are cultivated using intensive industrial farming that leads to massive soil erosion and loss of soil carbon, worsening climate change. In Iowa, the leading corn growing state, we lose 1 pound of topsoil for every pound of corn grown.[25] We lose almost

2 billion tons of topsoil a year.[26] That's about 200,000 tons every single hour. The cost of soil erosion from industrial agriculture is $44 billion a year.[27] We have lost a third of all our topsoil—which took billions of years to create—in the last 150 years. It is projected that in 60 years we may completely "mine" all our topsoil, making it almost impossible to grow food. Soil gone. No food. No people. What will your grandchildren eat?

Soil erosion and the loss of carbon in soil together lead to the massive global problem of desertification, the decline of farm- or rangeland into desert. Twelve million hectares of land, an area the size of Nicaragua or North Korea, are lost every year to desert. The land we lose every year could produce 20 million tons of grain.[28]

DIRT TO SOIL—FROM TRAGEDY TO TRIUMPH

Several farmers have shown that we can do better farming with cheaper production, better-quality food, fewer or no chemical inputs, more yields and more profits to the farmer, and lower costs to the consumer. Gabe Brown, a North Dakota farmer trained in land-grant colleges (funded in part by Big Ag) on the merits of industrial agriculture, assiduously applied these conventional methods to his 5,000-acre farm. After four seasons of crop failure from destructive hail, storms, and heat waves, he was about to go bankrupt.

Brown then discovered the principles of regenerative agriculture through reading Thomas Jefferson's journals, and now 15 years later he has created a thriving, highly profitable, diversified carbon farm that lets nature do the work. Brown's farm has created 29 inches of new topsoil, and his farm is healthier, more productive, and far more profitable than his neighbors' farms. He says that his soil used to hold only half an inch of rain per hour; now it can hold 8 inches. Rather than buying fertilizer, he instead plants nitrogen-fixing plants and grazes his cattle on those plants, which drives more nitrogen into the soil via the cattle's manure and urine. Brown said he actually makes money from his "fertilizer," instead of having to buy it. He produces 20 percent more food than his neighbors on the same land and makes up to twenty times more money from his diversified regenerative farm. Now he travels the country teaching other farmers about the false promise of industrial farming and the true power of regenerative agriculture to help farmer, nature, and eater. We were both featured in two films about regenerative agriculture now available on Amazon Prime Video, *Kiss the Ground* and *Common Ground*. They are worth watching to better understand the nuances.

Another farmer, Allen Williams, PhD, a sixth-generation Mississippi farmer, bought a depleted 100-year-old cotton plantation, which had been overgrazed by cattle, then turned into hunting grounds, then sold for pennies to Williams because there was no life on the land. In just five years, he created 5 inches of soil with regenerative agriculture. He has taught more than 4,000 farmers how to transition their farms and ranches. He is part of a group of ranchers and farmers known as the Soil Carbon Cowboys,[29] who make more money with less effort and time and fewer inputs, and in tougher conditions, and are more resistant to climate stress than conventional farmers.

WATER: ARE WE RUNNING OUT?

Water is something most of us in the developed world take for granted. Turn on the tap; buy a case of bottled water; take long, hot showers. Sadly, water is not so plentiful in much of the world. Cape Town, South Africa, almost completely ran out of water not too long ago.[30] Just a few years back, Californians faced a moratorium on watering their lawns and were forced to limit water use because of droughts. About 3 billion people[31] face water scarcity one month a year; half a billion face it all year round.[32] Half of all major cities experience water scarcity.[33]

But because of the lifelessness of our dirt, we now have to irrigate these crops because soil that has been depleted can't hold water (which also contributes to the increased number of floods and droughts we have seen in recent years). Seventy percent (!) of the human use of the world's fresh water is for agriculture.[34] About one-third of this—roughly 23 percent of total fresh water—is used for growing food for animals rather than humans or for ethanol.[35] The thing is, these animals evolved to eat grass, graze on rangelands, and drink rainwater or eat grass grown with rainwater, not eat corn irrigated by fresh water from precious aquifers and rivers.

Water is a limited resource; only 2.5 percent of water on the planet is fresh water,[36] and we are depleting our ancient aquifers faster than rainfall can replenish them. Irrigation of crops is the main cause, because again, dirt (unlike soil), cannot hold water. If we switched to range (grass)-fed regenerative livestock production, we would restore soils, draw down carbon (reversing climate change), and store massive amounts of water, which can prevent floods and droughts. No water, no food, no humans. *The solution is soil, not oil.* According to a 2019 UN report, $300 billion invested in regenerative agriculture—less than the amount the United States has sent to Ukraine in the past three years—would be enough to restore 900 hectares of the 2 billion hectares (5 million acres) of degraded land in the world, build soil, and slow down climate change enough to give us more than 20 years to innovate climate-change solutions. That is the total global military spending in just sixty days, or less than one-tenth the annual cost of obesity and diabetes in the United States.

Sucking the Earth Dry

Groundwater is drawn out from our aquifers for irrigation of agriculture faster than it can be replenished. Water overdraw from irrigated agriculture is expected to increase with growing populations. Overuse (such as through pumping for irrigation or fracking) can mean that sources that were previously renewable get so low that they can't recover. For instance, Saudi Arabia decided it wanted to grow its own food and used its ancient fossil aquifers. They were successful for a while, until their water nearly ran out.[37] Closer to home, the 174,000-square-mile Ogallala Aquifer lies underneath the Great Plains and irrigates America's breadbasket. It is also being pumped dry. We are currently taking out 1.3 trillion gallons a year more than can be replenished by rainfall.[38]

Fortunately, innovations in farming and regenerative agriculture build soil, which acts as a sponge for rain and reduces the need for irrigation. Some farmers are changing their practices. Kansas farmer Rodger Funk farmed without groundwater. As of 2024, he pumped almost no water on his 6,000 acres, which are planted largely with wheat and grain sorghum. "We decided to go dryland," he says.[39] "Dryland" means growing crops without irrigation. Instead of plowing his fields after harvest, he leaves the stubble in the ground and plants a new crop in the residue. Leaving the roots and stems intact not only reduces soil erosion but also decreases evaporation and catches more blowing snow than bare ground. Leaving crop residue in the field can reduce moisture loss by the equivalent of an inch or more of rainfall annually, scientists say.[40] Funk aims to capture every bit of the 18 inches of precipitation that fall on southwestern Kansas. "Got to," Funk says. "It's all we've got around here."

MAKING SOIL A GIANT SPONGE FOR WATER

In some regions the issue is not enough water, while in other areas it's too much. For example, in 2019 the Missouri and Mississippi Rivers flooded fields all the way from Minnesota to Louisiana. Some farms had millions of dollars in damage. While floods may sound like they create extra water for the farms, most of that water runs off or through the soil and can't be retained. Soil rich in organic matter can help farmers make their land more resilient to floods by improving the health and spongelike qualities of their soils. Although they can't prevent floods, they can do damage control. In fact, a 1 percent increase in organic matter in the soil can hold up to 27,000 gallons of water per acre.[41] Regenerative practices can increase soil organic matter 3 to 8 percent, creating a virtuous cycle.[42] More soil, more water retention, more drought resistance, more water in soil, more plant growth, more evaporation from plants, more rain. Ever wonder why it rains in the rain forest and not the desert? It's the evaporation of water from plants!

HOW INDUSTRIAL AGRICULTURE IS POISONING OUR WATER, LAND, AND FOOD

You probably don't realize that your burger isn't just made of beef—it's actually built from fossil fuels. The nitrogen fertilizer, pesticides, and herbicides used to grow cattle feed come straight from petroleum. Forty percent[43] of all fossil fuels extracted globally go into fertilizer production—more than the fuel used for every car, plane, and ship combined. So, consider that every time you bite into a factory-farmed burger, you're literally eating petroleum.

What happens to the fertilizer that doesn't end up on our food? It washes off industrial farms, runs into rivers, and dumps into lakes and oceans, where it suffocates marine life. The Gulf of Mexico alone now has a nearly 7,000-square-mile dead zone—a wasteland the size of New Jersey[44]—where nitrogen runoff kills 212,000 metric tons of seafood each year.[45] And it's not just the Gulf; there are nearly 400 similar dead zones worldwide,[46] covering an area the size of Europe that half a billion people depend on for their food. We're sacrificing one of the world's healthiest protein sources—seafood—just to keep factory-farmed meat, ethanol, and ultraprocessed food cheap.

The price tag? Two hundred ten billion dollars a year in nitrogen pollution damages.[47] And it doesn't just kill fish—it's in our drinking water. Runoff from industrial farms contaminates wells, lakes, and tap water with nitrates, pesticides, and toxic chemicals linked to cancer, birth defects, and preterm labor. In 2014, Lake Erie was suffocated by algal blooms, killing fish and turning Toledo's drinking water toxic, and costing the city almost $900 million just to clean it up.[48]

Animal factory farms dump nitrogen-loaded waste into giant manure lagoons that overflow into rivers and streams. Remember Hurricane Florence in 2018? More than fifty hog-waste lagoons in North Carolina flooded,[49] dumping E. coli, salmonella, cryptosporidium, and toxic waste[50] (all of which are poison to humans) into drinking water supplies. Just before this, Trump 1.0's EPA had rolled back water-quality regulations for CAFOs, leaving communities defenseless against this contamination.

Meanwhile, America's drinking water is already loaded with toxins—glyphosate,[51] pesticides, pharmaceuticals,[52] plastics,[53] and nitrates[54]—all linked to cancer, cardiovascular disease, and reproductive issues. The food industry's "solution"? Bottled water. But those plastic bottles leach hormone-disrupting chemicals like BPA, phthalates, and micro- and nanoplastics, and their waste fuels the Great Pacific Garbage Patch in the middle of the Pacific Ocean—twice the size of Texas, with 1.8 trillion pieces of plastic.[55]

We don't need more plastic—we need clean, safe public water. Regenerative farming, better water management, and stricter CAFO regulations can reverse this crisis. But until we stop subsidizing destruction, industrial agriculture will keep polluting the land, water, and food we rely on to survive.

THE LOSS OF BIODIVERSITY: WHY SHOULD YOU CARE?

In recent books like *Growing a Revolution* by David Montgomery, the film *Kiss the Ground* (and the latest iteration, *Common Ground*) by Josh Tickell, and films like *The Biggest Little Farm,* the importance of rebuilding soil is being shared with new audiences. What we are learning is the crucial biological elements of soil health: the critters living there. These critters include the familiar earthworm as well as ones that may be new to you: arbuscular mycorrhizal fungi, soil bacteria, protozoa, nematodes, and arthropods. Together they form complex ecosystems that build soil structure, prevent erosion, and absorb water and carbon from the atmosphere. Living creatures are central to decomposition, nutrient cycling, and plant growth. Working together, these ecosystems can nurture crops and protect them from pests and diseases. The soil is home to a large proportion of the world's genetic biodiversity. There are more microbes in a handful of soil than in all the humans who ever lived. The soil food web is the whole life cycle of the Earth. When soil is depleted, it causes a cascading effect: small insects die, then larger insects that eat the small ones die, and then the birds, small mammals, and amphibians that eat the insects die, which is why these populations are crashing around the world.

In 2019, the Intergovernmental Science-Policy Platform on Biodiversity and Ecosystem Services (IPBES) released the most comprehensive report on biodiversity to date, estimating that 1 million species are on the verge of extinction because of human activity. That includes 40 percent of amphibian species, 33 percent of coral reefs, and 10 percent of insects.[56] According to the Living Planet Index, we have seen a 60 percent decline in species since 1970 alone.[57]

Why should you care? Aside from just the idea of destroying the natural world, what does it really matter if we lose species, insects, forests, plants, and microbes and damage oceans and kill coral reefs, you might wonder? It matters because biodiversity is essential to grow nutrient-dense (or any) food, to have coral reefs that support our fisheries, to protect our coastlines and control floods, and to have fresh drinking water filtered by wetlands, medicines from wild plants, and even building materials and breathable air. Economists estimate these ecosystems provide services worth about $125 trillion a year.[58] In the end, saving nature is not about saving it for its own sake, but about saving it for our sake. As the quote often attributed to Albert Einstein goes, "If the bee disappeared from the face of the earth, man would have only four years to live."

According to the UN report on biodiversity, "The health of ecosystems on which we and all other species depend is deteriorating more rapidly than ever. We are eroding the very foundations of our economies, livelihoods, food security, health and quality of life worldwide," said former IPBES chair Sir Robert Watson. "The Report also tells us that it is not too late to make a difference, but only if we start now at every level from local to global. Through 'transformative change,' nature can still be conserved, restored and used sustainably—this is also key to meeting most other global goals."[59]

We are witnessing massive insect population collapses due to pesticides and land use changes such as converting land into monocrop agriculture.[60] But it is not just soy fields and cornfields that are the problem. On California almond orchards, local bee populations are dying because once the almonds are pollinated, there is no other food to eat, meaning that "slave" bees need to be imported from around the world. We have seen a 75 percent decline over 30 years in flying insect biomass.[61] Just the decline in pollinators is putting $577 billion of food crops at risk. Insects are crucial to the web of life, and their demise ripples up the food chain; bird populations are declining because they have less food. It also has huge economic implications for us. Bees, butterflies, and other insect pollinators contribute $29 billion to US farm income.[62] There is no doubt that our well-being is interconnected with biodiversity on farmland.

Many causes contribute to the biodiversity loss: climate change, pollution, invasive species, human encroachment on natural habitats, and excessive harvesting through fishing, hunting, and poaching. However, regenerative agricultural practices at scale can stop the destruction. This is not some hippie fad but the position of the UN, the European Union, and pretty much every major scientific and governmental assessment of our current state of affairs.

FOOD FIX: REGENERATIVE AGRICULTURE— WHAT IS IT?

But there is a way to fix all of this. We have the technology; it's low-cost, it's available globally, and it has been proven and tested (for billions of years). It is called photosynthesis, the magic cycle plants use to turn water and carbon dioxide (which they breathe from the air) into carbohydrates, which we eat (called "carbo" hydrates because they are built from carbon in the air), and that also feed the microbes in the soil, which in turn feed the plants nitrogen, phosphorus, and minerals. It's a great barter system that makes the world go around, and it's one of the foundations of regenerative agriculture.

On the Great Plains of North America, tens of millions of bison, elk, and deer used to feed on deep-rooted perennial grasses. As these bison moved through the landscape, their hooves pierced the soil and their waste nurtured the soil biology and their saliva increased the growth rate of grasses.[63] Native Americans participated in this process by periodically burning the prairie to encourage new growth (counter-intuitively, fires actually fertilize the ground). The plants, in turn, bartered some of the carbohydrates they made through photosynthesis with soil microbiology to make minerals and nutrients in the soil available to the plants.

Regenerative agriculture is a game-changing approach to farming that focuses on restoring soil health rather than depleting it. Instead of the industrial model that strips the land bare, this method works with nature—using no-till farming to protect soil structure, cover crops to prevent erosion and improve fertility, and crop rotations to naturally manage pests and weeds. But perhaps the most powerful tool? Livestock. When managed properly, grazing animals stimulate plant growth, strengthen root systems, and enrich the soil with manure, saliva, and urine—a biological jump start for the land.

The impact goes far beyond healthier farms. Some estimates suggest that regenerative agriculture could draw down between 15 percent and 100 percent of all carbon released[64] since the Industrial Revolution—potentially helping to even *reverse* global warming. That's up to 1 trillion tons of carbon[65]—just from fixing our soil. While the actual impact depends on how widely these methods are adopted across different ecosystems, experts agree on one thing: This is the most overlooked, low-cost, and scalable solution to climate change that we already have.

Remarkably, some major food monoliths are recognizing this too. The former vice chair of PepsiCo Mehmood Khan told me he was invited to speak at the USDA about regenerative agriculture. Big Food knows that if there is no soil and no water, they can't make their products. Danone, Nestlé, and Mondelēz are among nineteen food companies with revenues of $500 billion that formed a coalition called One Planet Business for Biodiversity, launched September 23, 2019, at the United Nations Climate Action Summit in New York to support regenerative agriculture, biodiversity, eliminating deforestation, and the restoration of ecosystems.

The international initiative "4 per 1000," launched in 2015 by Stéphane Le Foll, then French minister of agriculture, agri-food, and forestry, includes more than 367 partners (governments, NGOs, foundations, farmers, scientists, and industry). The goal is to increase carbon in the soil by 0.4 percent (4 per 1000) every year by scaling regenerative practices to the more than 500 million farms and 1 billion farmers worldwide.

This simple concept is relatively new to the zeitgeist, but is based on ancient principles to restore and enhance natural systems. While it can be organic (and ideally should be), it goes beyond organic by laying out the principles for building soil, enhancing biodiversity, and reducing outside inputs. Large-scale organic farms can use methods that, while better than conventional agriculture, still can deplete soil, require extensive inputs, and drain water resources. Michael Pollan refers to this as "industrial organic" in his book *The Omnivore's Dilemma*. Even small organic farms that don't use regenerative practices can contribute to the problem through tillage and leaving land bare instead of planting cover crops to protect the soil and build organic matter.

Regenerative agriculture on farms, grasslands, and rangelands is the most powerful force for fixing much of what's wrong with agriculture while producing more and better food. And the practice can be adapted across diverse and global environments. These are the foundational principles:

- Regenerative agriculture is a system of farming principles and practices that increases biodiversity, enriches soils, improves watersheds, and enhances ecosystem services.
- It aims to capture carbon in soil and aboveground biomass, reversing current global trends of atmospheric accumulation.
- It offers increased yields, more nutrient-dense foods, resilience to climate instability, and improved health and vitality for farming and ranching communities and consumers.

■ The system draws from decades of scientific and applied research by the global communities of organic farming, agroecology, holistic management, and agroforestry.

For animals, regenerative practices include rotational grazing, which mimics natural herd movements to prevent overgrazing, enrich soil carbon storage, and promote healthier pastures. For plants, techniques such as cover cropping, no-till farming, and polycultures foster nutrient-rich soils, reduce erosion, and minimize synthetic inputs like chemical fertilizers and pesticides. By working in harmony with nature, regenerative farming not only produces high-quality, nutrient-dense food but also combats climate change through carbon sequestration, strengthens local ecosystems, and supports long-term resilience for both the land and the farmers who steward it.

It even turns out that regenerative agriculture is more profitable (for farmers, not Big Ag or Big Food) and produces higher yields and better-quality food, even when used to grow commodity crops (soy, corn, wheat), all while reversing climate change, conserving water, and increasing biodiversity![66]

There are extraordinary examples of conventional farmers who turned to regenerative agriculture to save their farms after hail and drought destroyed them and now have more productive and profitable farms than their conventional-farming neighbors. There are "soil farmers" like Joel Salatin (formerly from Polyface Farm), who use animals as a method for building soil, increasing productivity and the nutrient density of food. Their mission statement is to "develop environmentally, economically, and emotionally enhancing agricultural prototypes and facilitate their duplication throughout the world." They say they are in the redemption business, healing the land, food, economy, and culture.

As leaders in this movement, three longtime farmers—Gabe Brown, Allen Williams, and the late Dave Brandt—teamed up with the government's Natural Resources Conservation Service soil champion Ray Archuleta to help farmers and ranchers across the world apply soil-health-focused regenerative-agriculture systems.[67] Their consulting focuses on ecological principles that can be applied practically and profitably in any farming operation:

- Limiting the amount of soil disturbance, preferably using no-till methods. Tilling turns over soil, disturbs root structures, and leads to soil erosion and loss. A number of effective alternatives to digging up the soil, such as seed drills or strip-till plows, minimize soil disturbance.
- Leaving no bare soil. This means leaving some plant material, such as roots and stalks, on top of the soil or planting cover crops during fallow periods, which help reduce soil and water loss and increase soil organic matter, soil biodiversity, and nutrient content.
- Maintaining diversity in what is planted in the fields. Rotating between crops prevents diseases and pests. In fact, regenerative farms have far fewer invasive insect pests than conventional farms that use insecticides. Using diverse cover crops can help break up soil compaction and bring nutrients like nitrogen into the soil.
- Integrating livestock into the farming operation. Cycling animals through the land means that their manure, urine, and saliva fertilize the soil, building soil the fastest. This must be done correctly by moving a diversity of animals around the farm ecosystem. If it's done incorrectly, overgrazing can harm the farm. There is no regenerative agriculture without animals as part of the ecological cycle.

FOOD FIX: THE GUATEMALAN AND THE COWBOYS—FOREST-FED CHICKENS!

In a room full of cowboy hats, Regi Haslett-Marroquin cuts a contrasting figure. As the native Guatemalan takes the stage to address the hundreds of farmers and ranchers who have gathered in Albuquerque, New Mexico, for the 2018 Regenerate conference, his humble brilliance electrifies the room. "We are not food producers," he says, softly smiling at his paradoxical challenge. "We are energy managers."

Regi is one of the original architects of the Main Street Project (MSP), a poultry-centered regenerative agroforestry system that aims to equip farmers to solve our nation's food crisis. It's not enough to just blame Big Ag, he says; we need to create new ways of thinking and doing when it comes to food production.

MSP starts with a regenerative farming model that is built not on a nearsighted drive toward maximum profit but on a *triple* bottom line. Agriculture must be ecologically, economically, and socially viable.

Regi says MSP's methods are informed by indigenous knowledge, supplemented by farmers' own experiential learning, and validated by scientific testing. When he tells the story of chicken, he speaks of their origin as jungle fowl, living under the canopies of forests. This origin is a long way from the cages of today's factory farms. Regi and MSP are designing a system that mimics this origin by raising chickens in food forests that produce the food sources that the chickens eat. MSP's free-range poultry are raised in paddocks planted with a "stacking function" combination. This type of farming is called "silvopasture," or raising animals in forests or trees. Hazelnut trees provide shade, food for the chickens, and an additional source of income from selling the nuts. And the trees protect the chickens from aerial predators such as hawks. Cover crops like legumes, along with the manure from the chickens, help to put nitrogen into the soil. A variety of grains grown on-site provide more chicken feed, which reduces the amount of money farmers have to spend on outside feed sources. The chickens also eat tons of insects. The farm is built as a living ecosystem, and Regi jokes that it's easier to work with nature rather than fight it.

With their quick growth, chickens, whether for meat or eggs, provide a positive revenue stream at a low cost of entry. Think of this type of farming as a mutual fund versus an individual stock. There are multiple crops, livestock, and multiple streams of revenue, creating a healthier farm and more stable economics for the farmers. Chickens are at the center of MSP's system because they work so well with the crops, farmers, and environment. They are a one-stop weed-eating, bug-killing, soil-enhancing replacement for the counter-productive synthetic pesticides, herbicides, and fertilizers destroying conventional farms and their communities. This type of agriculture—diversified, intensive, integrating animals, trees, and plants in a natural ecological restorative cycle—is resilient and low-impact, protects and builds soils, conserves water, and draws down carbon from the atmosphere, all while producing healthy, nutrient-dense food. It's also how nature works.

This is quite a contrast to the factory-farmed horror show that is the majority of American chicken production: massive buildings where thousands of chickens are crammed into cages, are fed imported grain and antibiotics, and pollute the environment. Did you know that Tyson Foods (one of the largest poultry producers) has dumped 104 million pounds of pollutants into waterways—more than fossil fuel company Exxon—and is the second-biggest industrial polluter after Big Steel?[68] Which chicken would you prefer to feed your family? The antibiotic- and arsenic-laced industrial chickens? Eggs that are pale yellow, devoid of nutrients? Or forest- and bug-fed chickens, and eggs with deep orange yolks dense in phytochemicals and nutrients?

MSP helps farmers incubate their own enterprises with a goal of developing regional food systems. They are building a poultry-production system that can also help immigrant communities move from laboring in an exploitative system to owning a small business. At the same time, the community benefits from the increased access to local, healthy food and the economic boost of thriving local markets. After years of proving their concept, MSP is expanding from its central farm into a regional cluster of farms in southeast Minnesota. The MSP blueprint is also being applied to partner farms in Mexico, Guatemala, Honduras, and South Dakota. Everybody wins when the goal is regenerating human and environmental health rather than simply extracting a profit at any cost. If the true costs of food production were included in the price, these methods would provide much cheaper food.

Regi's story is one thread in an expanding tapestry of regenerative agricultural innovation that is occurring across the world. Efforts are under way to convert millions of acres of land to these types of integrated regenerative farms and ranches. While this innovation has developed on the margins, it's making its way to the mainstream. General Mills, one of the nation's largest food companies, has pledged to "advance regenerative agricultural practices" on 1 million acres of farmland by 2030.[69] That's a huge step in the right direction. Other companies such as Danone and Nestlé are also committing to shift their supply chain to regenerative agriculture. Purdue Farms has also responded to consumer demand by removing all antibiotics from their chicken farms and shifting toward more organic, regenerative, and pasture-raised animal farming.

FOOD FIX: THE ROLE OF GOVERNMENT AND POLICYMAKERS

As individuals we can advocate for change, drive changes in the marketplace, hold our representatives accountable, elect members with values we share, and engage in individual choices that don't contribute to the problems we face.

"The only remedy for the threats we face at the scale at which they confront us is massive political and economic change," Dr. Daniel Aldana Cohen, assistant professor of sociology at the University of California, Berkeley, says. "By far the most meaningful thing an individual person can do is join a social, political, or cultural movement aimed at transforming our political economy. No individual's consumer choices and no group's consumer choices are significant in the absence [of] structural change."[70]

Here are key policy levers that can move us to a more sensible approach to our agriculture and food system. In the United States these reforms must happen across agencies, but the most important instrument of change is the USDA's Farm Bill. Much more has been mapped out in the reports I have mentioned in this chapter, among others.

1. **Establish a national food policy and a national food policy adviser**[71] **and reinvent the USDA as the US Department of Food, Health, and Well-Being** to align our agricultural and food

policies with economic and public health goals, coordinating policy across all agencies that touch any aspect of our food system, from seed to fork to landfill. Much can be done with regulation, executive action, and enforcing existing laws, even in the absence of legislative changes (which are desperately needed). We need to stop incentives for growing the wrong stuff, which makes us sick and poisons the planet, and start supporting the growth of food that focuses on quality of calories rather than quantity.

2. **Re-solarize agricultural production.** Shift the energy input to farms from fossil fuels to the solar inputs of photosynthesis, which will improve our diets and reverse climate change.

3. **Increase publicly funded research on sustainable, regenerative agriculture to improve practices, build soil, determine best regional practices, and address water issues.** Much research is done through publicly funded land-grant agricultural colleges, which now receive funding from Big Ag, helping them generate private profits from public investment. That needs to stop. Future studies should focus on reductions in concentrations of toxic runoff such as nitrogen, phosphate, and organic carbon from integrated crop and livestock systems.[72]

4. **Start a Farmers Corps to enlist a new generation of farmers in regenerative agriculture** and help them overcome the financial and education barriers to joining our food production system. Provide training and funding to access land and resources for converting conventional farms to regenerative farms. Think of it as a Peace Corps for regenerative agriculture.

5. **Create incentives and support for regenerative agriculture through the USDA** (and global agriculture ministries and departments) including financial support for farmers to transition from industrial, chemical-intense agriculture and to integrate animals into farm ecosystems. New Zealand ended all agricultural subsidies, and as a result, its farms are more diverse, productive, and profitable.[73] Support for regenerative agriculture will increase productivity, reduce soil and water loss, reduce fertilizer, pesticide, herbicide, and antibiotic use, and promote the production of healthier foods and the creation of healthier

ecosystems. Kiss the Ground is an education and advocacy nonprofit advancing initiatives across four distinct programs: advocacy, farmland, education, and media. One of its programs provides training and support for farmers to transition to regenerative agriculture. I was able to connect Kiss the Ground with a venture philanthropist who could provide up to $1 billion in funding for farmers to transition to regenerative agriculture.

6. **End the ethanol mandate. The Energy Independence and Security Act of 2007 mandated that US farms grow corn for ethanol to decrease reliance on foreign energy sources.** This led to 33 million acres producing 40 percent of our corn crops that are used for ethanol.[74] It takes more energy to produce ethanol (from all the fossil fuel inputs needed to grow corn from fertilizer, pesticides, herbicides, etc.) than the energy that is provided by the ethanol, according to the late Cornell scientist David Pimentel.[75] Environmentalists and oil companies both oppose the ethanol mandate. Agricultural policies could be implemented that simultaneously protect the farmers who grow the corn and convert those 33 million acres to regenerative agriculture, creating more and better food, restoring ecosystems, and helping reverse climate change.

7. **Create a safety net of credit and risk management tools for farmers who practice sustainable and regenerative agriculture,** not just for commodity farmers who produce corn and soy. The farmers are pawns in the big game of agribusiness and food conglomerates. If we reduce or eliminate subsidies for commodity crops, it won't be enough to protect farmers. The subsidies encourage overproduction of corn, soy, and wheat, leading to low prices, which hurt farmers. The real beneficiaries of the subsidies are the factory farms, food processors (like Cargill and Archer Daniels Midland), manufacturers, and meatpackers that buy the cheap raw materials from the farmers. Rather than taxpayers helping Big Food and Big Ag buy cheap food, farmers should be protected, and industry should pay the true cost of the food. I once asked the vice chair of PepsiCo why the company uses high-fructose corn syrup in their beverages. "Mark," he told me, "it's because the government makes it too cheap for us not to."

8. **Pay for ecosystem services.** Many countries have created systems to support farmers and corporations that restore ecosystems through reforestation, soil restoration, better water management practices, and improvements in biodiversity. Costa Rica has been a pioneer in this. Payment for ecosystem services incentivizes farmers and corporations to solve the problem of climate change, water shortages, biodiversity loss, and soil degradation rather than contribute to it.

9. **Consider a "nitrogen tax" levied on fertilizer companies to account for the greenhouse gases and the destruction of our soils, waterways, and fisheries** and provide funds for the cleanup of our lakes, rivers, and oceans and the transition to regenerative practices. Shouldn't big fertilizer companies be accountable for the harm they cause?

10. **Implement mandatory municipal and institutional (and even personal) composting and provide the compost to farmers and ranchers.**

11. **Have Congress fund, and the USDA implement, programs that help farmers grow more fruits and vegetables, or actual food.** Support the development of "specialty crops" such as fruits and vegetables, whole grains, beans, nuts, and seeds. This could create 189,000 new jobs and $9.5 billion in new revenue for healthy foods.[76]

12. **End penalties for farmers who receive crop insurance so they can create diverse farms that include fruits and vegetables.** Research has shown that if farmers in six midwestern states shifted some of their cropland to fruits and vegetables, it would create 6,724 new jobs and $336 million in additional income.[77]

13. **Include environmental and sustainability guidelines in the US Dietary Guidelines.** The 2015 scientific advisory group recommended including this in the guidelines, but the politicians took it out under pressure from Big Ag and Big Food.[78]

14. **Ensure that the next farm bill helps break up monopolies and addresses consolidation of seed companies, seed patents, grain trading, animal feeding, meatpacking, agrochemical companies, and supermarkets.**[79] This will create a fairer and more

sustainable marketplace. Antitrust legislation would break up these monopolies, encouraging open access to and use of seeds, supporting local farming systems, and increasing the diversity of our food by supporting diverse seed libraries. Remember that 75 percent of our food comes from just twelve plants (all controlled by Big Ag and chemical companies) and 60 percent comes just from rice, corn, and wheat. This is not good for humans or the planet.

We need to enforce and strengthen antitrust laws to establish fair and functioning markets by breaking up the massive consolidation in the seed, agricultural chemical, fertilizer, and food industries. There is enormous control of the food system by a few dozen companies across these sectors, with very little oversight, which prevents fair competition in the marketplace. They control what is grown, how it is grown, what seeds and chemicals are used, what's manufactured, and even what ends up where on the grocery store shelves. The first antitrust laws were established to break up the railroad, oil, and steel conglomerates in the 1890s. Senator John Sherman, author of the first antitrust law, said, "If we will not endure a king as a political power we should not endure a king over the production, transportation, and sale of any of the necessaries of life."[80] These laws were established to protect consumers, ensure fair competition, and rebuild the infrastructure to link farmers to eaters in their region. The harm done by today's monopolization of the food industry is far greater than any impact of the railroad, oil, and steel industries 100 years ago. Yet the laws are not enforced.

15. **Build local and regional capacity to transition the food system from extractive agriculture to regenerative agriculture.** While it could take years for land reform and a new farm bill to go into effect, consumers, farmers, and state governments can still do plenty to stem the tide of the environmental fallout and build better farming and better food. As you'll see in Chapter 18, regenerative agriculture is absolutely essential. And it will take more than farmers to make that transformation.

16. **Align all agricultural and public health policies by providing incentives for purchasing healthy foods and limiting harmful foods in all federal, state, and local programs.**

17. **Support urban agriculture and vertical farming to both improve food access and food quality and revive impoverished urban communities.** A real food fix will align agriculture with nourishing people, repairing our environment, stabilizing our climate, and taking hidden costs out of the system. This alignment is one of the most important challenges of our lifetime.

18. **Create federal, state, and local food procurement standards and practices** to ensure that tax dollars are spent only on health-promoting foods. This initiative could be modeled after the Good Food Purchasing Program, whose mission is to transform "the way public institutions purchase food by creating a transparent and equitable food system built on five core values: local economies, health, valued workforce, animal welfare, and environmental sustainability. The Center for Good Food Purchasing provides a comprehensive set of tools, technical support, and verification systems to assist institutions in meeting their Program goals and commitments." This should also apply to public hospitals and health care institutions with any government funding (which essentially includes every health care institution that receives money from Medicare or Medicaid). And of course, it must apply to all schools and universities with government funding, the military, prisons, universities, community colleges, day care centers, government offices, and any other government organization or organization that receives government funds.

FOOD FIX: GRASSROOTS AND CITIZEN ACTION

Never doubt that a small group of thoughtful, committed citizens can change the world: indeed, it's the only thing that ever has.

—MARGARET MEAD (ATTRIBUTED)

If we're not farmers or policymakers, or don't run a Big Ag or Big Food company, can we influence change in agriculture and our food system?

The deck *is* stacked against us by the corporate control of government. But that doesn't mean our actions, our voices, and our votes don't matter. They do. Change happens from the margins, before they gradually reach the center. Did Harriet Tubman believe that ferrying a few enslaved people to freedom was fruitless? Did Emma Goldman believe there was no point marching because the Equal Rights Amendment would not pass even decades after women got the right to vote? They were radicals, on the sidelines, but their voices and actions carried, inspired, and changed an entire entrenched agriculture system based on slavery and delivered women from second-class citizenship.

Your daily food choices absolutely matter, and we all must work together to make agriculture work for producers, consumers, animals, and the land that grows everything we eat.

Here's a list, by no means exhaustive, of what you can do to be part of the solution.

1. **Look for the regenerative organic certified label.** In 2019, a coalition of groups launched a pilot program to develop Regenerative Organic Certification.[81] These guidelines should seem self-evident but are not; they are aspirational. Regenerative Organic Certification is a "beyond organic" certification that involves three areas: soil health, animal welfare, and social fairness.

2. **Join a community-supported agriculture (CSA) program in your area for local organic produce.** Go to www.localharvest.org to find one in your area. They will deliver a box of organic vegetables every week at low prices. Get a cow share from a regenerative farm. For example, you can get grass-fed meat for an average of $10 a pound from Mariposa Ranch and other regenerative farms and ranches across the country.[82] That's $2 for a 4-ounce serving or about half the price of a Big Mac. Certainly, this is doable for most families.

3. **Shop at farmers' markets.** Farmers' markets support local food systems, and their popularity is resurging. While the impact may

be small, it provides a foothold into innovations in agriculture that eventually will spread.

4. **Start a home garden (even a windowsill of herbs is great).** Or reserve a plot in a local community garden. Turn your lawn into an edible garden or orchard. Plant fruit trees and avoid the use of glyphosate herbicides like Roundup and pesticides.

5. **Create a community garden.** Do it with your church, school, or company or as a family project. Even the Centers for Disease Control and Prevention determined that community gardens can help rebuild broken communities and reduce violence in urban areas.[83]

6. **Educate yourself and your community about regenerative agriculture.** Films like *Kiss the Ground, Common Ground,* and *The Biggest Little Farm* are a good start. Check out the Carbon Underground to learn more.[84] Take a tour of a regenerative farm to see how it all works.

7. **Change your banking and investment strategy to support regenerative and sustainable business solutions.** Seek out social investment companies and options. Most big investment firms now offer this. The Jeremy Coller Foundation in the United Kingdom aggregated institutional investors with $75 trillion in assets[85] and got them to agree to change their investment policies to end factory farming of animals.[86] Their first step was to get the largest twenty fast-food companies to agree to end the use of antibiotics in animal feed by a certain date. They simply told those companies they would divest all their investments if they didn't do what they asked. Who knows? Their next target may be to force Big Food to source from regenerative agriculture. That would be a game changer. Not all of us have that power, but all our little choices matter.

8. **Avoid GMO foods as much as possible.** Everyone can do this to some degree. In Chapter 6, I mentioned buying non-GMO foods as a way to support grassroots efforts to implement non-GMO labeling, but it's also a way to support better agricultural practices through your food choices and avoid potential health issues from the pesticides and herbicides like glyphosate used on GMO foods. You may want to check

your urine levels of glyphosate. One test is offered by a company formerly known as Great Plains Laboratory (now Mosaic Diagnostics); ask your health care provider to order one for you.

9. **Vote with your vote.** The truth is that if we had an active voting citizenship, much could change. Only 55 percent of Americans vote in presidential elections, and even fewer do in midterm elections, while an average of 70 percent vote in most other democracies. The Food Policy Action network created "An Eater's Guide to Congress" scorecard, rating each member on how they vote on food and agriculture policies. In the 2018 election, two congressmen with dismal scores on food policy were defeated by a targeted social media campaign focused on low-turnout voters.

These are a few ways to push the rock up the hill. Buying local, organic, and regenerative food is a start. Consider joining or starting a food policy council, through which local people can educate one another and advocate for better food policies.[87] Petition anchor institutions like hospitals and schools to buy locally sourced, regenerative food.[88] Support farmworkers and the organizations, such as the HEAL Alliance, fighting for their rights.[89]

Small steps add up to big change if we all participate.

For a quick reference guide on the Food Fixes and resources to help you restore our natural resources and promote regenerative agriculture, go to www.foodfixuncensored.com.

CHAPTER 18

HOW INDUSTRIAL AGRICULTURE BECAME A CLIMATE CRISIS

Globally, agriculture and its related deforestation are directly responsible for about a quarter of greenhouse gases (GHGs).[1] But when every aspect of the food chain is included, it may add up to more like 50 percent![2] This is in part why we must transform our agriculture and food. In fact, our very survival as a species just may depend on it.

Industrial agriculture contributes to climate degradation through the overproduction of the three main GHGs: methane, nitrous oxide, and carbon dioxide. Here's how:

- Carbon dioxide is released into the atmosphere when soil is disturbed—primarily through tilling, which depletes organic matter, and through deforestation to make way for massive soy and corn production used in CAFOs (confined animal feeding operations). Yet, the irony is staggering: The world's soils hold *three times more carbon* than the entire atmosphere[3]—and with the right practices, they have the potential to absorb even more.
- Methane is released by cattle on factory farms—and yes, also by grass-finished cattle. Some critics argue that grass-fed cattle may emit more total methane because they take longer to reach market weight. But that view is overly simplistic and ignores critical factors: grass-fed cattle consume a higher-quality, natural diet that can lead to lower methane production per day; healthy, well-managed grasslands often contain methane-oxidizing bacteria that absorb

methane from the air. And, most importantly, regenerative ranching systems can actually result in net-negative GHG emissions—meaning they sequester more carbon than they emit, actively helping to reverse climate change rather than contribute to it.[4]

- Synthetic nitrogen fertilizers used in industrial agriculture don't just pollute waterways—they also release nitrous oxide, a GHG that is nearly 300 times[5] more potent than carbon dioxide at trapping heat in the atmosphere. This invisible gas is a major driver of climate change, yet it's rarely discussed. The overuse of nitrogen fertilizers in conventional farming isn't just an environmental issue—it's a climate emergency. Reducing our reliance on synthetic fertilizers through regenerative practices isn't optional; it's essential for any serious climate solution.

- Food waste in landfills is responsible for off-gassing of GHGs (methane).

- Food transportation, processing, and refrigeration use fossil fuels all along the food chain.

SO...SHOULD WE ALL JUST BE VEGAN?

Veganism has been trending recently. But let me take you back in history a bit to anchor the philosophy of a plant-based diet.

If you're reading this, you most certainly are familiar with the Kellogg's brand. But I bet you don't know the figure behind the brand—the OG vegan warrior—Dr. John Harvey Kellogg. An influential and eccentric doctor at the turn of the twentieth century, Kellogg was a Seventh-day Adventist[6] who became the original plant-based crusader. He ran the world-famous Battle Creek Sanitarium in the late 1800s and early 1900s, where he treated presidents and celebrities alike with a regimen of fiber-rich vegetarianism, enemas, and a strict abstinence from meat, alcohol, and even sexual activity.[7]

Long before "wellness" was a buzzword, Kellogg was preaching the gospel of gut health, bowel regularity, and moral purity through food. He fundamentally reshaped the trajectory of nutrition science and

American food culture—not by way of rigorous science but through a potent mix of moral conviction, religious fervor, medical authority, and visionary marketing.

At a time when mainstream medicine paid little attention to diet, Kellogg built an empire on the radical idea that food was central not only to health but also to morality, behavior, and even salvation. His focus was on red meat, which he believed stimulated excess desire (translation: sexual urges). The bland, grain-based breakfast cereals he invented were intended to tame the body's "passions" (curb sexual desire) and promote spiritual health. By promoting a low-fat, plant-based diet as a path to moral and physical purity, Kellogg helped birth a nutritional worldview that framed meat as not only unhealthy but also unclean—an idea that would echo through dietary guidelines for the next century.

His invention of the breakfast cereal—and his brother Will's decision to commercialize it—transformed how the world starts its day. Cereal wasn't just a convenient meal; it was Kellogg's attempt to replace meat-laden breakfasts with a bland, digestible, and "clean" alternative, marking a profound cultural shift: For the first time, breakfast became a grain-based ritual rather than a hearty, protein-rich feast. The cereal aisle became a symbol of modern health, despite later iterations being heavily processed and sugar-laden.

But Kellogg's legacy goes far beyond what we eat for breakfast. Perhaps most importantly, he helped entrench the idea that nutrition should be morally prescriptive—that certain foods make you a better person. He blurred the lines between wellness and virtue, seeding the legacy that still shapes today's most heated food debates. Whether it's plant-based movements or the vilification of red meat, Kellogg's ideology has echoed in our collective unconscious for more than a century.

His legacy persists in today's cultural zeitgeist around veganism—the narrative that meat is destroying the planet (and our health) and that a plant-based diet is the ultimate path to redemption. The itch is everywhere: ditch meat, save the world, and cleanse your body and soul in one virtuous, kale-filled swoop. Meatless Mondays, cow farts, lab-grown meat, and Impossible brand GMO soy burgers have dominated the mainstream headlines.

As a doctor, I'm all for eating more vegetables—in fact, we are almost all deficient in them—and I've spent much of my career encouraging exactly that. There's no question a plant-rich diet is essential for health. And there's no defending the environmental and ethical catastrophe of feedlot-finished beef. Case closed, right?

Well, like most things in health (and science), it's a bit more nuanced than that.

It is a common conception that the farming of animals, especially cows, is *causing* climate change. Activists (of the variety that throw paint on priceless art pieces) claim that eating meat will destroy our health and that cattle are the carbon equivalent of the atomic bomb. That a meatless diet is the only way to save our health and the planet. That animal products should not be part of a healthy diet. That vegan and vegetarian diets prevent disease and prolong life.

While this topic could merit its own book entirely, I'll try to provide the basics for you here. Compared to our standard ultraprocessed and CAFO diet, plant-based diets *are* better. Factory farming of animals is bad for you, for them, and for the planet. Steer clear. Full agreement on all sides.

But this is an incomplete narrative. The reality, like most things, is a bit more nuanced than that. Let me unpack it.

This "plants are good, meat is bad" argument lacks essential nuance. What plants? What meat? Industrial soy, no. Vegetables from a regenerative farm, yes. Factory-farmed steak, no. Regeneratively raised steak, yes. A recent independent life-cycle analysis by the sustainability experts at Quantis of regeneratively raised beef versus GMO soy burger (Impossible Burger) showed that the soy burger *is* far better than feedlot beef, but it still adds 1.7 kilograms of CO_2 to the environment,[8] while the regeneratively raised beef burger removes 3.5 kilograms of CO_2. Soy is the main staple of "healthy vegan" meat replacements and plant-based burgers, so this means that your soy burger or pea protein shake may not be so good for you or the planet after all. Since the soy from the Impossible Burger is made with GMO soy sprayed with Roundup, it has 11 parts per billion (ppb) more glyphosate than the BeyondBurger, made from pea protein.[9] Research shows that just 0.1 ppb of glyphosate is enough to harm the gut bacteria or microbiome.[10] Just one Impossible Burger has 110 times that much!

You may be confused reading that as someone writing about fixing the food system, I recommend animal protein. This is, admittedly, a fairly touchy topic.

In terms of the philosophy of nutrition, I firmly believe that we sound the alarm on anyone pushing a one-size-fits-all food ideology, especially when it involves eliminating meat entirely and replacing it with ultraprocessed, lab-grown alternatives like the Impossible Burger and Beyond Burger sans any longitudinal studies (since they're so new). The idea that we can simply cut out meat without consequences is not just misguided—it's actually dangerous.

But the TL;DR is that meat is the highest bioavailable protein (pound for pound, you get the most bang for your nutrition buck) and, farmed properly, is a major environmental protector. *BUT,* and this is a big "but," CAFO meat—meat produced in the industrial farmed feedlots you see in photos on environmentalists' websites—not only is harmful to the planet but is actually quite toxic to your body.

Meat provides essential amino acids, high-quality protein, and highly bioavailable nutrients like preformed vitamins A, K_2, D_3, and B_{12}—nutrients that plant-based diets either lack entirely or provide in far less absorbable forms. If we removed meat, where exactly would our protein come from? The answer, for most, would be industrially processed soy, pea protein isolates, and synthetic additives, stripped of real nutrition and designed to mimic the very thing they claim to replace.

My personal view is that pushing a mandatory plant-based diet, especially one reliant on corporate-engineered meat substitutes, isn't just a health risk—it's a social disservice. It prioritizes ideology over biology, ignoring the fact that animal foods have sustained human life for millennia, while ultraprocessed plant-based substitutes have barely been around a decade. Instead of banning cows, we should be rethinking industrial food production—starting with the very fake foods being marketed as "progress."

So yes, you, as an omnivore species, want to eat animals, but you want the wild kind, also known as "free range," "grass-fed," or "regeneratively raised." Look for those labels and you'll be getting the highest-quality fuel for your body.

It's Not the Cow; It's the How!

According to a UN Food and Agriculture Organization figure, using a full life-cycle assessment, livestock are responsible for 14.5 percent of human GHG emissions, more than all transportation emissions.[11] Eighty percent of these emissions come from ruminants (e.g., cattle, sheep, goats), half being methane, a quarter nitrous oxide, and the rest carbon dioxide.[12] The feed required for these operations is often grown using the worst agricultural practices: annual tilling combined with pesticides and fertilizers, often accompanied by deforestation and use of native grasslands to grow food for the animals.

A report released by the Institute for Agriculture and Trade Policy calculated emissions from the entire supply chain, finding that the world's top five meat and dairy producers combined—Brazil's JBS, New Zealand's Fonterra, Dairy Farmers of America, Tyson Foods, and Cargill—emit more GHGs than the combined emissions of oil giants ExxonMobil, Shell, and BP. If these meat and dairy companies continue to grow conventional meat and dairy based on current projections, by 2050 they will be responsible for 81 percent of global emissions.[13]

Seventy percent of available agricultural lands are used to grow feed for animals being raised on farms and ranches for human consumption.[14] But not all farms and ranches are the same, nor are all cattle. Nicolette Hahn Niman, the vegetarian cattle rancher who wrote *Defending Beef,* put it this way: "It's not the cow; it's the how," a catchphrase she borrowed from Russ Conser, one of the Soil Carbon Cowboys.

Grass-fed and grass-finished beef, managed the right way, is actually deeply healthy for the animals, the humans, the environment, and the climate. In fact, properly managed livestock on grasslands and in diversified farms can convert inedible grasses on land unsuitable for crops into healthy protein and nutrients for humans. Well-managed grazing is possibly *the* most important strategy to create the new soil required to suck carbon out of the atmosphere and save us from extinction.

The regenerative-agriculture movement suggests that animals are not just a luxury for our human diets but are actually an *essential* part of the natural biological cycle necessary to create sustainable ecosystems, that animals must be integrated into farms to regenerate soil, enabling it to store massive amounts of carbon and water. These practices can reduce the need for factory-farmed meat and its overuse of antibiotics, pesticides, herbicides, and farming practices that deplete the soil, and they can be done at scale more profitably than feedlots. With 40 percent of agricultural lands suited only for grazing, this seems like a good idea. Even if you wanted to grow vegetables or grains on them, you couldn't.

Other research claims that the amount of methane released into the air from ruminants such as cattle surpasses the amount of carbon those animals sequester on rangelands. The *Grazed and Confused?* report, written by Tara Garnett, a vegetarian from the Food Climate Research Network (now called TABLE),[15] found that methane emissions outweigh the carbon sequestration capacity of grasslands.[16] This is important because methane is a powerful GHG and over the last decade, methane emissions have been rising. Rice cultivation accounts for 10 percent of GHG emissions globally and up to 19 percent of methane emissions, but I've yet to hear demands for cutting our rice consumption by 90 percent, although innovative methods of rice cultivation *can* dramatically reduce those emissions. Methane is also produced from poor manure management on CAFOs, and, yes, cow burps (actually it's technically the fermentation from bacteria in ruminants' guts, which result when they eat non-native foods). Turns out that fracking for natural gas along with the production of synthetic nitrogen used to fertilize commodity crops (like corn) releases more methane than animal agriculture.[17]

Many cite *Grazed and Confused?* as proof that even grass-fed cows are harmful to the environment. However, while many of Garnett's findings are accurate, there are major flaws in the report.[18] Sadly, often when ideology mixes with science, the average reader or policymaker is left dazed and confused. The flaws in Garnett's report were detailed in a report from the Sustainable Food Trust.[19]

Studies debunking the idea that grass-fed beef can help reverse climate change focus on old-style continuous grazing, which damages the land, not on holistic management, which uses adaptive multi-paddock grazing. Short-term studies Garnett relied on didn't study a long enough period for the benefits of increasing soil carbon to be measured. It takes time to regenerate land and bring it back to life. Looking at carbon cycles over four years, a recent study in the Midwest found that an adaptive multi-paddock grazing model (rotating livestock around multiple paddocks to avoid overgrazing and stimulate plant growth) put more carbon back into the soil (where we need it) than into the air (where it does harm).[20] The few papers on which Garnett's assessment was based didn't even review holistic management approaches, automatically rendering her assessment of the climate impact of grass-fed cows irrelevant.[21]

Another recent life-cycle analysis of regenerative methods on the White Oak Pastures farm in Georgia also found net carbon sequestration, meaning that their farming practices might actually *reverse* climate change.[22]

The degree of carbon sequestration depends on the quality of the soil to start with. Poor soils, when rehabilitated, will sequester more carbon than soils already in good shape. The fact that much of our soil is depleted to varying degrees makes the promise of regenerative agriculture at scale significant.[23]

The moral of the story is that holistically managed animals actually *should* be part of a regenerative system that draws carbon out of the atmosphere by building healthy soil and offsets methane emissions as well. When cattle are managed through techniques like mob grazing, which mimics the natural behavior of herd animals, they eat some of the grass and then are moved, giving the grass a chance to regenerate. This regeneration draws down carbon through photosynthesis and pushes it through the grass's roots to stimulate the soil biology. Additionally, high-quality forage in these actively managed pastures is easier

---

THE BENEFITS OF GRAZING

For the geeks among you, I refer you to twenty-six papers documenting the benefits of the right kind of grazing and regenerative farming for restoring the environment, water retention, increased biodiversity, and soil carbon sequestration, among other benefits.[24] These are known as ecosystem or environmental services. In the report *Greening Livestock,* the benefits are so great that they suggest payment to farmers for providing these services, much like carbon credits, enabling more farmers to transition to regenerative agriculture.[25]

---

for cattle to digest, which reduces methane production. So, contrary to the vegan propaganda you're most likely seeing in ideologically driven media outlets, these cows are actually *contributing* to environmental regeneration and carbon sequestration.

UC Berkeley studies "carbon farming" and through meticulous research on grasslands in California also proved that properly managed grasslands remove carbon from the atmosphere.[26] It's a complicated ecosystem, so failing to account for the full cycle and all the players could easily lead to a misinterpretation of the data. In a robust study comparing feedlot beef to adaptive-multi-paddock-raised grass-fed cattle, including all the outside inputs and methane, the grass-fed operations reduced net carbon by 170 percent and the feedlots increased net carbon emissions.[27]

Reducing emissions through regenerative operations like White Oak Pastures is a far more sustainable and healthier alternative than removing all animals from the land and converting it to the monocrop soy manipulated to create the plant-based alternatives pumped with synthetic chemicals. While there have been some studies that seem to show that regenerative agriculture doesn't produce a net benefit, they studied parameters including only conventional (over)grazing and assumed 50 percent of the land was irrigated—which is not how regenerative agriculture works.[28] True holistic management doesn't require irrigation and builds more soil that holds more water and more carbon. In fact, a comparative analysis of true regenerative practices (from White Oak Pastures) compared to those used to grow GMO monocrop soy for Impossible Burgers found that one 100 percent grass-fed burger would offset the GHG emissions produced by one Impossible Burger.[29] The life-cycle analyses for both the grass-fed burger and the Impossible Burger were done by the same research organization, Quantis.

CARBON FOOTPRINT BREAKDOWN FOR WOP BEEF

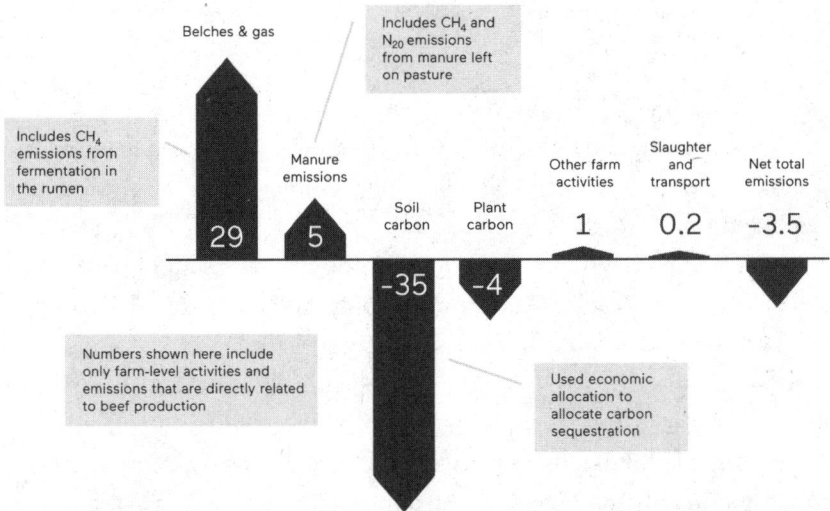

Belches & gas

Includes CH_4 and N_{20} emissions from manure left on pasture

Includes CH_4 emissions from fermentation in the rumen

Manure emissions

Soil carbon

Plant carbon

Other farm activities

Slaughter and transport

Net total emissions

29   5   -35   -4   1   0.2   -3.5

Numbers shown here include only farm-level activities and emissions that are directly related to beef production

Used economic allocation to allocate carbon sequestration

Courtesy of White Oak Pastures

Complicating the meat debate further is the fact that much of the rangeland used for livestock grazing is considered "marginal" land—unsuitable for crop production due to poor soil quality, low moisture, or challenging terrain. Attempting to convert this land into cropland often requires intensive tilling and irrigation, which not only fails to yield viable crops but also results in significantly higher carbon emissions through soil disturbance and water use. In many cases, the effort to replace grazing with crop production—especially for more soy, corn, and wheat—can actually increase CO_2 output, not reduce it.

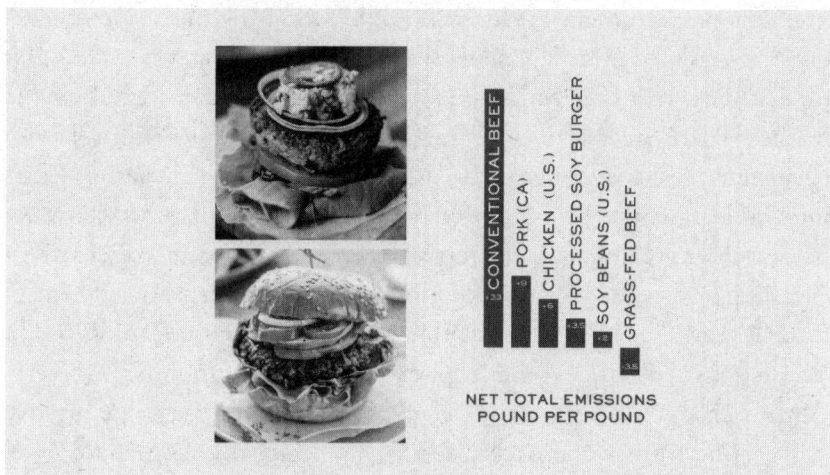

NET TOTAL EMISSIONS
POUND PER POUND

Courtesy of White Oak Pastures

So, without livestock, we would forgo the use of rangeland that could do two very important things: (1) generate high-quality, nutrient-dense protein and (2) restore ecosystems and biodiversity and store large amounts of rainwater and carbon, creating a virtuous cycle of fertility, food, and environmental restoration.

The best solution for rangelands is managing livestock in ways that sequester carbon, help prevent floods and droughts, and promote biodiversity. On top of that, water consumption by animals on rangelands is mostly rainwater, so it doesn't contribute to depletion of the earth's fresh water the way the irrigation required to grow feed for feedlot cattle does.

Regenerative grazing restores the land and supports livestock and all forms of wildlife—a beautiful ecological cycle. Land regenerates as the soil is restored. With better grazing practices, where cattle eat only half the forage before being moved, the root mass is retained. And the roots continuously pump carbon into the ground. This causes the soil structure to improve and thus more water infiltrates and is retained. The nutrients from the soil are more available. There's more plant growth and forage, which in turn transpire both water vapor and monoterpenes, molecules created by forests that form aerosols, which create clouds, create more rain, and cool the climate.

A counterargument to this philosophy of raising meat often points out that grass-fed meats are expensive and elitist and can't be scaled. But models show that they can, *and then some.* Allen Williams has done the math.[30] There are 29 million grain-fed cattle consumed from factory farms in America every year. By using idle grasslands, including existing USDA Conservation Reserve Program land unsuitable for farming but good for grazing, and converting corn and soy monocrops used for fattening feedlot cattle, we could produce 52.9 million grass-fed head of cattle a year, which is almost double what's produced in feedlots today. Those grass-fed cattle would help revitalize rural communities, reverse climate change, increase biodiversity, reduce water use, and improve soil health. Similar approaches can be used globally. While we don't need that much meat, the argument that this is simply an elitist, limited strategy is clearly erroneous.

Nevertheless, we should not deceive ourselves: All agriculture *is* massively destructive—and not just factory farms. Even growing beans, grains, and vegetables is inherently harmful because the natural ecosystem and animal habitat supporting wild animals such as rabbits, rodents, turkeys, bees, earthworms, and insects is destroyed, not to mention the living, breathing system that is soil and all its trillions of inhabitants. Growing plants kills 7 billion animals a year. I respect the moral choice of being a vegan, but the idea that it is saving animals and the planet and even improving our health is actually quite misguided. Turns out a cornfield is much more destructive than a grass-fed beef regenerative ranch.

THE EAT-LANCET COMMISSION REPORT ON HEALTHY DIETS AND SUSTAINABLE FOOD SYSTEMS

The good news is that there is increasing awareness and extensive science on the links between our current food system, how and what food it produces, and the links to health, the environment, and climate. The

EAT-Lancet Commission report[31] was a notable attempt to highlight these issues.

The report got a lot right:

- The need for plant-rich diets
- Reductions in sugar and processed foods
- Reduction or elimination of factory-farmed meat
- Highlighting the importance of transitioning to sustainable agricultural systems that address environmental degradation and climate change and the need to feed a population of 9.8 billion by 2050 in a sustainable way for the planet
- Providing flexible guidelines for diet that match cultural and geographical needs
- Providing the first-ever scientific modeling connecting diet, environment, and climate to create healthy humans, environment, and climate

While there are always challenges in modeling and the underlying science that informs any attempt at developing guidelines, the report takes a big leap forward in defining the issues and spurring further research and policy actions. However, many scientists have taken issue with the science, the omissions, and the conclusion that we should dramatically reduce meat consumption (the average American man consumes 68 grams of meat a day, or about 10 ounces, while the EAT-Lancet advises only 7 grams a day, or 1 ounce), which can produce a nutritionally deficient diet.[32] Even the EAT-Lancet Commission, one of the biggest promoters of plant-based diets, quietly admits a massive flaw in its own recommendations: a plant-based diet isn't sufficient for some of the most vulnerable people in society. They acknowledge that the sick, elderly, malnourished, and young require more protein than plants alone can provide and that low animal food consumption in children leads to stunting, anemia, and malnutrition—while higher consumption improves growth, cognitive function, motor skills, and overall health.

So, if even EAT-Lancet agrees that cutting out animal foods can damage human development, why are they still pushing for a global reduction in meat consumption? Are we really willing to risk childhood malnutrition and long-term health consequences to satisfy an agenda that prioritizes ideology over biology? This isn't about sustainability—it's about ignoring science to push a narrative.

The data on the harmful effects of meat used in their analysis is from population-based studies fraught with problems, the most stunning of which is that cause and effect cannot be determined from those studies. It is an association that can and does have many other explanations. In rigorous reviews, up to 80 percent of these conclusions from population-based studies turn out to be false when subjected to proper clinical trials (as shown by the Reproducibility Project).[33] These are the other issues that have been identified with the EAT-Lancet Commission report:

- No explicit recognition that well-managed holistic farm and rangeland ecosystems require animals to sequester carbon.
- Calls for increased use of chemical inputs, which is perplexing considering the toxicity of nitrogen pollution to the soil, water, and climate, to support growth in developing countries, which may be better served by more local, regenerative practices that don't depend on outside chemical and seed inputs.
- Contradictory mention of managed grazing and the use of manure as part of the solution but no acknowledgment of the profound difference between CAFO meat and grass-fed regeneratively raised meat.[34]
- Thirty-one out of thirty-seven scientists behind the report have published records in favor of vegan or vegetarian diets or against meat.[35]
- No external peer review.[36]
- Conflicts of interest went unreported.[37]
- Members of their corporate partner FReSH (Food Reform for Sustainability and Health)[38] hail from big seed monopolies, fertilizer giants, agrochemical companies, Big Pharma (a handful of companies), and food behemoths including Bayer (which now owns Monsanto), DuPont, Syngenta, Yara (the biggest nitrogen fertilizer company), PepsiCo, and Cargill.[39]

Twenty of the largest Big Food companies signed up to support the report. Why would they be supporting this platform? Hidden within it is the implicit need to grow more grains and beans and food products using industrial agriculture, seeds, fertilizer, and chemicals that drive profits for all these companies.

Physicist and agroecologist Dr. Vandana Shiva says that the EAT-Lancet report evades the "glaring chronic disease epidemic related to pesticides and toxins in food, imposed by chemically intensive industrial agriculture and food systems."[40] She says, "Instead of recognizing the role of organic farming and agroecology for providing sustainable ways for repairing the broken nitrogen cycle, the report recommends 'redistribution of global use of nitrogen and phosphorus,' which in effect is saying chemicals should be spread in the Third World."[41] We've already exported our ultraprocessed foods to developing countries to the detriment of their health. Should we really harm them even more by exporting our chemicals and expanding extractive, fossil-fuel, and chemical-industrial agriculture to grow more grains and beans?

It is true that the developed world eats too much meat, and the wrong meat. But eating less but better-quality meat is much better for you and the planet.

BUT ISN'T MEAT BAD FOR OUR HEALTH?

The question of whether meat is bad for our health has been extensively debated, sadly mostly along ideological lines, not with accurate scientific data. Nearly all studies on the harm of meat studied *only* factory-farmed meat (which is obviously toxic), and they are population-based studies that categorically cannot prove cause and effect. Many of the studies vilifying meat conveniently ignore a critical detail: The meat eaters they analyzed weren't exactly health-conscious individuals. They smoked more, drank more, exercised less, ate fewer fruits and vegetables, and consumed an extra 800 calories a day compared to non–meat eaters.[42]

So, are these studies really proving that meat itself is harmful—or that people with generally unhealthy lifestyles tend to eat more burgers and processed junk? Correlation is not causation, but that hasn't stopped anti-meat advocates from using these flawed studies as ammunition to push their agenda. When you isolate the data and compare health-conscious meat eaters to health-conscious vegetarians, the so-called harms of meat suddenly disappear. Funny how that works.

Many other studies contradict those findings as well. The PURE study of 135,000 people found those who ate animal protein and fat had *fewer* heart attacks and deaths than those who ate more cereal grains.[43] Another study of food consumption patterns in forty-two countries showed a lower risk of heart disease and death in those who ate animal fat and protein and higher risk in those who ate cereal grains and potatoes.[44] A 17-year study of vegetarians and meat eaters who shopped at health food stores found mortality dropped in half for both groups.[45] Other studies point to the nutritional benefits of grass-fed meat, including higher levels of omega-3 fats and CLA (a metabolism-boosting anti-cancer fat) and high levels of minerals, vitamins, and antioxidants.[46] I can understand why you might be confused!

I have reviewed this subject extensively in my book *Food: What the Heck Should I Eat?* I also recommend, for those who want to take a deep dive into the research, Chris Kresser's online review of the science, called "Why Eating Meat Is Good for You."[47] Read the data and decide for yourself. But if I could make any suggestion: Try to avoid relying on inflammatory documentaries or others' interpretation of the science (including mine). Do your own research.

FOOD FIX: ADAPTING FOOD SYSTEMS TO CLIMATE CHANGE

The data is clear: Our food system as a whole is the number one cause of and the number one solution to climate change. The worse the environmental degradation becomes, the harder it will be to grow crops in hotter, more unstable climate conditions. The faster we can transform the food system, the better we will be in terms of buffering the effects of climate chaos.

It may seem complex to transform agriculture. And it is. We need overall change of the economic, political, and agricultural systems that cause environmental destruction. We need to build systems that can address regeneration of soil, water, climate, biodiversity, and human communities. Luckily, efforts are already under way.

You may have heard about Project Drawdown, a quantified study of ninety-three of the most effective solutions to climate change. Because no other plan has been proposed, my friend Paul Hawken started Project Drawdown to change the climate narrative from doom and gloom and to focus on solutions that currently exist. *Drawdown: The Most Comprehensive Plan Ever Proposed to Reverse Global Warming* lays out all the solutions that are scientifically established. This is not just about slowing emissions, converting to renewable energy, climate mitigation, or carbon taxes or credits, which are most of the solutions proposed in the Paris Accord. Those measures are necessary but not sufficient. What's required is literally to massively reduce or draw down carbon from the atmosphere.

Project Drawdown collected proven, data-driven, economically viable, commonly available solutions that remove carbon from the atmosphere while saving billions of dollars, far offsetting the costs of implementing the solutions. Nothing new needs to be invented, though innovation will drive more solutions over time.

Hawken brought together a team of seventy scientists from twenty-two countries to analyze the data and mathematically modeled the most effective ways to reduce GHG emissions as well as take carbon out of the atmosphere and put it back into the soil. Each solution is measured by gigatons of CO_2 reduced, the cost to implement, and the billions saved. Guess what tops the list: Though we also need to draw down fossil fuel extraction worldwide while scaling up renewable energy, food-related solutions collectively were the number one solution to reverse global warming.

Project Drawdown outlines the food-based strategies that collectively will make the biggest difference for human and planetary health.[48]

- Support regenerative agriculture, optimizing farmland irrigation and managed grazing, which is estimated to reduce CO_2 by 23 gigatons and save $1.93 trillion on an investment of $57 billion.

■ Shift agriculture to support a plant-rich diet that is ideally regeneratively grown (which doesn't mean going vegan, just eating mostly plants).

■ Restore depleted farmland and protect the Amazon rain forest from expanding cattle ranching and monocrop soy production for CAFOs. Deforestation is also driven by land speculation because land without trees is worth 100 to 200 times more than land with forest.

■ Address food waste, including mandated food composting. Composting addresses food waste while improving soil health.

■ Reduce fertilizer use and improve nutrient management to draw down 1.8 gigatons of CO_2 and save farmers $102 billion.

■ Improve rice cultivation (which now accounts for 10 percent of GHG emissions and 19 to 29 percent of global methane emissions).

■ Intercrop trees and crops to reduce inputs and create healthier crops and higher yields.

■ Develop silvopasture, lands that integrate trees with pastures for cattle or livestock that forage in the forests.

■ Scale no-till farming and conservation agriculture.

■ Plant more tropical staple food trees such as avocados, coconuts, and tree legumes to provide food and sequester carbon.

■ Create government financial incentives for new enzyme and algal technologies that greatly reduce methane emissions from cows.

All these practices have been scientifically quantified in both cost savings and gigatons of carbon that would be reduced.

ENDING FOOD WASTE: A SOLUTION FOR HUNGER AND CLIMATE CHANGE

Imagine throwing away a third of your paycheck. Ridiculous, right? Well, somewhere between a third and a half of the food we grow does not make it from the farm to your fork or your belly. To grow just the food that we waste in the United States, it would take 780 million pounds of pesticides and 4.2 trillion gallons of water on 30 million acres of cropland.[49] To grow all the food we waste *around the world*—about

1.3 billion pounds' worth[50]—it would take the entire landmass of China![51] And the loss of all that food costs our economy $2.6 trillion a year, or about 4 percent of global world product.[52]

This is an obvious waste of resources at every stage. Think of the labor, seeds, water, energy, land, fertilizer, and money that end up in the landfill. Even worse, when this wasted food sits in the landfill, it undergoes anaerobic decomposition (decomposition without oxygen) and generates methane gas—a powerful GHG. If you are worried about cow burps, you should be much more worried about the consequences of your veggies ending up in a landfill. The current food we waste is responsible for roughly *8 percent* of global emissions;[53] if food waste were a country, it would be the third-largest emitter of GHGs, just after the United States and China.

The new UN Sustainable Development Goals have called for cutting food waste in half by 2030.[54] Food waste can happen because prices are too low and farmers leave food to rot in the fields because it is not worth selling even though it is perfectly good. Food waste can also come from food that is ugly, misshapen, or not "perfect," like the 800 million pounds of sun-bleached watermelons that are thrown out every year.[55] Food service companies, restaurants, retailers, and consumers waste food at each step, and much ends up in landfills. Grocery chains police their garbage to make sure dumpster divers don't get their slightly overripe food—which, by the way, is still safe to eat. Restaurants overorder to be sure not to run out of anything and disappoint their customers.

It is true that rich and poor countries waste food for different reasons and need different solutions; while poor countries struggle with lack of refrigeration, poor roads and infrastructure, heat, humidity, and lack of proper packaging, they waste almost no food once it enters the home. But rich countries throw out massive quantities of food for reasons closer to inconvenience and poor planning. Americans throw out 35 percent of the food *in their fridge*. "Best by" and "sell by" dates are unintuitively not related to food safety but to when the food will *taste* best, which only confuses customers and leads to massive food waste.

Illustratively, a family of four throws away on average, $1,800 in food every year,[56] and in the United States we spend $218 billion a year, or 1.3 percent of our GDP, growing, processing, transporting, and disposing of food that is never eaten.[57] We have more than enough food to feed all 8.3 billion humans.[58] We even grow enough food for the projected 9.8 billion. But more than 40 percent (some estimate more!) is wasted at every step in the food chain.[59]

METABOLIC FOOD WASTE: HOW THE OBESITY EPIDEMIC CONTRIBUTES TO CLIMATE CHANGE

Is there an environmental and climate cost to obesity? It turns out the answer is yes, and it's a big cost. Ten percent of the world's population doesn't have enough food to eat, while 30 percent of the population is overweight. Big Food and Big Ag have produced about 500 calories more a day per person in the United States than in the 1970s, and we have eaten them. That's about 170 billion extra calories a day just in the United States. The energy, water, and soil needed, and GHGs produced, in growing all that excess food (which makes us sick and fat and has been pushed on us by the food industry) globally equates to about 140 gigatons of carbon a year.[60] To put that in perspective, the total annual emissions of CO_2 from the fossil fuel industry is 9.7 gigatons. The explosion of obesity across the globe, it turns out, is not only damaging human health but also driving climate change.

For a quick reference guide on the Food Fixes and resources to help you restore our natural resources and promote regenerative agriculture, go to www.foodfixuncensored.com.

THE FUTURE OF FOOD: SUSTENANCE OR SURVIVAL?

Facing the facts of our food system is sobering. But after years of research and after speaking to dozens of experts, scientists, and policy-makers about the solutions, I am left with a sense of hope and possibility. Understanding the problems and challenges we face sets the foundation for the solutions. It is also the beginning of reimagining a food system that provides real, whole, nutrient-dense food across the globe, address-ing hunger and obesity. A food system that saves trillions of wasted dollars every year that could be redirected to solving our most intracta-ble problems of disease, poverty, violence, lack of education, and social injustice. A food system that restores ecosystems, builds soil, protects our scarce water resources, reduces pollution, increases biodiversity, and reverses climate change. A food system that builds rather than destroys communities. A food system that is not extractive and destruc-tive to everything that matters but is restorative and regenerative. A food system that is redemptive rather than rapacious.

The inspiration I found during my investigation for this book led me to create a nonprofit and lobbying entity designed to counter the dark forces of the Toxic Triad and beyond. For too long, the good guys had no repre-sentation in Washington, and I knew that had to change. Americans deserve an advocate—someone fighting for our health, our children's futures, and a food system that prioritizes people over corporate profits. It is time to push back against the corruption that repeatedly puts industry bot-tom lines above public well-being.

A DOCTOR GOES TO WASHINGTON

In the five years since I wrote the first edition of this book, some really exciting progress has emerged.

While the release of the 1.0 version of this book in March 2020 was sadly eclipsed by a far noisier public health crisis—COVID-19—we still managed to pull together a pretty exciting feat. We launched a nonprofit as an education and advocacy campaign committed to fighting the chronic disease epidemic in the United States. Our work is designed to educate policymakers and the public about the root causes of illness and advocate for systemic solutions from field to fork. We are long past due to rethink how we produce and consume food by incentivizing regenerative organic agriculture and realizing the potential of food as medicine.

We set up this initiative to help us advance our proposals to clean up America's health care, food system, and agricultural complex. Though this has been a massive undertaking, we have made significant strides in educating influential members of Congress, along with coauthoring bills and proposals to reform some of our most egregiously anti-health policies.

We were just getting started when in the spring of 2021, on a Sunday afternoon overlooking the ocean at my COVID escape in Maui, I got an unexpected call from a senator from New Jersey. Cory Booker had read *Food Fix* and told me that, categorically, it was the most important book he'd ever read. He believed in the movement I was launching, and he wanted to help.

Booker—an open-minded, high-integrity politician—indicated that he was willing to work with all political persuasions to move the needle on our most pressing social issues. By then, he was cutting his teeth as an advocate for comprehensive food and health policy reforms, focusing on creating a more equitable and sustainable food system in the United States. Recognizing the urgency of the issues outlined in my book, he leveraged his network to help drive meaningful conversations and advance solutions that prioritize public health and food security.

Because much of this book critiques the political-industrial complex, I feel it is important to also highlight the leaders working to change the system from within. Senator Cory Booker has been a dedicated advocate for a healthier, more sustainable food system, championing policy reforms that align with many of the issues raised in this book—often independently of my work, but also certainly informed by it.

In 2020, Booker introduced the Farm System Reform Act to address the dominance of large-scale CAFOs. The legislation proposes a moratorium on new CAFOs and aims to phase out existing large operations by 2040, promoting more sustainable and ethical farming practices. In 2021, as chair of the Senate Subcommittee on Food and Nutrition, Specialty Crops, Organics, and Research, he led hearings on the concept of "Food as Medicine," emphasizing nutrition's role in health care.

With our support, Booker has called on the FDA to use its authority to regulate ultraprocessed foods, highlighting their direct link to America's worsening nutrition crisis. Most recently, in September 2024, he introduced the Safe School Meals Act, aimed at protecting children from harmful toxins in school meals. The legislation proposes limits on heavy metals, bans certain pesticide residues, and calls for the reassessment of food additives, including artificial dyes linked to behavioral and developmental health issues. It also seeks to eliminate harmful substances like PFAS, phthalates, and bisphenols from school meal packaging.

And as a true plot twist, Senator Roger Marshall, the Kansas Republican and former physician I cited earlier due to his conflicts of interest, has recently demonstrated a notable shift in his legislative focus by founding the Make America Healthy Again (MAHA) Caucus. This bipartisan initiative aims to address critical health issues such as nutrition, access to affordable, nutrient-dense foods, and the root causes of chronic diseases.

While, historically, Senator Marshall's campaigns received substantial contributions from the food and beverage industry, his recent actions indicate a departure from industry-aligned positions. By launching the MAHA Caucus, Senator Marshall has aligned himself with advocates for public health reforms, including Robert F. Kennedy Jr., the new secretary of Health and Human Services. This collaboration underscores a commitment to policies that prioritize health initiatives over previous industry affiliations, as well as a growing bipartisan effort to tackle pressing health challenges.

Having allies in Congress who oversee food and nutrition policy, specialty crops, and organics is invaluable. Senators Booker and Marshall, among many others, continue to push for healthier food systems and support regenerative farming practices, amplifying the movement to transform the way we grow, distribute, and consume food.

PROGRESS REPORT: TRANSFORMING FOOD POLICY FOR A HEALTHIER FUTURE

So, with Cory's help, among many, *many* others, we have gradually made strides with members of Congress on both sides of the aisle.

I have begun working with Florida's representative, Vern Buchanan, who serves as the vice chair of the House Ways and Means Committee (and the chair of the Health Subcommittee)—which has jurisdiction over health care, welfare, Social Security, and Medicare, among others. Through his support, we have made inroads with many key members of Congress who are equally motivated to address our crushing health and food crisis.

The momentum for food and health policy reform has never been stronger, and the past year has been a landmark period in driving legislative, regulatory, and cultural change. From shaping national policy to engaging top government officials, we are making significant strides toward a food system that prioritizes health, sustainability, and equity. Following are some of our major wins in the past few years.

Major Policy Achievements

Bringing Food to the Center of Government Action

- Landmark Government Accountability Office (GAO) report issued on improving federal diet-related programs, recognizing the need for systemic change.
- Legislation enacted unifying more than 200 diet-related programs across twenty-one federal agencies, ensuring a coordinated approach to food policy.
- Historic federal Food as Medicine pilot program created and funded, integrating nutrition into health care.
- Appropriations legislation passed emphasizing nutrition and securing funding for Food as Medicine programs.
- First-ever Preventive Health and Wellness Caucus established in Congress to drive legislative action on food, nutrition, and wellness.
- Passage of a Medicare medically tailored meal delivery demonstration program, bringing nutrition-based treatment into federal health care.
- Defense legislation passed, recognizing obesity as a disease and improving provider training on nutrition.

Regulatory and Policy Advancements

- Launch of USDA Climate-Smart Agriculture and Forestry Partnership, funding grants, incentives, and research for regenerative farming.
- Development of Creating Reduced Overhead for Producers (CROP), a Farm Bill reform package supporting regenerative and organic farmers.
- Engagement with lawmakers on reforms advancing regenerative and organic agriculture.
- Formal regulatory comments submitted, and educational outreach launched on federal dietary guidelines reform.
- Engagement with FDA officials on front-of-package food labeling, food additives, and GRAS regulations improving consumer awareness of food choices and improving our food supply.

High-Level Government Engagement

- Dr. Hyman invited to the White House Conference on Hunger, Nutrition, and Health, a pivotal event shaping the future of food policy.
- Food Fix Listening Session hosted—producing detailed policy recommendations for the White House.
- Meetings with the surgeon general and top Health and Human Services and USDA officials on embedding nutrition in health care delivery.
- Submission of formal recommendations to federal agencies and congressional committees on priority topics such as ultraprocessed food regulation, ending ultraprocessed food marketing, regenerative agriculture, and food-as-medicine programs.

Advancing Public Awareness and Advocacy

- Ultra-Processed Food: Eating Ourselves to Death initiative launched, targeting one of the biggest drivers of chronic disease.
- Bipartisan letter to ACGME (Accreditation Council for Graduate Medical Education) urging clinician training on nutrition in medical treatment, to which they subsequently agreed.
- Strategic media placement and social outreach amplifying the dangers of ultraprocessed food and the power of real nutrition.
- Dr. Hyman testified before the Ways and Means Health Subcommittee, exposing America's food crisis and charting a path forward.

As of August 2025, meaningful momentum has continued to build. The US Department of Health and Human Services (HHS) has begun reshaping federal food policy in ways that reflect a growing national awareness: What we eat is fueling not just chronic disease but deep health inequities. In a major shift, the FDA has turned its attention to food additives—especially synthetic dyes increasingly linked to developmental and behavioral issues in children—signaling a more precautionary approach to what ends up in our food supply.

At the same time, HHS has launched a groundbreaking interagency initiative between the FDA and NIH to supercharge nutrition science. The goal is to close the gap between emerging research and regulatory action, and ensure future policies are grounded in robust, up-to-date evidence.

Meanwhile, the FDA has *finally* issued a formal Request for Information (RFI) on ultraprocessed foods, laying the groundwork for potential new definitions, warning labels, or limits based not just on nutrient profiles, but on how food is made. And as the Dietary Guidelines for Americans go through their latest overhaul, there is a clear shift toward transparency and inclusivity, and a reckoning with the chronic disease burden affecting millions. Together, these changes represent more than incremental progress—they signal a cultural and political tipping point where nutrition policy may finally start catching up with modern science and public demand.

LOOKING AHEAD

Working alongside members of Congress I might never have crossed paths with has been eye-opening. Regardless of party lines, we all recognize that this issue transcends politics. The future of our children and our nation hinges on the state of our health, and that's not Democratic or Republican—it's a fundamental, bipartisan truth.

As Robert F. Kennedy Jr. states, "We must love our children more than we hate each other."

Indeed, chronic disease and the related mental health epidemic affect every single American, regardless of political affiliation, ideology, beliefs, or sect—and the solutions *must* be apolitical. Your body doesn't have a political ideology. I believe deeply that we must not sacrifice the mission of healing the health of our nation at the behest of politics; rather, I see an opportunity for this cause, this deeply equalizing, humanizing cause, to become a source of unity and compassion for our country. It transcends ideology, and I hope we can see the forest through the trees on this one such that we can collaborate with opposing parties.

The chronic disease epidemic and the mental health crisis are issues that need all voices at the table, and I look forward to extending this dialogue further, welcoming anyone who is willing to step up and engage. I believe and hope that it is one of the few equalizing forces that can withstand the pressure of political rhetoric.

The groundwork laid this year is just the beginning. As we continue pushing for legislative victories, medical training reforms, and corporate accountability, the focus remains on shifting the national food system from one that fuels disease to one that fosters health and resilience.

With bipartisan support growing, regenerative agriculture gaining traction, and nutrition becoming a mainstream health care priority, the future of food is finally changing—for the better. This is the moment to accelerate progress and demand a food system that works for people, not profits.

But we are not just talking about policy. We are building a movement. And to make real, lasting change, we need you.

One of the biggest lessons we've learned in DC is that even the most engaged, curious, and well-intentioned leaders in Congress are limited by one thing: you, their constituents. Their careers, their decisions, their votes—they all depend on the voices of the people they represent.

That's where YOU come in.

If we want a food system that nourishes instead of poisons, if we want health over profit, if we want to reclaim our right to real, clean food—we have to demand it. Loudly. Relentlessly. Unapologetically.

That means knocking on the doors of your representatives and demanding that they listen. That means writing, calling, and showing up. That means marching in the streets, refusing to be ignored, and making it impossible for them to turn away from this crisis.

We are at a crossroads. Do we accept a system designed to keep us sick and dependent, or do we fight for something better? The power is in our hands—but only if we use it. Check out the Food Fix Action Guide for more on how to get involved in an initiative that's meaningful to you: www.foodfixactionguide.com.

Let's rise up. Let's take action. Let's make history.

Acknowledgments

This book was inspired by the work of an endless list of individuals dedicated to transforming the food system starting from the farm and extending all the way to our forks and beyond. There are thousands of people who are fighting this good fight along with me, and I would like to take this opportunity to thank them, specifically those who helped to bring this labor of love to life. And to any whom I didn't mention, all the tireless workers, warriors, farmers, health activists, food leaders, and voices of truth, without your inspiration, teaching, and support, this book would never have come to be: Thank you.

I'd like to thank my patients, who will always be my greatest teachers and the reason behind my passion for creating a happier and healthier world.

I'd also like to thank my book team: Andrea Vinley Converse for her insights and for keeping this project organized while constantly keeping my vision in mind. Anahad O'Connor was instrumental to this book in many ways, including providing a deep understanding of food politics and policy. My daughter, Rachel Hess, MD, who gathered research and provided insight into the effects of our food system on the environment and workers' rights.

And of course, my friends Drs. Dariush Mozaffarian, David Ludwig, Robert Lustig, Aseem Malhotra, and Chris van Tulleken, whose rigorous science, public health advocacy, food activism, and political vision for a better future of health for all of us have guided my way for a long, long time.

A special thank-you to everyone we interviewed and who contributed their wealth of knowledge to this project. Lisel Loy, Barry Popkin,

Chris Kresser, Gunhild Stordalen, Congressman Vern Buchanan, Tim Ryan, Jim McGovern, Congresswoman Chellie Pingree, Senators Cory Booker and Roger Marshall, Larry Summers, Dan Glickman, Ann Veneman, Michele Simon, Jerold Mande, Laura Schmidt, John Robbins, Lance Price, Steven Druker, Kelly Brownell, Nina Teicholz, John Ioannidis, Vani Hari, Pamela Koch, Hawk Newsome, Navina Khanna, Dr. David Montgomery, Paul Hawken, Walter Robb, William Li, Leah Pennimen, Kimbal Musk, Christiana Musk, Danielle Nierenberg, Kavita Shukla, Mark Bittman, Dan Barber, Tom Colicchio, David Wallace-Wells, Sonia Angell, Marco Canora, David Bouley, Thomas Newmark, Rain Henderson, Chilean senator Guido Girardi, Stephen Ritz, Robert Egger, and Ben Simon—thank you for all that you do and allowing us to share it with the world. And a special thank you to Casey and Calley Means for carrying the torch and making a better world possible.

I'd also like to thank my teams at Function Health and the UltraWellness Center. I especially want to thank Denise Morrisey for her relentless commitment to improving our health care and food system and now as the First Lady of West Virginia for her mission to make West Virginia the healthiest state in America and David Bryant for being a fierce ally at Food Fix along with the rest of the Food Fix team. These teams are dedicated to transforming health care, and I am so grateful to get to work with every single one of these folks in our joint mission.

A huge thank-you to the Hyman Health team. Thank you for making my life so much easier and for nurturing and expanding our platform so that we can spread our message far and wide. And an extra-special thank-you to Meredith Jones, who helps me keep all of my projects and life in order so that I get to do what I love to do every single day, and Taylor Groff, for her support with research.

All of my success over the last twenty years would not have been possible without the support and guidance of my publishing team, who believed in me and gave me the chance to publish so many books. My editor, Tracy Behar, made every word and story better and was beyond patient with me. Richard Pine, my agent, made all my dreams come true. My team at Little, Brown is fabulously talented at getting my books out in the world. Without them, my hopes and dreams would still be in my head and not making the impact they are. Thank you.

And finally, I'd like to thank my wife, my Human, the CEO of Hyman Health, and the coauthor of this revised book, Brianna Bella–Hyman. Thank you for your unfettered support, for showing up through it all, and for being my fiercest advocate and ally. Thank you for being *all the things*. I really, seriously, couldn't do it without you.

Notes

INTRODUCTION

1. World Health Organization. (2024, December 23). "Noncommunicable Diseases." https://www.who.int/news-room/fact-sheets/detail/noncommunicable-diseases.
2. Ibid.
3. World Health Organization. (2025, May 7). "Obesity and Overweight." https://www.who.int/news-room/fact-sheets/detail/obesity-and-overweight.
4. Hayes TO, Gillian S. (2020, September 10). "Chronic Disease in the United States: A Worsening Health and Economic Crisis." American Action Forum. https://www.americanactionforum.org/research/chronic-disease-in-the-united-states-a-worsening-health-and-economic-crisis.
5. Office of People Analytics, Department of Defense. (2022, March). *Qualified Military Available (QMA): Technical Report.* OPA Report No. 2022-085. https://www.esd.whs.mil/Portals/54/Documents/FOID/Reading%20Room/Personnel_Related/23-F-1060_QMA_Technical_Report_Mar_2022.pdf.
6. Centers for Disease Control and Prevention. (2022, July). "Unfit to Serve: Obesity and Physical Inactivity Are Impacting National Security." https://www.cdc.gov/physicalactivity/downloads/unfit-to-serve-062322-508.pdf.
7. World Health Organization. (2005, August 11). "The Bangkok Charter for Health Promotion in a Globalized World." https://www.afro.who.int/sites/default/files/2017-06/hpr%20The%20Bangkok%20Charter.pdf.
8. World Health Organization. (2023, March 21). "Commercial Determinants of Health." https://www.who.int/news-room/fact-sheets/detail/commercial-determinants-of-health.
9. World Health Organization. (n.d.). "SAFER: Raise Prices on Alcohol Through Excise Taxes and Pricing Policies." https://www.who.int/initiatives/SAFER/pricing-policies. Accessed August 19, 2025.
10. Planet Tracker. (2022, December 14). "How Much Is Your Food Worth?" https://planet-tracker.org/how-much-is-your-food-worth/.
11. Market Research Future. (2025, August.) "Food Processing Market Summary." https://www.marketresearchfuture.com/reports/food-processing-market-8588; International Monetary Fund. (2024, January). "World Economic Outlook Update: Moderating Inflation and Steady Growth Open Path to Soft Landing." https://www.imf.org/en/Publications/WEO/Issues/2024/01/30/world-economic-outlook-update-january-2024.
12. Philpott T. (2012, August 15). "80 Percent of Public Schools Have Contracts with Coke or Pepsi." *Mother Jones.* https://www.motherjones.com/food/2012/08/schools-limit-campus-junk-food-have-lower-obesity-rates/.
13. Morgan K. (2025). *Serving the Public: The Good Food Revolution in Schools, Hospitals, and Prisons.* Manchester University Press.
14. Koons K. (2025, July 24). "Federal Agencies Say Ultraprocessed Foods 'Driving' Chronic Disease Rates." *Iowa Capital Dispatch.* https://iowacapitaldispatch.com/briefs/federal-agencies-say-ultraprocessed-foods-driving-chronic-disease-rates/.

15. Organisation for Economic Co-operation and Development. (n.d.). "Health Spending." https://www.oecd.org/en/data/indicators/health-spending.html. Accessed June 26, 2025.

16. World Health Organization. (n.d.). "Obesity Among Adults, BMI ≥ 30, Prevalence (Age-Standardized Estimate) (%). https://www.who.int/data/gho/data/indicators/indicator-details /GHO/prevalence-of-obesity-among-adults-bmi-=-30-(age-standardized-estimate)-(-). Accessed June 27, 2025.

17. Murphy SL, Kochanek KD, Xu J, et al. (2024, December). "Mortality in the United States, 2023." NCHS Data Brief No. 521. National Center for Health Statistics. https://www.cdc .gov/nchs/products/databriefs/db521.htm.

18. World Health Organization. (n.d.). "Number of COVID-19 Deaths Reported to WHO." https://data.who.int/dashboards/covid19/deaths. Accessed June 27, 2025.

19. US Department of Agriculture, Food and Nutrition Service. (n.d.). "Supplemental Nutrition Assistance Program (SNAP)." https://www.fns.usda.gov/snap. Accessed August 19, 2025.

20. USDA Department of Agriculture, Food and Nutrition Service. (2016, November). "Foods Typically Purchased by Supplemental Nutrition Assistance Program (SNAP) Households (Summary)." https://fns-prod.azureedge.us/sites/default/files/ops/SNAPFoodsTypicallyPurchased -Summary.pdf.

21. US Department of Health and Human Services. (n.d.). "Celebrating Big Wins of the Trump Administration." https://www.hhs.gov/hhs-big-wins-maha/index.html. Accessed August 19, 2025.

CHAPTER 1

1. Waters H, Graf M. (2018, August.) "The Costs of Chronic Disease in the U.S." Milken Institute. https://milkeninstitute.org/sites/default/files/reports-pdf/ChronicDiseases-HighRes -FINAL_0.pdf.

2. Trading Economics. (n.d.). "World GDP." https://tradingeconomics.com/world/gdp. Accessed January 25, 2025.

3. Waters H, Graf M. (2018, August.) "The Costs of Chronic Disease in the U.S." Milken Institute. https://milkeninstitute.org/sites/default/files/reports-pdf/ChronicDiseases-HighRes -FINAL_0.pdf.

4. Lane MM, Gamage E, Du S, et al. (2024, February 28). "Ultra-Processed Food Exposure and Adverse Health Outcomes: Umbrella Review of Epidemiological Meta-Analyses." *BMJ*. 384:e077310. https://doi.org/10.1136/bmj-2023-077310.

5. Department of the Treasury. (n.d.) "How Much Revenue Has the U.S. Government Collected This Year?" https://fiscaldata.treasury.gov/americas-finance-guide/government -revenue/. Accessed August 19, 2025.

6. Centers for Medicare and Medicaid Services. (2024, November). *CMS Financial Report: Fiscal Year 2024 Financial Report*. Publication no. 12074. https://www.cms.gov/files/document /cms-financial-report-fiscal-year-2024.pdf.

7. Centers for Disease Control and Prevention. (2024, July 12). "Fast Facts: Health and Economic Costs of Chronic Conditions." https://www.cdc.gov/chronic-disease/data-research /facts-stats/index.html.

8. Centers for Medicare and Medicaid Services. (2025, June 24). "NHE Fact Sheet." https:// www.cms.gov/data-research/statistics-trends-and-reports/national-health-expenditure -data/nhe-fact-sheet.

9. Centers for Medicare and Medicaid Services. (2024, December 18). "Historical." https:// www.cms.gov/data-research/statistics-trends-and-reports/national-health-expenditure -data/historical.

10. GBD 2017 Diet Collaborators. (2019, May 11). "Health Effects of Dietary Risks in 195 Countries, 1990–2017: A Systematic Analysis for the Global Burden of Disease Study 2017." *The Lancet*. 393(10184):P1958–72. https://doi.org/10.1016/S0140-6736(19)30041-8.

11. World Obesity Foundation. (n.d.) "Prevalence of Obesity." https://www.worldobesity.org/about/about-obesity/prevalence-of-obesity. Accessed August 19, 2025.

12. Centers for Disease Control and Prevention. (2024, July 12). "Fast Facts: Health and Economic Costs of Chronic Conditions." https://www.cdc.gov/chronic-disease/data-research/facts-stats/index.html.

13. Centers for Medicare and Medicaid Services. (2025, June 24). "NHE Fact Sheet." https://www.cms.gov/data-research/statistics-trends-and-reports/national-health-expenditure-data/nhe-fact-sheet.

14. Centers for Medicare and Medicaid Services. (2004, January 8). "Health Care Spending Reaches $1.6 Trillion in 2002." https://www.cms.gov/newsroom/press-releases/health-care-spending-reaches-16-trillion-2002.

15. Waters H, Graf M. (2018, August.) "The Costs of Chronic Disease in the U.S." Milken Institute. https://milkeninstitute.org/sites/default/files/reports-pdf/ChronicDiseases-HighRes-FINAL_0.pdf.

16. Ansah JP, Chiu C-T. (2022). "Projecting the Chronic Disease Burden Among the Adult Population in the United States Using a Multi-State Population Model." *Frontiers in Public Health* 10. https://www.frontiersin.org/journals/public-health/articles/10.3389/fpubh.2022.1082183/full.

17. Watson KB, Wiltz JL, Nhim K, et al. (2025, April 17). "Trends in Multiple Chronic Conditions Among US Adults, by Life Stage, Behavioral Risk Factor Surveillance System, 2013–2023." *Preventing Chronic Disease* 22:E15. https://doi.org/10.5888/pcd22.240539.

18. Emmerich SD, Fryar CD, Stierman B, et al. (2024, September). "Obesity and Severe Obesity Prevalence in Adults: United States, August 2021–August 2023." NCHS Data Brief no. 508. National Center for Health Statistics, Centers for Disease Control and Prevention. https://www.cdc.gov/nchs/products/databriefs/db508.htm.

19. Fryar CD, Carroll MD, Ogden CL. (2014, September). "Prevalence of Overweight, Obesity, and Extreme Obesity Among Adults: United States, 1960–1962 Through 2011–2012." National Center for Health Statistics, Centers for Disease Control and Prevention. https://www.cdc.gov/nchs/data/hestat/obesity_adult_11_12/obesity_adult_11_12.pdf.

20. National Agricultural Statistics Service, US Department of Agriculture. (2024, March). "Farms and Farmland." ACH22-3. https://www.nass.usda.gov/Publications/Highlights/2024/Census22_HL_FarmsFarmland.pdf.

21. Austin DA. (2023, November 7)."Trends in Mandatory Spending." Congressional Research Service, R44641. https://sgp.fas.org/crs/misc/R44641.pdf.

22. Levit MR, Austin DA, Stupak JM. (2015, March 18). "Mandatory Spending Since 1962." Congressional Research Service, RL33074. https://fas.org/sgp/crs/misc/RL33074.pdf.

23. Centers for Medicare and Medicaid Services. (2025, June 24). "NHE Fact Sheet." https://www.cms.gov/data-research/statistics-trends-and-reports/national-health-expenditure-data/nhe-fact-sheet.

24. Centers for Medicare and Medicaid Services. (2024, June 12). "CMS Releases 2023–2032 National Health Expenditure Projections." https://www.cms.gov/newsroom/press-releases/cms-releases-2023-2032-national-health-expenditure-projections.

25. Department of the Treasury. (n.d.) "How Much Revenue Has the U.S. Government Collected This Year?" https://fiscaldata.treasury.gov/americas-finance-guide/government-revenue/. Accessed August 19, 2025.

26. Hyman M. (2024, September 18). "Written Statement of Mark Hyman, M.D." Testimony before the House Ways and Means Health Subcommittee. https://www.congress.gov/118/meeting/house/117660/witnesses/HHRG-118-WM02-Wstate-HymanM-20240918.pdf.

27. World Economic Forum. (2013). *Global Risks 2013: Eighth Edition.* https://www3.weforum.org/docs/WEF_GlobalRisks_Report_2013.pdf.

28. Finlay S. (2004, March 1). "GM Is Getting Sick of High Health-Care Costs." WardsAuto. https://www.wardsauto.com/general-motors/gm-is-getting-sick-of-high-health-care-costs.

29. Kowitt B. (2010, June 7). "Starbucks CEO: 'We Spend More on Health Care than Coffee.'" CNN Money. https://web.archive.org/web/20250316104720/https://money.cnn.com/2010/06/07/news/companies/starbucks_schultz_healthcare.fortune/index.htm.

30. Lobstein T, Jackson-Leach R, Powis J, et al. (2023, March). *World Obesity Atlas 2023.* World Obesity Federation. https://s3-eu-west-1.amazonaws.com/wof-files/World_Obesity_Atlas_2023_Report.pdf.

31. Dobbs R, Sawers C, Thompson F, et al. (2014, November 1). "How the World Could Better Fight Obesity." McKinsey Global Institute. https://www.mckinsey.com/industries/healthcare/our-insights/how-the-world-could-better-fight-obesity.

32. Higuchi M. (2010, July 28). "Lifestyle Diseases: Access to Chronic Disease Care in Low- and Middle-Income Countries." *UN Chronicle.* https://www.un.org/en/chronicle/article/lifestyle-diseases-access-chronic-disease-care-low-and-middle-income-countries.

33. World Health Organization. (2017). "The Double Burden of Malnutrition: Policy Brief." WHO/NMH/NHD/17.3. https://iris.who.int/bitstream/handle/10665/255413/WHO-NMH-NHD-17.3-eng.pdf.

34. Rockefeller Foundation. (2021, July). "True Cost of Food: Measuring What Matters to Transform the U.S. Food System." https://www.rockefellerfoundation.org/wp-content/uploads/2021/07/True-Cost-of-Food-Full-Report-Final.pdf.

35. Environmental Protection Agency. (2016, February 22). "Just the Facts—Cleaning Up Hudson River PCBs." https://www3.epa.gov/hudson/just_facts_08_04.htm.

36. Riverkeeper. (2024, June 28). "Honoring Our Foundation in Science." https://www.riverkeeper.org/news-and-events/news-and-updates/honoring-our-foundation-in-science.

37. Reuters. (2018, October 1). "New York sues EPA over GE's Hudson River PCB cleanup", https://www.reuters.com/article/business/environment/new-york-sues-epa-over-ges-hudson-river-pcb-cleanup-idUSKCN1VB1YJ.

38. Mindock C. (2023, June 23). "3M Reaches Tentative $10.3 Billion Deal over U.S. 'Forever Chemicals' Claims." Reuters. https://www.reuters.com/legal/3m-reaches-tentative-103-billion-deal-over-us-forever-chemicals-claims-2023-06-22/.

39. Mindock C. (2023, June 2). "Chemical Makers Settle PFAS-Related Claims for $1.19 Billion." Reuters. https://www.reuters.com/business/chemical-makers-reach-pfas-related-settlement-us-2023-06-02/.

40. DuPont. (2023, June 2). "Chemours, DuPont, and Corteva Reach Comprehensive PFAS Settlement with U.S. Water Systems." Press release. https://www.dupont.com/news/chemours-dupont-and-corteva-reach-comprehensive-pfas-settlement-with-us-water-systems.html.

41. Eilperin J. (2004, September 10). "DuPont Settles Water-Contamination Lawsuit." *Washington Post.* https://www.washingtonpost.com/archive/business/2004/09/10/dupont-settles-water-contamination-lawsuit/a66ab42a-c24b-4d0d-b13e-daaf17758858/.

42. Nair AS. (2017, February 13). "DuPont Settles Lawsuits over Leak of Chemical Used to Make Teflon." Reuters. https://www.reuters.com/article/business/dupont-settles-lawsuits-over-leak-of-chemical-used-to-make-teflon-idUSKBN15S18T/.

43. Chase R. (2006, April 19). "Lawsuit Alleges DuPont Contamination of New Jersey Drinking Water." Associated Press. https://www.liebermanblecher.com/aop/toxic-torts-including-drinking-water-litigation/lieberman-blecher-serves-as-new-jersey-counsel-in-a-class-action/.

44. Lehner P. (2017, August 16). "The Hidden Costs of Food." *HuffPost*. https://www.huffpost.com/entry/the-hidden-costs-of-food_b_11492520.

45. Pimentel D. (2005). "Environmental and Economic Costs of the Application of Pesticides Primarily in the United States." In Peshin R, Dhawan AK (Eds.), *Integrated Pest Management: Innovation-Development Process*. Springer. https://scispace.com/pdf/environmental-and-economic-costs-of-the-application-of-yii0xqz03v.pdf.

46. Pimentel D. (2005). "Environmental and Economic Costs of the Application of Pesticides Primarily in the United States." In Peshin R, Dhawan AK (Eds.), *Integrated Pest Management: Innovation-Development Process*. Springer. https://scispace.com/pdf/environmental-and-economic-costs-of-the-application-of-yii0xqz03v.pdf.

47. Gurian-Sherman D. (2008). "CAFOs Uncovered: The Untold Costs of Confined Animal Feeding Operations." Union of Concerned Scientists. https://www.ucs.org/sites/default/files/2019-10/cafos-uncovered-full-report.pdf.

48. Ibid.

49. Hayes TO, Kerska K. (2021, November 3). "Primer: Agriculture Subsidies and Their Influence on the Composition of U.S. Food Supply and Consumption." American Action Forum. https://www.americanactionforum.org/research/primer-agriculture-subsidies-and-their-influence-on-the-composition-of-u-s-food-supply-and-consumption/.

50. US Congress. (2024, December 21). American Relief Act, 2025. Pub. L. No. 118-158. https://www.congress.gov/118/plaws/publ158/PLAW-118publ158.pdf.

51. Hook B. (2023, May 31). "Phenomenal Phytoplankton: Scientists Uncover Cellular Process behind Oxygen Production." Scripps Institution of Oceanography. https://scripps.ucsd.edu/news/phenomenal-phytoplankton-scientists-uncover-cellular-process-behind-oxygen-production.

52. World Health Organization. (2023, November 21). "Antimicrobial Resistance." https://www.who.int/news-room/fact-sheets/detail/antimicrobial-resistance.

53. Institute for Economics and Peace. (2020, September 9). "Over One Billion People at Threat of Being Displaced by 2050 Due to Environmental Change, Conflict and Civil Unrest." Press release. https://www.economicsandpeace.org/wp-content/uploads/2020/09/Ecological-Threat-Register-Press-Release-27.08-FINAL.pdf.

54. Swiss Re Institute. (2024, December 5). "Hurricanes, Severe Thunderstorms and Floods Drive Insured Losses Above USD 100 Billion for 5th Consecutive Year, Says Swiss Re Institute." Press release. https://www.swissre.com/press-release/Hurricanes-severe-thunderstorms-and-floods-drive-insured-losses-above-USD-100-billion-for-5th-consecutive-year-says-Swiss-Re-Institute/f8424512-e46b-4db7-a1b1-ad6034306352.

55. Danielle M. (2025, January 13). "AccuWeather Estimates More than $250 Billion in Damages and Economic Loss from LA Wildfires." AccuWeather. https://www.accuweather.com/en/weather-news/accuweather-estimates-more-than-250-billion-in-damages-and-economic-loss-from-la-wildfires/1733821.

56. Romanello M, Walawender M, Hsu S-C, et al. (2024, November 9). "The 2024 Report of the *Lancet* Countdown on Health and Climate Change: Facing Record-Breaking Threats from Delayed Action." *The Lancet* 404(10465):1847–96. https://doi.org/10.1016/S0140-6736(24)01822-1.

57. Intergovernmental Panel on Climate Change. (2023). "Climate Change 2023 Synthesis Report: Summary for Policymakers." https://www.ipcc.ch/report/ar6/syr/downloads/report/IPCC_AR6_SYR_SPM.pdf.

58. Lowe P. (2014, July 16). "Lobbyists of All Kinds Flock to Farm Bill." Investigate Midwest. https://investigatemidwest.org/2014/07/16/lobbyists-of-all-kinds-flock-to-farm-bill/.

59. Bayer AG. (2018, June 7). "Bayer Closes Monsanto Acquisition." https://www.bayer.com/media/en-us/bayer-closes-monsanto-acquisition/.

60. Deconinck K. (2019, February 27). "From Big Six to Big Four: New OECD Study Sheds Light on Concentration and Competition in Seed Markets." Seed World. https://www .seedworld.com/europe/2019/02/27/from-big-six-to-big-four-new-oecd-study -sheds-light-on-concentration-and-competition-in-seed-markets.

61. UN Conference on Trade and Development. (2015, October 5). "Policy, Not Technical Challenges, Is the Real Hurdle for Smallholder Farmers, Says Civil Society." https://unctad .org/news/policy-not-technical-challenges-real-hurdle-smallholder-farmers-says-civil -society.

62. Penn State Extension. (2023, June 6). "Why We Need to Keep Talking about Farm Stress." https://extension.psu.edu/why-we-need-to-keep-talking-about-farm-stress.

63. Lara-Castor L, O'Hearn M, Cudhea F, et al. (2025, January 6). "Burdens of Type 2 Diabetes and Cardiovascular Disease Attributable to Sugar-Sweetened Beverages in 184 Countries." *Nature Medicine* 31:552–64. https://www.nature.com/articles/s41591-024-03345-4.

64. Malik VS, Li Y, Pan A, et al. (2019, March 8). "Long-Term Consumption of Sugar-Sweetened and Artificially Sweetened Beverages and Risk of Mortality in US Adults." *Circulation* 39(18):2113-2125. doi: 10.1161/CIRCULATIONAHA.118.037401.

65. USDA Department of Agriculture, Food and Nutrition Service. (2016, November). "Foods Typically Purchased by Supplemental Nutrition Assistance Program (SNAP) House-holds (Summary)." https://fns-prod.azureedge.us/sites/default/files/ops/SNAPFoodsTypically Purchased-Summary.pdf.

66. Higham A. (2025, January 30). "SNAP Benefits Face Major Change Under New Proposal." *Newsweek*. https://www.newsweek.com/snap-benefits-major-change-fizz-no-act-2022855.

67. Bleich SN, Vercammen KA. (2018, February 20). "The Negative Impact of Sugar-Sweetened Beverages on Children's Health: An Update of the Literature." *BMC Obesity* 5:6. doi:10.1186 /s40608-017-0178-9; Harvard T. H. Chan School of Public Health. (2023, August). "Sugary Drinks." https://www.hsph.harvard.edu/nutritionsource/healthy-drinks/sugary-drinks/.

68. Hayes TO, Kerska K. (2021, November 3). "Primer: Agriculture Subsidies and Their Influ-ence on the Composition of U.S. Food Supply and Consumption." American Action Forum. https://www.americanactionforum.org/research/primer-agriculture-subsidies-and -their-influence-on-the-composition-of-u-s-food-supply-and-consumption/.

69. US Department of Energy. (n.d.). "U.S. Corn Use by Market Year" [dataset]. Alternative Fuels Data Center. https://afdc.energy.gov/data/10340. Accessed June 25, 2025.

70. US Department of Agriculture. (2015, February). "USDA Coexistence Fact Sheets: Corn." https://www.usda.gov/sites/default/files/documents/coexistence-corn-factsheet.pdf.

71. Dickerson M. (2024, May 8). "EPIC Report: Food Stamps: A Culture of Dependency." Economic Policy Innovation Center. https://epicforamerica.org/social-programs/food-stamps -a-culture-of-dependency/.

72. Dickerson M. (2023, July 20). "The Percentage of Americans on Food Stamps Has Doubled Since 2001." Economic Policy Innovation Center. https://epicforamerica.org/social-programs /the-percentage-of-americans-on-food-stamps-has-doubled-since-2001.

73. USAFacts. (n.d.). "How Much Does the Federal Government Spend on SNAP Every Year?" https://usafacts.org/answers/how-much-does-the-federal-government-spend-on-snap -every-year/country/united-states. Accessed June 9, 2025.

74. Mares J. (2022, November 10). "NIH-Funded 'Food Pyramid' Rates Lucky Charms Healthier Than Steak." Pirate Wires. https://www.piratewires.com/p/tufts-food-compass.

75. Global Nutrition Report. "The Burden of Malnutrition at a Glance." https://globalnutrition report.org/resources/nutrition-profiles/north-america/northern-america/united-states -america/. Accessed September 29, 2025.

76. US Supreme Court. (2019, June 24). *Food Marketing Institute v. Argus Leader Media.* 588 US_ (2019). https://www.supremecourt.gov/opinions/18pdf/18-481_5426.pdf.

77. Evans S, Idicula I. (2019). "Food Marking Institute v. Argus Leader Media." Legal Information Institute, Cornell Law School. https://www.law.cornell.edu/supct/cert/18-481.

78. Faria J. (2025, March 25). "Food Advertising in the United States—Statistics and Facts." Statista. https://www.statista.com/topics/2223/food-advertising/.

79. US Government Accountability Office. (2021, August). "Chronic Health Conditions: Federal Strategy Needed to Coordinate Diet-Related Efforts." https://www.gao.gov/assets/gao-21-593.pdf.

80. US Department of Health and Human Services. (2025, March 27). "HHS Announces Transformation to Make America Healthy Again." Press release. https://www.hhs.gov/press-room/hhs-restructuring-doge.html.

CHAPTER 2

1. Javers E, Breuninger K. (2025, January 21). "Trump Announces AI Infrastructure Investment Backed by Oracle, OpenAI and SoftBank." CNBC. https://www.cnbc.com/2025/01/21/trump-ai-openai-oracle-softbank.html.

2. Forbes Breaking News. (2025, January 23). "Larry Ellison: This Is How AI Can Help Create a 'Cancer Vaccine.'" YouTube. https://www.youtube.com/watch?v=ON-uS-S9cDU.

3. Lane MM, Gamage E, Du S, et al. (2024, February 28). "Ultra-Processed Food Exposure and Adverse Health Outcomes: Umbrella Review of Epidemiological Meta-Analyses." *BMJ* 384:e077310. https://doi.org/10.1136/bmj-2023-077310.

4. Siegel KR, McKeever Bullard K, Imperatore G, et al. (2016, August 1). "Association of Higher Consumption of Foods Derived from Subsidized Commodities with Adverse Cardiometabolic Risk Among US Adults." *JAMA Internal Medicine* 176(8):1124–32. doi: 10.1001/jamainternmed.2016.2410.

5. Murphy SL, Kochanek KD, Xu J, et al. (2024, December). "Mortality in the United States, 2023." NCHS Data Brief No. 521. National Center for Health Statistics. https://www.cdc.gov/nchs/products/databriefs/db521.htm.

6. World Health Organization. (n.d.). "GHE: Life Expectancy and Healthy Life Expectancy." Global Health Observatory. https://www.who.int/data/gho/data/themes/mortality-and-global-health-estimates/ghe-life-expectancy-and-healthy-life-expectancy. Accessed August 5, 2025.

7. Black SE, Duzett N, Lleras-Muney A, et al. (2024, May). "Intergenerational Transmission of Lifespan in the US." Working Paper no. 31034. National Bureau of Economic Research. https://doi.org/10.3386/w31034.

8. Ney J. (2023, April 12). "Americans Are Dying Younger—But Where You Live Makes a Big Difference." *Time.* https://time.com/6270808/americas-life-expectancy-divide/.

9. National Institute on Drug Abuse. (2024, August). "Drug Overdose Deaths: Facts and Figures." https://www.nida.nih.gov/research-topics/trends-statistics/overdose-death-rates.

10. Centers for Disease Control and Prevention. (2024, October 24). "Heart Disease Facts." https://www.cdc.gov/heart-disease/data-research/facts-stats/index.html.

11. US Department of Health and Human Services. (2025, July 22). "Mortality Dashboard." National Center for Health Statistics. https://www.cdc.gov/nchs/nvss/vsrr/mortality-dashboard.htm.

12. Dwyer-Lindgren L, Bertozzi-Villa A, Stubbs RW, et al. (2017, July). "Inequalities in Life Expectancy Among US Counties, 1980 to 2014: Temporal Trends and Key Drivers." *JAMA Internal Medicine* 177(7):1003–11. doi:10.1001/jamainternmed.2017.0918.

13. Manzel A, Muller DN, Hafler DA, et al. (2014, January). "Role of 'Western Diet' in Inflammatory Autoimmune Diseases." *Current Allergy and Asthma Reports* 14(1):404. doi: 10.1007/s11882-013-0404-6.

14. Li Y, Lv MR, Wei YJ, et al. (2017, July). "Dietary Patterns and Depression Risk: A Meta-Analysis." *Psychiatry Research* 253:373–82.

15. Firth J, Marx W, Dash S, et al. (2019, April). "The Effects of Dietary Improvement on Symptoms of Depression and Anxiety: A Meta-Analysis of Randomized Controlled Trials." *Psychosom Med.* 2019 Apr;81(3):265–80. doi: 10.1016/j.psychres.2017.04.020.

16. Afshin A, Sur PJ, Fay K, et al. "Health Effects of Dietary Risks in 195 Countries, 1990–2017: A Systematic Analysis for the Global Burden of Disease Study 2017." *The Lancet.* 2019 Apr 4. https://www.thelancet.com/journals/lancet/article/PIIS0140-6736(19)30041-8/fulltext.

17. Worldometer. (2024, April 13). "COVID-19 Coronavirus Pandemic." https://www.worldometers.info/coronavirus.

18. World Health Organization. (2024, December 23). "Noncommunicable Diseases." https://www.who.int/news-room/fact-sheets/detail/noncommunicable-diseases.

19. Christakis NA, Fowler JH. (2007, July 26). "The Spread of Obesity in a Large Social Network Over 32 Years." *New England Journal of Medicine* 357(4):370–79. DOI: 10.1056/NEJMsa066082; Powell K, Wilcox J, Clonan A, et al. (2015, September 30). "The Role of Social Networks in the Development of Overweight and Obesity Among Adults: A Scoping Review." *BMC Public Health* 15:996. https://doi.org/10.1186/s12889-015-2314-0.

20. Ludwig J, Sanbonmatsu L, Gennetian L, et al. (2011, October 20). "Neighborhoods, Obesity, and Diabetes—A Randomized Social Experiment." *New England Journal of Medicine.* 365(16):1509–19. DOI: 10.1056/NEJMsa1103216.

21. Centers for Disease Control and Prevention. (2006, September 14). "State-Specific Prevalence of Obesity Among Adults—United States, 2005." https://www.cdc.gov/mmwr/preview/mmwrhtml/mm5536a1.htm.

22. Centers for Disease Control and Prevention. (2006, September 14). "State-Specific Prevalence of Obesity Among Adults—United States, 2005." https://www.cdc.gov/mmwr/preview/mmwrhtml/mm5536a1.htm.

23. Hample SE, Hassink SG, Skinner AC, et al. (2023, January 9). "Executive Summary: Clinical Practice Guideline for the Evaluation and Treatment of Children and Adolescents with Obesity." American Academy of Pediatrics. https://publications.aap.org/pediatrics/article/151/2/e2022060641/190440/Executive-Summary-Clinical-Practice-Guideline-for.

24. O'Mary L. (2024, November 26). "White House Wants Medicare, Medicaid to Cover GLP-1 Drugs." WebMD. https://www.webmd.com/obesity/news/20241126/white-house-wants-medicare-medicaid-to-cover-glp-1-drugs.

25. Reed T. (2024, April 29). "Steep Ozempic, Wegovy Prices Face Fresh Scrutiny from Officials." Axios. https://www.axios.com/2024/04/29/weight-loss-drugs-cost-glp-1.

26. Centers for Medicare and Medicaid Services. (2025, June 24). "NHE Fact Sheet." https://www.cms.gov/data-research/statistics-trends-and-reports/national-health-expenditure-data/nhe-fact-sheet.

27. Baraldi LG, Martinez SE, Cannella DS, et al. (2018, March 9). "Consumption of Ultra-Processed Foods and Associated Sociodemographic Factors in the USA Between 2007 and 2012: Evidence from a Nationally Representative Cross-Sectional Study." *BMJ Open* 8:e020574. https://doi.org/10.1136/bmjopen-2017-020574.

28. Bird JK, Murphy RA, Ciappio ED, et al. (2017, June 24). "Risk of Deficiency in Multiple Concurrent Micronutrients in Children and Adults in the United States." *Nutrients* 9(7):655. https://doi.org/10.3390/nu9070655.

29. Via M. (2012, March 15). "The Malnutrition of Obesity: Micronutrient Deficiencies That Promote Diabetes." *ISRN Endocrinology* 2012:103472. doi:10.5402/2012/103472.

30. Feeding the Economy. (n.d). "What Is the Food and Agriculture Sector's Impact in Your Community?" https://feedingtheeconomy.com/. Accessed August 19, 2025.

31. World Bank. (n.d.). "Agriculture and Food." https://www.worldbank.org/en/topic/agriculture/overview. Accessed May 27, 2018.

32. Holt-Gimenez E. (2014, December 18). "We Already Grow Enough Food for 10 Billion People—and Still Can't End Hunger." *HuffPost*. https://www.huffpost.com/entry/world -hunger_n_1463429.

33. US Department of Agriculture, Economic Research Service. (2025, January 8). "Food Security in the U.S.—Key Statistics and Graphics." https://www.ers.usda.gov/topics/food -nutrition-assistance/food-security-in-the-us/key-statistics-graphics.aspx.

34. Center on Budget and Policy Priorities. (2024, November 25). "Policy Basics: The Supplemental Nutrition Assistance Program (SNAP)." ERR-256. https://www.cbpp.org/research /food-assistance/the-supplemental-nutrition-assistance-program-snap.

35. Coleman-Jensen A, Rabbitt MP, Gregory CA, et al. (2018, September 5). "Household Food Security in the United States in 2017." US Department of Agriculture, Economic Research Service. https://www.ers.usda.gov/publications/pub-details?pubid=90022.

36. Innovative Health Initiative. (2023, March 3). "Better Understanding the Genetic Link Between Obesity and Type 2 Diabetes." https://www.ihi.europa.eu/news-events/newsroom /better-understanding-genetic-link-between-obesity-and-type-2-diabetes.

37. Schnabel L, Kesse-Guyot E, Allès B, et al. (2019, February 11). "Association Between Ultraprocessed Food Consumption and Risk of Mortality Among Middle-Aged Adults in France." *JAMA Internal Medicine* 179(4):490–98. doi:10.1001/jamainternmed.2018.728.

38. Park A. (2019, February 21). "Why Food Could Be the Best Medicine of All." *Time*. http:// time.com/longform/food-best-medicine/.

39. Feinberg AT, Hess A, Passaretti M, et al. (2018, April 10). "Prescribing Food as a Specialty Drug." *NJEM Catalyst*. https://catalyst.nejm.org/prescribing-fresh-food-farmacy/.

40. Athinarayanan SJ, Adams RN, Hallberg SJ, et al. (2019, June 4). "Long-Term Effects of a Novel Continuous Remote Care Intervention Including Nutritional Ketosis for the Management of Type 2 Diabetes: A 2-Year Non-Randomized Clinical Trial." *Frontiers in Endocrinology* 10. https://www.frontiersin.org/journals/endocrinology/articles/10.3389/fendo.2019 .00348/full.

41. Hayes TO, Kerska K. (2021, November 3). "Primer: Agriculture Subsidies and Their Influence on the Composition of U.S. Food Supply and Consumption." American Action Forum. https://www.americanactionforum.org/research/primer-agriculture-subsidies-and -their-influence-on-the-composition-of-u-s-food-supply-and-consumption/.

42. Berkowitz SA, Terranova J, Hill C, et al. (2018, April). "Meal Delivery Programs Reduce the Use of Costly Health Care in Dually Eligible Medicare and Medicaid Beneficiaries." *Health Affairs* 37(4). https://www.doi.org/10.1377/hlthaff.2017.0999.

43. Gurvey J, Rand K, Daugherty S, et al. (2013, October). "Examining Health Care Costs Among MANNA Clients and a Comparison Group." *Journal of Primary Care and Community Health* 4(4):311–17. doi: 10.1177/2150131913490737.

44. Cohen SB, Yu W. (2012, January). "Statistical Brief #354: The Concentration and Persistence in the Level of Health Expenditures over Time: Estimates for the U.S. Population, 2008–2009." Agency for Healthcare Research and Quality. https://meps.ahrq.gov/data_files /publications/st354/stat354.shtml.

45. California Food Is Medicine Coalition. (n.d.). "Who We Are." https://calfimc.org/. Accessed August 19, 2025.

46. Ibid.

47. Hallberg SJ, McKenzie AL, Williams PT, et al. (2018, February 7). "Effectiveness and Safety of a Novel Care Model for the Management of Type 2 Diabetes at 1 Year: An Open-Label, Non-Randomized, Controlled Study." *Diabetes Therapy* 9(2):583–612. https://doi .org/10.1007/s13300-018-0373-9.

48. Virta Health. (n.d.). Website. https://www.virtahealth.com/. Accessed August 19, 2025.

CHAPTER 3

1. Regmi A, Gehlhar M. (2005, February 1). "New Directions in Global Food Markets." AIB-794. US Department of Agriculture, Economic Research Service. https://www.ers.usda.gov/publications/pub-details?pubid=42591.

2. Scapin T, Romaniuk H, Feeley A, et al. (2025, March 3). "Global Food Retail Environments Are Increasingly Dominated by Large Chains and Linked to the Rising Prevalence of Obesity." *Nature Food* 6(3):283–295. https://doi.org/10.1038/s43016-025-01134-x.

3. Jacobs A, Richtel M. (2017, September 16). "How Big Business Got Brazil Hooked on Junk Food." *New York Times*. https://www.nytimes.com/interactive/2017/09/16/health/brazil-obesity-nestle.html.

4. Dunlop S. (2025, February 27). "Yum's Digital Strategy, Strong International Footprint Underpin Robust Long-Term Growth Prospects." Morningstar. https://www.morningstar.com/company-reports/1267078-yums-digital-strategy-strong-international-footprint-underpin-robust-long-term-growth-prospects.

5. Dhanjal SS, Tandon S. (2015, September 29). "With Sapphire Foods Franchisee, Yum Reorganizes India Business." *Mint*. https://www.livemint.com/Companies/jChCarxfXopS8iiI5X4E7H/With-Sapphire-Foods-franchisee-Yum-reorganizes-India-busine.html.

6. Searcey D, Richtel M. (2017, October 2). "Obesity Was Rising as Ghana Embraced Fast Food. Then Came KFC." *New York Times*. https://www.nytimes.com/2017/10/02/health/ghana-kfc-obesity.html.

7. Pereira MA, Kartashov AI, Ebbeling CB, et al. (2005, January). "Fast-Food Habits, Weight Gain, and Insulin Resistance (The CARDIA Study): 15-Year Prospective Analysis." *The Lancet* 365(9453):36–42. https://doi.org/10.1016/s0140-6736(04)17663-0.

8. Seeking Alpha. (2018, December 7). "Yum! Brands, Inc. (YUM) CEO Greg Creed Hosts 2018 Investor and Analyst Day Conference (Transcript)." https://seekingalpha.com/article/4227124-yum-brands-inc-yum-ceo-greg-creed-hosts-2018-investor-analyst-day-conference-transcript.

9. World Health Organization. (n.d.). "Obesity." https://www.who.int/health-topics/obesity#tab=tab_1. Accessed August 5, 2025.

10. Ibid.

11. NCD Risk Factor Collaboration. (2024, March 16). "Worldwide Trends in Underweight and Obesity from 1990 to 2022: A Pooled Analysis of 3663 Population-Representative Studies with 222 Million Children, Adolescents, and Adults." *The Lancet* 403(10431):1027–50. https://www.thelancet.com/journals/lancet/article/PIIS0140-6736(23)02750-2/fulltext.

12. Doak CM, Adair LS, Bentley M, et al. (2005, January). "The Dual Burden Household and the Nutrition Transition Paradox." *International Journal of Obesity* 29(1):129–36. https://doi.org/10.1038/sj.ijo.0802824.

13. Khan M. (2006, March 1). "The Dual Burden of Overweight and Underweight in Developing Countries." Population Reference Bureau. https://www.prb.org/resources/the-dual-burden-of-overweight-and-underweight-in-developing-countries/.

14. Dunkin may no longer operate in China, so this is a retrospective observation.

15. NCD Risk Factor Collaboration. (2024, November 23). "Worldwide Trends in Diabetes Prevalence and Treatment from 1990 to 2022: A Pooled Analysis of 1,108 Population-Representative Studies with 141 Million Participants." *The Lancet* 404(10467):2077–93. https://www.thelancet.com/journals/lancet/article/PIIS0140-6736(24)02317-1/fulltext.

16. Muralidharan S. (2024, January–March). "Diabetes and Current Indian Scenario: A Narrative Review." *Journal of Diabetology* 15:12–17. https://journals.lww.com/jodb/fulltext/2024/15010/diabetes_and_current_indian_scenario__a_narrative.3.aspx.

17. Anand G. (2017, December 26). "One Man's Stand Against Junk Food as Diabetes Climbs Across India." *New York Times*. https://www.nytimes.com/2017/12/26/health/india-diabetes -junk-food.html.

18. Apollo Hospitals. (2025, February 18). "How Obesity in India is the Rising Cause of Heart Diseases." https://www.apollohospitals.com/health-library/how-obesity-in-india-is-the-rising -cause-of-heart-diseases.

19. Ali MK, Narayan KMV, Tandon N. (2010, November). "Diabetes and Coronary Heart Disease: Current Perspectives." *Indian Journal of Medical Research* 132(5):584–97. https:// pubmed.ncbi.nlm.nih.gov/21150011/.

20. Shrivastav S. (2015, April 8). "Heart, Lung Diseases Now Leading Killers in India." *Times of India*. https://timesofindia.indiatimes.com/india/heart-lung-diseases-now-leading-killers-in -india/articleshow/46843861.cms.

21. Dhamnetiya D, Patel P, Jha RP, et al. (2021, November 16). "Trends in Incidence and Mortality of Tuberculosis in India over Past Three Decades: A Joinpoint and Age-Period-Cohort Analysis." *BMC Pulmonary Medicine* 21(1):375. https://doi.org/10.1186/s12890-021-01740-y.

22. Rukmini S. (2025, July 30). "India's Disease Transition." Data for India. https://www .dataforindia.com/indias-disease-transition/.

23. International Diabetes Federation. (2025). *IDF Diabetes Atlas 2025*. https://diabetesatlas.org /resources/idf-diabetes-atlas-2025/.

24. Centers for Disease Control and Prevention. (2024, May 15). "1 in 3 Americans Have Prediabetes Social Media Graphic." https://www.cdc.gov/diabetes/communication-resources /1-in-3-americans.html.

25. Abuyassin B, Laher I. (2016, April 25). "Diabetes Epidemic Sweeping the Arab World." *World Journal of Diabetes* 7(8):165–74. https://doi.org/10.4239/wjd.v7.i8.165.

26. Ibid.

27. Ibid.

28. Al-Daghri NM, Alharbi NS, Jones A, et al. (2014). "Trends in the Prevalence of Type 2 Diabetes Mellitus and Obesity in the Arabian Gulf States: A Systematic Review and Meta-Analysis." *Diabetes Research and Clinical Practice* 106(2):e30–e33. https://doi.org/10.1016 /j.diabres.2014.08.019.

29. Jacobs A, Richtel M. (2017, December 11). "A Nasty, Nafta-Related Surprise: Mexico's Soaring Obesity." *New York Times*. https://www.nytimes.com/2017/12/11/health/obesity -mexico-nafta.html.

30. Suhartono M. (2018, August 12). "In Thailand, 'Obesity in Our Monks Is a Ticking Time Bomb.'" *New York Times*. https://www.nytimes.com/2018/08/12/world/asia/thailand-monks -obesity.html.

31. Cochrane L, Vimonsuknopparat S. "Thai Buddhist Monks' Health Suffering from Sugary Drinks." ABC News Australia. May 27, 2018. https://www.abc.net.au/news/2018-05-28 /thai-buddhist-monks-health-ruined-by-sugary-drinks/9711412.

32. Dinu M, Pagliai G, Sofi F, et al. (2022, April 22). "Consumption of Ultra-Processed Foods Is Inversely Associated with Adherence to the Mediterranean Diet: A Cross-Sectional Study." *Nutrients* 14(10):2073. https://doi.org/10.3390/nu14102073.

33. European Association for the Study of Obesity and World Health Organization. (2021, May 11). "WHO Joint Session Including the Results of the Latest Childhood Obesity Surveillance Initiative (COSI) Report." https://easo.org/who-joint-session-including-the-results -of-the-latest-childhood-obesity-surveillance-initiative-cosi-report.

34. Committee on the Evaluation of the Addition of Ingredients New to Infant Formula, Food and Nutrition Board, Institute of Medicine. (2004). "Comparing Infant Formulas with Human Milk." In *Infant Formula: Evaluating the Safety of New Ingredients*. National Academies Press. https://www.ncbi.nlm.nih.gov/books/NBK215837/.

35. Farmer JJ. (2015, November 27). "My 40-Year History with *Cronobacter/Enterobacter sakazakii*—Lessons Learned, Myths Debunked, and Recommendations." *Frontiers in Pediatrics* 3:84. https://pmc.ncbi.nlm.nih.gov/articles/PMC4662064/.

36. US Food and Drug Administration. (2005, May). "CPG Sec. 555.425 Foods, Adulteration Involving Hard or Sharp Foreign Objects." https://www.fda.gov/media/71953/download.

37. Kappes W. (2025, March 19). "Baby Formula Under Scrutiny as Study Finds Heavy-Metal Contamination." The Bump. https://www.thebump.com/news/baby-formula-contaminants-study.

38. Greenhouse L. (1986, May 31). "Consumer Saturday: Safeguards on Baby Formula." *New York Times.* https://www.nytimes.com/1986/05/31/style/consumer-saturday-safeguards-on-baby-formula.html.

39. Anttila-Hughes JK, Fernald LCH, Gertler PJ, et al. (2025, January). "Mortality from Nestlé's Marketing of Infant Formula in Low and Middle-Income Countries." Working Paper no. 24452. National Bureau of Economic Research. https://www.nber.org/system/files/working_papers/w24452/w24452.pdf.

40. UNICEF and World Health Organization. (2022). "How the Marketing of Formula Milk Influences Our Decisions on Infant Feeding." https://www.unicef.org/media/115916/file/Multi-country.

41. Dunford EK, Scully M, Coyle D. (2024, August 12). "Commercially-Produced Infant and Toddler Foods—How Healthy Are They? An Evaluation of Products Sold in Australian Supermarkets." *Maternal and Child Nutrition* 20(4):e13709. https://doi.org/10.1111/mcn.13709.

42. World Health Organization. (1981, January 27). *International Code of Marketing of Breast-Milk Substitutes.* https://www.who.int/publications/i/item/9241541601.

43. Rips-Goodwin AR, Jun D, Griebel-Thompson A, et al. (2025, May). "US Infant Formulas Contain Primarily Added Sugars: An Analysis of Infant Formulas on the US Market." *Journal of Food Composition and Analysis* 141:107369. https://www.sciencedirect.com/science/article/pii/S0889157525001838.

44. Ferdinand P. (2025, May 11). "Most U.S. Infant Formulas Contain Mainly Added Sugars, Posing a Serious Risk to Babies' Health." Green Social Thought. https://www.greensocialthought.org/less-what-we-dont-need/most-u-s-infant-formulas-contain-mainly-added-sugars-posing-a-serious-risk-to-babies-health.

45. Jacobs A, Richtel M. (2017, September 16). "How Big Business Got Brazil Hooked on Junk Food." *New York Times.* https://www.nytimes.com/interactive/2017/09/16/health/brazil-obesity-nestle.html.

46. Ibid.

47. Ibid.

48. Jacobs A. (2018, February 7). "In Sweeping War on Obesity, Chile Slays Tony the Tiger." *New York Times.* https://www.nytimes.com/2018/02/07/health/obesity-chile-sugar-regulations.html.

49. Ibid.

50. Denecken AA. (2018, July). "Development and Implementation Processes of the Food Labeling and Advertising Law in Chile." Global Delivery Initiative. https://www.effectivecooperation.org/system/files/2021-06/GDI%20Case%20Study%20-%20Food%20Labeling%20and%20Advertising%20Law%20in%20Chile.pdf.

51. Kolker C. (2024, March 13). "A Decade After Its Pioneering Food Law, Where Does Chile's Obesity Crisis Stand?" The Examination. https://www.theexamination.org/articles/a-decade-after-its-pioneering-food-law-where-does-chile-s-obesity-crisis-stand.

52. Denecken AA. (2018, July). "Development and Implementation Processes of the Food Labeling and Advertising Law in Chile." Global Delivery Initiative. https://www

.effectivecooperation.org/system/files/2021-06/GDI%20Case%20Study%20-%20Food%20 Labeling%20and%20Advertising%20Law%20in%20Chile.pdf.

53. Ibid.

54. Jacobs A. (2018, February 7). "In Sweeping War on Obesity, Chile Slays Tony the Tiger." *New York Times.* https://www.nytimes.com/2018/02/07/health/obesity-chile-sugar-regulations .html.

55. Denecken AA. (2018, July). "Development and Implementation Processes of the Food Labeling and Advertising Law in Chile." Global Delivery Initiative. https://www.effective cooperation.org/system/files/2021-06/GDI%20Case%20Study%20-%20Food%20Labeling %20and%20Advertising%20Law%20in%20Chile.pdf.

56. Jacobs A. (2018, February 7). "In Sweeping War on Obesity, Chile Slays Tony the Tiger." *New York Times.* https://www.nytimes.com/2018/02/07/health/obesity-chile-sugar-regulations .html.

57. Denecken AA. (2018, July). "Development and Implementation Processes of the Food Labeling and Advertising Law in Chile." Global Delivery Initiative. https://www.effective cooperation.org/system/files/2021-06/GDI%20Case%20Study%20-%20Food%20Labeling %20and%20Advertising%20Law%20in%20Chile.pdf.

58. Swinburn BA, Kraak V, Allender S, et al. (2019, February 23). "The Global Syndemic of Obesity, Undernutrition, and Climate Change: *The Lancet* Commission Report." *The Lancet.* January 27, 2019. https://www.thelancet.com/journals/lancet/article/PIIS0140-6736 (18)32822-8/fulltext.

59. Environmental Working Group. (2016, February 25). "Food Lobby Spends $101 Million in 2015 to Avert GMO Labeling." https://www.ewg.org/research/food-lobby-spends-101 -million-2015-avert-gmo-labeling.

60. Global Food Research Program at UNC Chapel Hill. (2025, March). "Front-of-Package Labels Around the World." https://www.globalfoodresearchprogram.org/wp-content/uploads /2025/03/GFRP-UNC_FOPL_maps_2025_3.pdf.

61. Global Food Research Program at UNC Chapel Hill. (2025, March). "Front-of-Package Labels Around the World." https://www.globalfoodresearchprogram.org/wp-content/uploads /2025/03/GFRP-UNC_FOPL_maps_2025_3.pdf.

62. Pineda E, Beaney TE. (2025, June). "Potassium-Enriched Salt: A New Era for UK Salt Reduction?" *The Lancet Public Health* 10(6):E436–37. https://doi.org/10.1016/S2468-2667 (25)00074-X.

63. U.S. Food and Drug Administration. (2025, January 14). "FDA Proposes Requiring At-a-Glance Nutrition Information on the Front of Packaged Foods." Press release. https:// www.fda.gov/news-events/press-announcements/fda-proposes-requiring-glance-nutrition -information-front-packaged-foods.

CHAPTER 4

1. Khemlani A. (2021, May 1). "Buffett on Failed Health Care Venture Haven: 'We Were Fighting a Tapeworm in the American Economy, and the Tapeworm Won.'" Yahoo Finance. https://finance.yahoo.com/news/buffett-on-failed-health-care-venture-haven-we -were-fighting-a-tapeworm-in-the-american-economy-and-the-tapeworm-won -220812439.html.

2. Centers for Medicare and Medicaid Services. (2024, December 18). "National Health Expenditure Data: Historical." https://www.cms.gov/data-research/statistics-trends-and -reports/national-health-expenditure-data/historical.

3. Task Force on Fiscal Policy for Health. (2024). "Health Taxes: A Compelling Policy for the Crises of Today." Bloomberg Philanthropies. https://assets.bbhub.io/dotorg/sites/64/2024 /09/Health-Taxes-A-Compelling-Policy-for-the-Crises-of-Today.pdf.

4. World Health Organization. (2022). *WHO Manual on Sugar-Sweetened Beverage Taxation Policies to Promote Healthy Diets.* https://iris.who.int/bitstream/handle/10665/365285/9789240 056299-eng.pdf.

5. City of Philadelphia, Department of Revenue. (n.d.). "Philadelphia Beverage Tax (PBT)." https://www.phila.gov/services/payments-assistance-taxes/taxes/business-taxes/business -taxes-by-type/philadelphia-beverage-tax-pbt/. Accessed August 5, 2025.

6. City Controller, City of Philadelphia. (2024, March). "Philadelphia Beverage Tax Eclipses $500 Million in Revenue." https://controller.phila.gov/wp-content/uploads/2024/03/MMM -March-.pdf-new.pdf.

7. San Francisco Department of Public Health. (2023, March). "San Francisco Sugary Drinks Distributor Tax (SDDT): Evaluation Report 2021–2022." https://www.sf.gov/sites/default /files/2023-03/21-22_SDDT_EvalReport_final_2_28_23.pdf.

8. Ibid.

9. Bishari NS. (2018, May 29). "Soda Tax Starts Paying Off." *SF Weekly.* https://www.sfweekly .com/archives/soda-tax-starts-paying-off/article_06c7b515-78d7-5117-92a4 -a7bc3a759bd5.html.

10. Patel AI, Schmidt LA. (2017, September). "Water Access in the United States: Health Disparities Abound and Solutions Are Urgently Needed." *American Journal of Public Health* 107(9):1354–56. https://doi.org/10.2105/AJPH.2017.303972.

11. Gibbs S. (2016, November 8). "Putting Sugary Soda out of Reach." *New York Times.* https:// www.nytimes.com/2016/11/08/well/eat/putting-sugary-soda-out-of-reach.html.

12. Epel ES, Hartman A, Jacobs LM, et al. (2020, January 1). "Association of a Workplace Sales Ban on Sugar-Sweetened Beverages with Employee Consumption of Sugar-Sweetened Beverages and Health." *JAMA Internal Medicine* 180(1):9–16. doi: 10.1001/jamainternmed .2019.4434.

13. Malhotra A, Lustig R. (2018, May 10). "Tax Sugary Foods to Reverse Type 2 Diabetes Epidemic Within 3 Years." Press release. https://www.dietdoctor.com/wp-content/uploads /2018/05/Press-Release-Tax-Sugary-Food-To-Reverse-Type-2-Diabetes.pdf.

14. Bhushan R. (2017, June 3). "Virat Kohli Not Keen on Endorsing Pepsi Any More, May Pick Another Healthier Brand." *Economic Times* (India). https://economictimes.indiatimes.com /industry/services/advertising/virat-kohli-not-keen-on-endorsing-pepsi-any-more-may -pick-another-healthier-brand-from-pepsico/articleshow/58969143.cms.

15. Valinksy J. (2025, March 26). "Steph Curry and Michelle Obama Team Up to Create a Sports Drink." CNN Business. https://www.cnn.com/2025/03/26/food/steph-curry-sports -drink-plezi.

16. Leasca S. (2017, October 19). "Tom Brady Follows a Super-Strict Diet, So Why Is He Promoting a Candy Company?" *Men's Health.* https://www.menshealth.com/trending-news /a19539041/tom-brady-diet-unreal-candy/.

17. US Department of Agriculture and US Department of Health and Human Services. (2020, December). *Dietary Guidelines for Americans, 2020–2025* (9th ed.). https://www.dietary guidelines.gov/sites/default/files/2021-03/Dietary_Guidelines_for_Americans-2020 -2025.pdf.

18. Emmert-Fees KM, Amies-Cull B, Wawro N, et al. (2023, November 21). "Projected Health and Economic Impacts of Sugar-Sweetened Beverage Taxation Scenarios in Germany: A Cross-Validation Modelling Study." *PLOS Medicine* 20(11). https://doi.org/10.1371 /journal.pmed.1004311; Zhao F, Gidwani R, Wang MC, et al. (2025, January 13). "Evaluation of the Soda Tax on Obesity and Diabetes in California: A Cost-Effectiveness Analysis." *MDM Policy and Practice,* 10(1):e25814683241309669. https://doi.org/10.1177/2381468324 1309669; Lee MM, Barrett JL, Kenney EL, et al. (2024, January). "A Sugar-Sweetened Beverage Excise Tax in California: Projected Benefits for Population Obesity and Health

Equity." *American Journal of Preventive Medicine* 66(1):94–103. https://doi.org/10.1016/j.amepre.2023.08.004.

19. Lee Y, Mozaffarian D, Sy S, et al. (2020, June 22). "Health Impact and Cost-effectiveness of Volume, Tiered, and Absolute Sugar Content Sugar-Sweetened Beverage Tax Policies in the United States: A Microsimulation Study." *Circulation* 142(6):523–34. https://doi.org/10.1161/CIRCULATIONAHA.119.042956.

20. World Bank. (2023, October). "Global SSB Tax Database." https://ssbtax.worldbank.org/.

21. Al-Jawaldeh A, Perucic A-M, Hammerich A, et al. (2024, December 3). "A Review of Sugar-Sweetened Beverages Taxation in Saudi Arabia and United Arab Emirates." *Eastern Mediterranean Health Journal* 30(11):746–56. https://doi.org/10.26719/2024.30.11.746.

22. World Bank. (2023, October). "Global SSB Tax Database." https://ssbtax.worldbank.org/.

23. Onagan FCC, Ho BLC, Chua KKT. (2018, December 1). "Development of a Sweetened Beverage Tax, Philippines." *Bulletin of the World Health Organization* 97(2):154–59. https://doi.org/10.2471/BLT.18.220459.

24. O'Connor A. (2016, January 7). "Mexican Soda Tax Followed by Drop in Sugary Drink Sales." *New York Times.* https://www.nytimes.com/2016/01/07/health/mexican-soda-tax-followed-by-drop-in-sugary-drink-sales.html.

25. Colchero MA, Molina M, Guerrero-López CM. (2017, June 14). "After Mexico Implemented a Tax, Purchases of Sugar-Sweetened Beverages Decreased and Water Increased: Difference by Place of Residence, Household Composition and Income Level." *Journal of Nutrition* 147(8):1552–57. https://doi.org/10.3945/jn.117.251892.

26. Sánchez-Romero LM, Penko J, Coxson PG, et al. (2016, November 1.) "Projected Impact of Mexico's Sugar-Sweetened Beverage Tax Policy on Diabetes and Cardiovascular Disease: A Modeling Study." *PLOS Medicine* 13(11):e1002158. https://www.ncbi.nlm.nih.gov/pubmed/27802278.

27. World Bank. (2023, October). "Global SSB Tax Database." https://ssbtax.worldbank.org/.

28. Lee MM, Falbe J, Schillinger D, et al. (2019, March 13). "Sugar-Sweetened Beverage Consumption 3 Years After the Berkeley, California, Sugar-Sweetened Beverage Tax." *American Journal of Public Health* 109(4):637–39. https://doi.org/10.2105/AJPH.2019.304971.

29. Langellier BA, Lê-Scherban F, Purtle J, et al. (2017, September). "Funding Quality Pre-Kindergarten Slots with Philadelphia's New 'Sugary Drink Tax': Simulating Effects of Using an Excise Tax to Address a Social Determinant of Health." *Public Health Nutrition* 20(13):2450–58. https://doi.org/10.1017/s1368980017001756.

30. Bailey M. (2016, October 24). "More Hospitals Are Refusing to Sell Sugary Drinks. And That's Angering Some Workers." *Stat.* https://www.statnews.com/2016/10/24/hospitals-selling-sugary-drinks.

31. Rudavsky S. (2013, May 16). "Ind. Hospitals' Rx: No Sugary Drinks." *USA Today.* https://www.usatoday.com/story/news/nation/2013/05/16/hospitals-no-sugary-drinks/2192673.

32. Partnership for a Healthier America. (n.d.) "Hospital Healthier Food Initiative." https://www.ahealthieramerica.org/articles/hospital-healthier-food-initiative-4. Accessed August 19, 2025.

33. Spector K. (2010, July 24). "Sugar-Sweetened Food, Beverages No Longer Will Be Sold at the Cleveland Clinic." Cleveland *Plain Dealer.* https://www.cleveland.com/healthfit/2010/07/sugar-sweetened_food_beverages.html.

CHAPTER 5

1. US House Committee on Agriculture. (2017, February 16). "Pros and Cons of Restricting SNAP Purchases." Hearing Before the Committee on Agriculture, 115th Congress, 2nd session. https://agriculture.house.gov/uploadedfiles/115-02_-_24325.pdf.

2. The report showed that about 7 percent of SNAP dollars are spent on sugar-sweetened beverages. At the 2023 SNAP funding level of $112 billion, that works out to more than $7 billion per year.

3. O'Connor A. (2017, January 13). "In the Shopping Cart of a Food Stamp Household: Lots of Soda." *New York Times.* https://www.nytimes.com/2017/01/13/well/eat/food-stamp-snap -soda.html; Carpenter M. (2025, May 2). "Why It's Still Unclear Exactly How Much Banning Soda from SNAP Could Improve Health." *Stat.* https://www.statnews.com/2025 /05/02/snap-soda-restrictions-expert-calls-for-pilot-program-testing-before-outright -bans.

4. Hyman M. (2018, April 9). "Our Food System: An Invisible Form of Oppression." https:// drhyman.com/blog/2018/04/09/our-food-system-an-invisible-form-of-oppression/.

5. USDA Department of Agriculture, Food and Nutrition Service. (2016, November). "Foods Typically Purchased by Supplemental Nutrition Assistance Program (SNAP) House-holds (Summary)." https://fns-prod.azureedge.us/sites/default/files/ops/SNAPFoodsTypically Purchased-Summary.pdf.

6. Conrad Z, Rehm CD, Wilde P, et al. (2017, March). "Cardiometabolic Mortality by Sup-plemental Nutrition Assistance Program Participation and Eligibility in the United States." *American Journal of Public Health* 107(3):466–74. https://doi.org/10.2105/ajph.2016.303608.

7. US Department of Agriculture, Economic Research Service. (2025, July 24). "Supplemen-tal Nutrition Assistance Program (SNAP)—Key Statistics and Research." https://www.ers .usda.gov/topics/food-nutrition-assistance/supplemental-nutrition-assistance-program -snap/key-statistics-and-research.

8. Hacıoğlu Hoke S. (2025, February 28). "How Were Extra SNAP Benefits Spent?" Board of Governors of the Federal Reserve System. https://doi.org/10.17016/2380-7172.3655

9. US Department of Agriculture, Food and Nutrition Service. (2025, January 24). *Characteris-tics of SNAP Households: FY 2014.* https://www.fns.usda.gov/research/snap/characteristics -households-fy-2014.

10. Ibid.

11. Leung CW, Ding EL, Catalano PJ, et al. (2012, November). "Dietary Intake and Dietary Quality of Low-Income Adults in the Supplemental Nutrition Assistance Program." *Ameri-can Journal of Clinical Nutrition*;96(5):977–88. https://doi.org/10.3945/ajcn.112.040014.

12. Aussenberg RA, Billings KC. (2025, January 7). "Farm Bill Primer: SNAP and Nutrition Title Programs." IF12255. Congressional Research Service. https://www.congress.gov/crs -product/IF12255.

13. Moran AJ, Musicus A, Gorski Findling MT, et al. (2018, July). "Increases in Sugary Drink Marketing During Supplemental Nutrition Assistance Program Benefit Issuance in New York." *American Journal of Preventive Medicine* 55(1):P55–62. https://doi.org/10.1016/j.amepre .2018.03.012.

14. Conrad Z, Rehm CD, Wilde P, et al. (2017, March). "Cardiometabolic Mortality by Supple-mental Nutrition Assistance Program Participation and Eligibility in the United States." *Ameri-can Journal of Public Health* 107(3):466–74. https://doi.org/10.2105/ajph.2016.303608.

15. Tufts University. (2017, January 19). "Americans in the Supplemental Nutrition Assistance Program (SNAP) Have Higher Mortality." https://now.tufts.edu/news-releases/americans -supplemental-nutrition-assistance-program-snap-have-higher-mortality.

16. Mozaffarian D, Liu J, Sy S, et al. (2018, October 2). "Cost-Effectiveness of Financial Incen-tives and Disincentives for Improving Food Purchases and Health Through the US Supple-mental Nutrition Assistance Program (SNAP): A Microsimulation Study." *PLOS Medicine* 15(10):e1002661. https://doi.org/10.1371/journal.pmed.1002661.

17. US Department of Agriculture, Food and Nutrition Service. (2025, June 4.) "What Can SNAP Buy?" https://www.fns.usda.gov/snap/eligible-food-items.

18. Roberte L. (2025, July 30). "15 Surprising Things You Can Buy with Your EBT Card (SNAP Benefits)." GoodRx Health. https://www.goodrx.com/health-topic/finance/surprising-things-you-can-buy-with-food-stamps.

19. US Department of Agriculture, Food and Nutrition Service. (2025, June 4.) "What Can SNAP Buy?" https://www.fns.usda.gov/snap/eligible-food-items.

20. US House Committee on Agriculture. (2017, February 16). "Pros and Cons of Restricting SNAP Purchases." Hearing Before the Committee on Agriculture, 115th Congress, 2nd session. https://agriculture.house.gov/uploadedfiles/115-02_-_24325.pdf.

21. His specific statement was: "You can't force them. You can't deny them their freedoms to be able to make choices without violating their pursuit of happiness."

22. US House Committee on Agriculture. (2017, February 16). "Pros and Cons of Restricting SNAP Purchases." Hearing Before the Committee on Agriculture, 115th Congress, 2nd session. https://agriculture.house.gov/uploadedfiles/115-02_-_24325.pdf.

23. Center for Responsive Politics. (2018). "David Scott: Contributors 2017–2018." https://www.opensecrets.org/members-of-congress/contributors?cid=N00024871&cycle=2018&type=I.

24. Center for Responsive Politics. (2018). "Roger Marshall: Contributors 2017–2018." https://www.opensecrets.org/members-of-congress/contributors?cid=N00037034&cycle=2018.

25. Merlin M. (2012, December 3). "Farm Bill Still Hanging: More Than 70 Groups Lobby on Food Stamps." Center for Responsive Politics. https://www.opensecrets.org/news/2012/12/more-than-70-groups-in-play-over-sn.

26. Sessa-Hawkins M. (2017, August 28). "Congress Could Cut Soda and Candy from SNAP, but Big Sugar Is Pushing Back." Civil Eats. https://civileats.com/2017/08/28/congress-could-cut-soda-and-candy-from-snap-but-big-sugar-is-pushing-back/.

27. Food Research and Action Center. (2018, February). "SNAP Benefits Need to Be Made Adequate, Not Cut or Restricted." https://frac.org/wp-content/uploads/snap-food-choice.pdf.

28. US Department of Agriculture, Food and Nutrition Service. (2015, May). "Diet Quality by SNAP Participation Status: Data from the National Health and Nutrition Examination Survey, 2007–2010." https://fns-prod.azureedge.us/sites/default/files/ops/NHANES-SNAP07-10-Summary.pdf.

29. Mande J, Flaherty G. (2022, November 11). "Supplemental Nutrition Assistance Program as a Health Intervention." *Current Opinion in Pediatrics* 35(1):S33–38. https://doi.org/10.1097/MOP.0000000000001192.

30. Harris A. (2024, January 24). "Congressman Harris Pens Op-Ed on the Need for Congress to Address SNAP's Contribution to Poor Health." https://harris.house.gov/media/press-releases/congressman-harris-pens-op-ed-need-congress-address-snaps-contribution-poor.

31. National Association of Convenience Stores. (2024, July 12). "Congress Blocks Language to Restrict SNAP Choice." https://www.convenience.org/Media/Daily/2024/July/12/4-Congress-Blocks-Language-SNAP-Choice_GR.

32. US Department of Agriculture. (2025, June 10). "Secretary Rollins signs state waivers to Make America Healthy Again by removing unhealthy foods from SNAP in Arkansas, Idaho, and Utah." https://www.usda.gov/about-usda/news/press-releases/2025/06/10/secretary-rollins-signs-state-waivers-make-america-healthy-again-removing-unhealthy-foods-snap.

33. Grassley C. (2025, April 11). [Letter to Robert F. Kennedy Jr. and Brooke Rollins from members of Congress.] https://www.grassley.senate.gov/imo/media/doc/maha-commission-integrity-final.pdf.

34. Harnack L, Oakes JM, Elbel B, et al. (2016, November 1). "Effects of Subsidies and Prohibitions on Nutrition in a Food Benefit Program: A Randomized Clinical Trial." *JAMA Internal Medicine* 176(11):1610–18. https://doi.org/10.1001/jamainternmed.2016.5633.

35. Massachusetts Public Health Alliance. (n.d.). "Massachusetts Healthy Incentives Program (HIP)." https://mapublichealth.org/wp-content/uploads/2019/01/HIP-Fact-Sheet-January -2019.pdf. Accessed August 19, 2025.

36. Ibid.

37. Virginia Farmers Market Association. (n.d.). "Virginia Fresh Match: Fair Access to Fresh Food." https://vafma.org/programs/virginia-fresh-match/. Accessed August 19, 2025.

38. Ibid.

39. For every dollar you spend on fruits and veggies with your Bridge Card, the grocery store will match it dollar for dollar, up to $20 a day. At the farmers market, for every $2 you spend with your Bridge Card, you will get $2 in Double Up Food Bucks, up to $20 a day.

40. Double Up National Network. (n.d.) "Bring Double Up to Your Community!" http:// www.doubleupfoodbucks.org/national-network/. Accessed August 19, 2025.

41. US Department of Agriculture, Economic Research Service. (2025, January 1). "2014 Farm Bill—Nutrition: Supplemental Nutrition Assistance Program (SNAP) Provisions." https:// www.ers.usda.gov/topics/farm-bill/2014-farm-bill/nutrition.

42. Chite RM. (2013, October 18). "The 2014 Farm Bill (P.L. 113-79): Summary and Side-by-Side." R43076. Congressional Research Service. https://www.congress.gov/crs -product/R43076.

43. Mozaffarian D, Liu J, Sy S, et al. (2018, October 2). "Cost-Effectiveness of Financial Incentives and Disincentives for Improving Food Purchases and Health Through the US Supplemental Nutrition Assistance Program (SNAP): A Microsimulation Study." *PLOS Medicine* 15(10):e1002661. https://doi.org/10.1371/journal.pmed.1002661.

44. Gallagher S. (2019, March 19). "Food as Medicine Prescriptions Could Be Good for Health and Budgets." Tufts University. https://now.tufts.edu/news-releases/prescribing-healthy -food-medicaremedicaid-cost-effective-could-improve-health-outcomes.

CHAPTER 6

1. Lowe P. (2014, July 16). "Lobbyists of All Kinds Flock to Farm Bill." Investigate Midwest. https://investigatemidwest.org/2014/07/16/lobbyists-of-all-kinds-flock-to-farm-bill/.

2. Riley Roche L, Dethman L. (2008, April 11). "Lobbyists' Reports Disclose Gifts to Lawmakers." *Deseret News.* https://www.deseret.com/2008/4/11/20081511/lobbyists-reports -disclose-gifts-to-lawmakers/.

3. Fix the Court. (2024, June 6). "A Staggering Tally: Supreme Court Justices Accepted Hundreds of Gifts Worth Millions of Dollars." https://fixthecourt.com/2024/06/a-staggering -tally-supreme-court-justices-accepted-hundreds-of-gifts-worth-millions-of-dollars/.

4. White House. (2009, January 21). "Executive Order 13490—Ethics Commitments by Executive Branch Personnel." https://obamawhitehouse.archives.gov/the-press-office/ethics -commitments-executive-branch-personnel.

5. Gerstein J. (2015, December 31). "How Obama Failed to Shut Washington's Revolving Door." *Politico.* https://www.politico.com/story/2015/12/barack-obama-revolving-door -lobbying-217042.

6. Holman C. (2017, June 26). "36 Former Lobbyists Working for Trump Have Clear Conflicts of Interest." Public Citizen. https://www.citizen.org/news/36-former-lobbyists-working -trump-clear-conflicts-interest/.

7. OpenSecrets. (n.d.). "Revolving Door: Administrations." https://www.opensecrets.org /revolving-door/administrations. Accessed August 5, 2025.

8. Egan M. (2021, January 4). "Janet Yellen Made Millions Giving Speeches to Wall Street Banks She'll Soon Regulate." CNN Business. https://www.cnn.com/2021/01/04/investing /janet-yellen-wall-street-speeches.

9. Guyer J, Grim R. (2021, July 6). "Meet the Consulting Firm That's Staffing the Biden Administration." *The American Prospect*. https://prospect.org/power/meet-the-consulting-firm -staffing-biden-administration-westexec/.

10. Moran M. (2021, March 22). "Jake Sullivan Advised Microsoft on Policy, and Now Coordinates with Microsoft on Policy. What Could Go Wrong?" The Revolving Door Project. https://therevolvingdoorproject.org/jake-sullivan-advised-microsoft-on-policy-and-now -coordinates-with-microsoft-on-policy-what-could-go-wrong/.

11. Speights K. (2024, April 28). "Former House Speaker Nancy Pelosi Nearly Tripled the S&P 500's Returns in 2023: Here Are the Stocks She's Been Buying." Yahoo Finance. https:// finance.yahoo.com/news/former-house-speaker-nancy-pelosi-095000785.html.

12. Reiley L. (2019, August 30). "How the Trump Administration Limited the Scope of the USDA's 2020 Dietary Guidelines." *Washington Post*. https://www.washingtonpost.com /business/2019/08/30/how-trump-administration-limited-scope-usdas-dietary -guidelines.

13. Corn Refiners Association. (2020, November 13). "CRA's Bode Comment on New ISEO President Kailee Tkacz Buller." https://corn.org/cra-alumn-new-president-iseo/.

14. Institute of Shortening and Edible Oils. (2020, December 14). "Kailee Tkacz Buller Named President of Institute of Shortening and Edible Oils; Robert Collette to Retire." https:// edibleoilproducers.org/kailee-tkacz-buller-named-president-of-institute-of-shortening -and-edible-oils-robert-collette-to-retire-1/.

15. McGahn DF. (2017, August 25). [Memorandum re Tkacz ethics pledge waiver.] https:// www.foodpolitics.com/wp-content/uploads/Tkacz_Ethics_Pledge_Waiver.pdf.

16. US Department of Agriculture. (2025, January 21). "U.S. Department of Agriculture Announces Key Slate of Presidential Appointments." https://www.usda.gov/about-usda /news/press-releases/2025/01/21/us-department-agriculture-announces-key-slate-presidential -appointments.

17. US Department of Agriculture. (2017, July 19). "Secretary Perdue Announces New Leadership for Food, Nutrition and Consumer Services." https://www.usda.gov/about-usda/news /press-releases/2017/07/19/secretary-perdue-announces-new-leadership-food-nutrition-and -consumer-services.

18. Office of Government Ethics. (n.d.) "Pledge Waivers (E.O. 13770)—Trump Administration." https://www.oge.gov/web/oge.nsf/Agency+Ethics+Pledge+Waivers+(EO+13770). Accessed August 19, 2025.

19. US Department of Agriculture. (2025, March 21). "USDA Announces New FPAC Leadership to Better Serve Farmers and Ranchers." https://www.usda.gov/about-usda/news/press -releases/2025/03/21/usda-announces-new-fpac-leadership-better-serve-farmers-and -ranchers.

20. McGahn DF. (2017, December 20). [Memorandum re Appleton ethics pledge waiver.] https://www.oge.gov/web/oge.nsf/0/163E08DB4BE33209852585B6005A1E2B/$FILE /USDA%20-%20Appleton%20(002)%205.pdf.

21. American Farm Bureau Federation. (2017, March 28). "#WomenInAg Spotlight: Kristi Boswell." https://www.fb.org/farm-bureau-news/womeninag-spotlight-kristi-boswell.

22. McGahn DF. (2017, May 16). [Memorandum re Boswell ethics pledge waiver.] https:// www.oge.gov/web/oge.nsf/0/8C275907A23BDA6C852585B6005A1E29/$FILE/USDA %20-%20Boswell%204.pdf.

23. Sunlight Foundation. (2009, May 26). "Brandeis and the History of Transparency." https:// sunlightfoundation.com/2009/05/26/brandeis-and-the-history-of-transparency/.

24. OpenSecrets. (n.d.). "Lobbying Data Summary." https://www.opensecrets.org/federal -lobbying. Accessed August 19, 2025.

25. Drutman L. (2015, April 20). "How Corporate Lobbyists Conquered American Democracy." *The Atlantic.* April 20, 2015. https://www.theatlantic.com/business/archive/2015/04/how -corporate-lobbyists-conquered-american-democracy/390822/.

26. Fang L. (2014, February 20). "The Shadow Lobbying Complex." Type Investigations. https://www.typeinvestigations.org/investigation/2014/02/20/shadow-lobbying -complex/.

27. OpenSecrets. (n.d.). "Lobbying Data Summary." https://www.opensecrets.org/federal -lobbying. Accessed August 19, 2025.

28. OpenSecrets. (n.d.). "Industry Profile: Food and Beverage." https://www.opensecrets.org /federal-lobbying/industries/summary?id=N01. Accessed August 5, 2025.

29. Aaron DG, Siegel MB. (2017, January). "Sponsorship of National Health Organizations by Two Major Soda Companies." *American Journal of Preventive Medicine* 52(1):20–30. https:// doi.org/10.1016/j.amepre.2016.08.010.

30. OpenSecrets. (n.d.). "Client Profile: American Beverage Assn." https://www.opensecrets.org /federal-lobbying/clients/issues?cycle=2009&id=d000000491. Accessed August 5, 2025.

31. Prins GS, Patisaul HB, Belcher SM, Vandenberg LN. "CLARITY-BPA Academic Labora- tory Studies Identify Consistent Low-Dose Bisphenol A Effects on Multiple Organ Systems." *Basic Clin Pharmacol Toxicol.* 2018 Sep 12.

32. Markey EJ. (2009, March 16). "H.R. 1523: To Ban the Use of Bisphenol A in Food Containers, and for Other Purposes." 111th Cong., 1st sess. https://www.govinfo.gov/content/pkg /BILLS-111hr1523ih/html/BILLS-111hr1523ih.htm.

33. Bardelline J. (2010, November 19). "BPA Ban Blocked from Food Safety Bill." *Green Biz.* https://web.archive.org/web/20230601075459/https://www.greenbiz.com/article/bpa -ban-blocked-food-safety-bill.

34. US Food and Drug Administration. (2023, April 20). "Bisphenol A (BPA): Use in Food Con- tact Applications." https://www.fda.gov/food/food-packaging-other-substances-come-contact -food-information-consumers/bisphenol-bpa-use-food-contact-application.

35. European Commission, Directorate-General for Health and Food Safety. (2024, December 19). "Commission Adopts Ban of Bisphenol A in Food Contact Materials." https://food .ec.europa.eu/food-safety-news-0/commission-adopts-ban-bisphenol-food-contact-materials -2024-12-19_en.

36. Guo J. (2015, May 28). "These 26 States Won't Let You Sue McDonald's for Making You Fat. The Surprising Consequence of Banning Obesity Lawsuits." *Washington Post.* https:// www.washingtonpost.com/blogs/govbeat/wp/2015/05/28/these-26-states-wont-let-you-sue -mcdonalds-for-making-you-fat-the-surprising-consequence-of-banning-obesity-lawsuits/.

37. Keller R. (2003, January 27). "H.R. 339—Personal Responsibility in Food Consumption Act." 108th Cong., 1st Sess. https://www.congress.gov/bill/108th-congress/house-bill/339.

38. Meier CF. (2003, August 1). "Keller, Kraft Weigh In on Obesity." https://heartland.org /opinion/keller-kraft-weigh-in-on-obesity/.

39. University of California, San Francisco. (n.d.). "Industry Documents Library." https:// www.industrydocuments.ucsf.edu/. Accessed August 5, 2025.

40. Simon M. (2006). *Appetite for Profit: How the Food Industry Undermines Our Health and How to Fight Back.* Bold Type Books.

41. Means C, Means C. (2024). *Good Energy: The Surprising Connection Between Metabolism and Limitless Health.* Avery, 70.

42. Means C, Means C. (2024). *Good Energy: The Surprising Connection Between Metabolism and Limitless Health.* Avery, 61.

43. *Martinez v. Kraft Heinz Company, Inc., et al.* (2025). Case No. 2:2025cv00377, U.S. District Court for the Eastern District of Pennsylvania. https://dockets.justia.com/docket/pennsylvania /paedce/2:2025cv00377/632523.

44. *Martinez v. Kraft Heinz Company, Inc., et al.* (2024). [Filed UPF Complaint.] Case No. 2:2025cv00377, U.S. District Court for the Eastern District of Pennsylvania. https://www.documentcloud.org/documents/25451650-filed-upf-complaint.

45. Wolfson R. (2016, July 14). "Congress Just Passed a GMO-Labeling Bill. Nobody's Super Happy About It." *The Salt.* https://www.npr.org/sections/thesalt/2016/07/14/486060866/congress-just-passed-a-gmo-labeling-bill-nobodys-super-happy-about-it.

46. Food and Water Watch. (2015, January). "How Much Will Labeling Genetically Engineered Foods Really Cost?" https://foodandwaterwatch.org/wp-content/uploads/2021/03/GMO-Labeling-Cost-FS-Jan-2015.pdf.

47. Faber S. (2016, February 22). "GMO Labeling Won't Increase Food Prices." Environmental Working Group. https://www.ewg.org/news-insights/news/gmo-labeling-wont-increase-food-prices.

48. Environmental Working Group. (2015, July 23). "DARK Act Passes, Fight for Americans' Right to Know Far from Over." https://www.ewg.org/news-insights/news-release/dark-act-passes-fight-americans-right-know-far-over.

49. Environmental Working Group. (2016, February 25). "Food Lobby Spends $101 Million in 2015 to Avert GMO Labeling." https://www.ewg.org/research/food-lobby-spends-101-million-2015-avert-gmo-labeling.

50. Kopicki A. (2013, July 27). "Strong Support for Labeling Modified Foods." *New York Times.* https://www.nytimes.com/2013/07/28/science/strong-support-for-labeling-modified-foods.html.

51. Center for Food Safety. (2016, March 1). "DARK Act Returns to Congress in Latest Industry Effort to Block GMO-Food Labeling." https://www.centerforfoodsafety.org/press-releases/4267/dark-act-returns-to-congress-in-latest-industry-effort-to-block-gmo-food-labeling.

52. Bickell EG. (2020, February 7). "The National Bioengineered Food Disclosure Standard: Overview and Selected Considerations." R46183. Congressional Research Service. https://www.congress.gov/crs-product/R46183.

53. Ibid.

54. Center for Food Safety. (n.d.). "International Labeling Laws: Genetically Engineered (GE) Food Labeling." https://www.centerforfoodsafety.org/issues/976/ge-food-labeling/international-labeling-laws. Accessed August 5, 2025.

55. Bickell EG. (2020, February 7). "The National Bioengineered Food Disclosure Standard: Overview and Selected Considerations." R46183. Congressional Research Service. https://www.congress.gov/crs-product/R46183.

56. Washington State Attorney General's Office. (2013, October 16). Complaint, *State of Washington v. Grocery Manufacturers Association.* Thurston County Superior Court Case No. 13-2-03258-34. https://agportal-s3bucket.s3.amazonaws.com/uploadedfiles/Complaint-20131016-Conformed.pdf.

57. Le P. (2013, October 19). "As Ad Claims Fly on GMO Labeling, Caveats Arise." Associated Press. https://komonews.com/news/local/as-ad-claims-fly-on-gmo-labeling-caveats-arise.

58. Simon M. (2012, July 31). "Big Food Puts Its Back into Fighting GMO Labeling in California." Grist. https://grist.org/food/big-food-puts-its-back-into-fighting-gmo-labeling-in-california/.

59. Washington State Attorney General's Office. (2013, October 16). Complaint, *State of Washington v. Grocery Manufacturers Association.* Thurston County Superior Court Case No. 13-2-03258-34. https://agportal-s3bucket.s3.amazonaws.com/uploadedfiles/Complaint-20131016-Conformed.pdf.

60. Ibid.

61. Legislative Analyst's Office, State of California. (2012, July 18). "Proposition 37: Genetically Engineered Foods. Mandatory Labeling. Initiative Statute." https://www.lao.ca.gov/ballot /2012/37_11_2012.aspx.

62. Peeples L. (2012, November 7). "Prop 37 GMO Labeling Law Defeated by Corporate Dollars and Deception, Proponents Say." *HuffPost.* https://www.huffpost.com/entry/proposition -37-gmo-labeling_n_2090112.

63. Washington State Attorney General's Office. (2013, October 16). Complaint, *State of Washington v. Grocery Manufacturers Association.* Thurston County Superior Court Case No. 13-2-03258-34. https://agportal-s3bucket.s3.amazonaws.com/uploadedfiles/Complaint -20131016-Conformed.pdf.

64. Office of the Attorney General, Washington State. (2016, November 2). "AG: Grocery Manufacturers Assoc. to Pay $18 Million—Largest Campaign Finance Penalty in U.S. History." https://www.atg.wa.gov/news/news-releases/ag-grocery-manufacturers-assoc-pay -18m-largest-campaign-finance-penalty-us.

65. Ibid.

66. Office of the Attorney General, Washington State. (2016, November 2). "AG: Grocery Manufacturers Assoc. to Pay $18 Million—Largest Campaign Finance Penalty in U.S. History." https://www.atg.wa.gov/news/news-releases/ag-grocery-manufacturers-assoc-pay -18m-largest-campaign-finance-penalty-us.

67. Office of the Attorney General, Washington State. (2016, February 16). "Documents Unsealed in GMA Lawsuit, Hearing Set for Friday." https://www.atg.wa.gov/news/news -releases/documents-unsealed-gma-lawsuit-hearing-set-Friday.

68. Office of the Attorney General, Washington State. (2016, November 2). "AG: Grocery Manufacturers Assoc. to Pay $18 Million—Largest Campaign Finance Penalty in U.S. History." https://www.atg.wa.gov/news/news-releases/ag-grocery-manufacturers-assoc-pay -18m-largest-campaign-finance-penalty-us.

69. Ballotpedia. (n.d.). "Washington Mandatory Labeling of Genetically Engineered Food Measure, Initiative 522 (2013)." https://ballotpedia.org/Washington_Mandatory_Labeling _of_Genetically_Engineered_Food_Measure,_Initiative_522_(2013). Accessed August 5, 2025.

70. Office of the Attorney General, Washington State. (2016, November 2). "AG: Grocery Manufacturers Assoc. to Pay $18 Million—Largest Campaign Finance Penalty in U.S. History." https://www.atg.wa.gov/news/news-releases/ag-grocery-manufacturers-assoc-pay -18m-largest-campaign-finance-penalty-us.

71. Connelly J. (2016, November 2). "Grocery Lobby Must Pay $18M for Laundering Campaign Money." *Seattle Post-Intelligencer.* https://www.seattlepi.com/local/politics/article /Grocery-manufacturers-told-Pay-millions-for-10531088.php.

72. Office of the Attorney General, Washington State. (2016, November 2). "AG: Grocery Manufacturers Assoc. to Pay $18 Million—Largest Campaign Finance Penalty in U.S. History." https://www.atg.wa.gov/news/news-releases/ag-grocery-manufacturers-assoc-pay -18m-largest-campaign-finance-penalty-us.

73. Office of the Attorney General, Washington State. (2016, November 2). "AG: Grocery Manufacturers Assoc. to Pay $18 Million—Largest Campaign Finance Penalty in U.S. History." https://www.atg.wa.gov/news/news-releases/ag-grocery-manufacturers-assoc-pay -18m-largest-campaign-finance-penalty-us.

74. Ibid.

75. Jenkins D. (2017, September 6). "Washington AG to Press for $18 Million Fine Against Foodmakers." *Capital Press.* https://www.capitalpress.com/state/washington/washington-ag-to -press-for-million-fine-against-foodmakers/article_7001b804-800d-5459-bcc3 -5787dbab9ea8.html; Office of the Attorney General, Washington State. (2020, November 9).

"Court of Appeals Unanimously Upholds $18M Penalty Against Grocery Manufacturer's Association in AG's Campaign Finance Lawsuit." https://www.atg.wa.gov/news/news-releases/court-appeals-unanimously-upholds-18m-penalty-against-grocery-manufacturer-s.

76. Brunner J. (2016, November 2). "Grocery Group Fined $18M in Fight Against GMO Food-Labeling Initiative." *Seattle Times.* https://www.seattletimes.com/seattle-news/politics/grocery-group-hit-with-18m-campaign-financing-fine-over-food-labeling-measure/.

77. Consumer Brands Association. (2019, September 26). "Bold New Agenda, New Name: GMA to Relaunch as Consumer Brands Association™ in 2020." Press release. https://consumerbrandsassociation.org/press-releases/bold-new-agenda-new-name-gma-to-relaunch-as-consumer-brands-association-in-2020.

78. Bottemiller Evich H, Boudreau C. (2017, November 26). "The Big Washington Food Fight: How the Food Lobby Is Splintering over Consumer Taste Preferences." *Politico.* https://www.politico.com/story/2017/11/26/food-lobby-consumer-tastes-washington-190528.

79. Sustainable Food Policy Alliance. (2018, July 12). "Four Major Food Companies Launch Sustainable Food Policy Alliance to Drive Progress in U.S. Public Policies That Shape What People Eat." https://foodpolicyalliance.org/news/four-major-food-companies-launch-the-sustainable-food-policy-alliance/.

80. Gaines R. (2025, March 22). "They offered to pay me to post…a big fat heck no." Twitter. https://x.com/Riley_Gaines_/status/1903467064712482881.

81. Cargill. (2024). "Corn Sweeteners: Making Your Products Better." https://www.cargill.com/food-beverage/na/corn-sweeteners.

82. Murphy A. (2024, November 25). "America's Top Private Companies." *Forbes.* https://www.forbes.com/lists/top-private-companies/.

83. Reuters. (2022, August 10). "Cargill Fiscal 2022 Revenue Jumps 23% to Record $165 Billion." https://www.reuters.com/markets/commodities/cargill-fiscal-2022-revenue-jumps-23-165-billion-2022-08-10/.

84. Forbes. (2023). "Cargill MacMillan, Jr." https://www.forbes.com/profile/cargill-macmillan/?sh=44fa93db4c0e.

85. Dent M. (2025, January 10). "How Corn Syrup Took over America." The Hustle. https://thehustle.co/originals/how-corn-syrup-took-over-america.

86. Jacques J. (2008, Winter). "A Not-So-Sweet Story—High Fructose Corn Syrup." Obesity Action Coalition. https://www.obesityaction.org/resources/a-not-so-sweet-story-high-fructose-corn-syrup/.

87. Basciano H, Federico L, Adeli K. (2005, February 21). "Fructose, Insulin Resistance, and Metabolic Dyslipidemia." *Nutrition and Metabolism* 2:article 5. https://doi.org/10.1186/1743-7075-2-5.

88. Lodge M, Dykes R, Kennedy A. (2024, July 13). "Regulation of Fructose Metabolism in Nonalcoholic Fatty Liver Disease." *Biomolecules* 14(7):845. https://doi.org/10.3390/biom14070845.

89. DiNicolantonio JJ, O'Keefe JH, Lucan SC. (2005, March). "Added Fructose: A Principal Driver of Type 2 Diabetes Mellitus and Its Consequences." *Mayo Clinic Proceedings* 90(3):P372–81. https://www.mayoclinicproceedings.org/article/s0025-6196(15)00040-3/fulltext.

90. Strom S. (2016, January 8). "Campbell Labels Will Disclose GMO Ingredients." *New York Times.* https://www.nytimes.com/2016/01/08/business/campbell-labels-will-disclose-gmo-ingredients.html.

91. Drutman L. (2011, June). "A Better Way to Fix Lobbying." *Issues in Governance Studies.* https://www.brookings.edu/wp-content/uploads/2016/06/06_lobbying_drutman.pdf.

92. Legislative Analyst's Office, State of California. (2012, July 18). "Proposition 37: Genetically Engineered Foods. Mandatory Labeling. Initiative Statute." https://www.lao.ca.gov/ballot /2012/37_11_2012.aspx.

CHAPTER 7

1. Garber J. (2019, November 6). "CDC 'Disclaimers' Hide Financial Conflicts of Interest." Lown Institute. https://lowninstitute.org/cdc-disclaimers-hide-financial-conflicts-of-interest/.
2. Iacobucci G. (2019, January 30). "Coca-Cola and Obesity: Study Shows Efforts to Influence US Centers for Disease Control." *BMJ* 364:l471. https://doi.org/10.1136/bmj.l471.
3. Maani Hessari N, Ruskin G, McKee M, et al. (2019). "Public Meets Private: Conversations Between Coca-Cola and the CDC." *Milbank Quarterly* 97(1):74–90. https://doi.org/10 .1111/1468-0009.12368.
4. Union of Concerned Scientists. (2019). "A Food and Farm Bill for Everyone." https://www .ucs.org/resources/food-and-farm-bill.
5. Congressional Budget Office. (2014, January 28). "H.R. 2642, Agricultural Act of 2014: Effects on Direct Spending and Revenues of the Conference Agreement on H.R. 2642, as Reported on January 27, 2014." Publication No. 45049. https://www.cbo.gov/publication/45049.
6. US Department of Agriculture. (n.d.). "Farm Bill." https://www.usda.gov/farming-and -ranching/farm-bill. Accessed August 5, 2025.
7. US Department of Agriculture and US Department of Health and Human Services. (n.d.). "Dietary Guidelines for Americans: Process." https://www.dietaryguidelines.gov/about -dietary-guidelines/process. Accessed August 5, 2025.
8. US Department of Agriculture and US Department of Health and Human Services. (n.d.). "Dietary Guidelines for Americans: History of the Dietary Guidelines." https://www .dietaryguidelines.gov/about-dietary-guidelines/history-dietary-guidelines. Accessed August 5, 2025.
9. McGandy RB, Hegsted DM, Stare FJ. (1967, July 27). "Dietary Fats, Carbohydrates and Atherosclerotic Vascular Disease." *New England Journal of Medicine* 277(4):186–92. https:// doi.org/10.1056/nejm196707272770405.
10. Pearce J. (2009, July 8). "D. Mark Hegsted, 95, Harvard Nutritionist, Is Dead." *New York Times.* https://www.nytimes.com/2009/07/09/health/09hegsted.html.
11. Kearns CE, Schmidt LA, Glantz SA. (2016). "Sugar Industry and Coronary Heart Disease Research: A Historical Analysis of Internal Industry Documents." *JAMA Internal Medicine* 176(11):1680–85. https://doi.org/10.1001/jamainternmed.2016.5394.
12. Ibid.
13. US Department of Agriculture. (2024, May). "A Brief History of the USDA Food Guides." https://myplate-prod.azureedge.us/sites/default/files/2024-05/A-Brief-History-of-the -USDA-Food-Guides.pdf.
14. Harvard T. H. Chan School of Public Health. (2016, January 7). "New Dietary Guidelines Remove Restriction on Total Fat and Set Limit for Added Sugars—But Censor Conclusions." https://nutritionsource.hsph.harvard.edu/2016/01/07/new-dietary-guidelines-remove -restriction-on-total-fat-and-set-limit-for-added-sugars-but-censor-conclusions/.
15. Lawrence DJ. (2004). "Policy Trumps Science in the Bush Administration." *Journal of the Canadian Chiropractic Association* 48(3):195–97. https://www.ncbi.nlm.nih.gov/pmc/articles /PMC1769461/.
16. Nutrition Coalition. (n.d.). "Impact." https://www.nutritioncoalition.us/impact. Accessed August 5, 2025.
17. Committee to Review the Process to Update the Dietary Guidelines for Americans. (2017). *Optimizing the Process for Establishing the Dietary Guidelines for Americans: The Selection Process.* Washington, DC: National Academies Press. https://doi.org/10.17226/24637.

18. Farrington C. (2022, August). "Take It with a Grain (or More) of Salt: Why Industry-Backed Dietary Guidelines Fail Americans and How to Fix Them." *Michigan Journal of Law Reform.* https://mjlr.org/journal/take-it-with-a-grain-or-more-of-salt-why-industry-backed-dietary-guidelines-fail-americans-and-how-to-fix-them.

19. Mialon M, Matos Serodio P, Crosbie E, et al. (2022, March 21). "Conflicts of Interest for Members of the US 2020 Dietary Guidelines Advisory Committee." *Public Health Nutrition* 27(1):e69. https://doi.org/10.1017/S1368980022000672.

20. US Department of Health and Human Services and US Department of Agriculture. (2020). "Dietary Guidelines for Americans, 2010." https://odphp.health.gov/sites/default/files/2020-01/DietaryGuidelines2010.pdf.

21. Monke J. (2024, December 27). "Farm Bill Primer: Budget Dynamics." IF12233. Congressional Research Service. https://www.congress.gov/crs-product/IF12233.

22. "For a Healthier Country, Overhaul Farm Subsidies." (2012, May 1). Editorial. *Scientific American.* https://www.scientificamerican.com/article/fresh-fruit-hold-the-insulin/.

23. Iowa Corn Growers Association. (n.d.). "Corn Facts and Fun." https://www.iowacorn.org/corn-facts-faq. Accessed August 5, 2025.

24. Mayo Clinic. (2025, February 1). "Trans Fat Is Double Trouble for Heart Health." https://www.mayoclinic.org/diseases-conditions/high-blood-cholesterol/in-depth/trans-fat/art-20046114.

25. American Soybean Association. (2025). "Soybean Oil: U.S. Vegetable Oils Consumption." https://soystats.com/soybean-oil-u-s-vegetable-oils-consumption/.

26. Nestle M. (2016, March 17). "The Farm Bill Drove Me Insane." *Politico.* https://www.politico.com/agenda/story/2016/03/farm-bill-congress-usda-food-policy-000070/.

27. Walsh B. (2009, August 21). "Getting Real About the High Price of Cheap Food." *Time.* https://time.com/archive/6689284/getting-real-about-the-high-price-of-cheap-food.

28. Elkadi N. (2024, April 8). "An Iowa Fertilizer Plant Purchase Spurs Antitrust Concerns." Civil Eats. https://civileats.com/2024/04/08/an-iowa-fertilizer-plant-purchase-spurs-antitrust-concerns/.

29. Don't Mess with Taxes. (2013, July 28). "Farm Bill Subsidies Feed America's Junk Food Appetite." https://www.dontmesswithtaxes.com/2013/07/farm-bill-subsidies-junk-food-pirg.html.

30. Russo M, Smith D. (2013, July). "Apples to Twinkies 2013: Comparing Taxpayer Subsidies for Fresh Produce and Junk Food." US PIRG. https://uspirg.org/reports/usp/apples-twinkies-2013. https://pirg.org/wp-content/uploads/2013/10/Apples_to_Twinkies_2013_USPIRG_0.pdf.

31. Siegel KR. (2016, August 1). "Association of Higher Consumption of Foods Derived from Subsidized Commodities with Adverse Cardiometabolic Risk Among US Adults." *JAMA Internal Medicine* 176(8):1124–32. https://doi.org/10.1001/jamainternmed.2016.2410.

32. Russo M, Smith D. (2013, July). "Apples to Twinkies 2013: Comparing Taxpayer Subsidies for Fresh Produce and Junk Food." US PIRG. https://uspirg.org/reports/usp/apples-twinkies-2013. https://pirg.org/wp-content/uploads/2013/10/Apples_to_Twinkies_2013_USPIRG_0.pdf.

33. Mulik K, O'Hara JK. (2013, October). "The Healthy Farmland Diet: How Growing Less Corn Would Improve Our Health and Help America's Heartland." Union of Concerned Scientists. https://www.ucs.org/sites/default/files/2019-09/healthy-farmland-diet.pdf.

34. Nestle M. (2016, March 17). "The Farm Bill Drove Me Insane." *Politico.* https://www.politico.com/agenda/story/2016/03/farm-bill-congress-usda-food-policy-000070/.

35. Ibid.

36. Bittman M, Pollan M, Salvador R, et al. (2014, November 7). "How a National Food Policy Could Save Millions of American Lives." *Washington Post.* November 7, 2014. https://www.washingtonpost.com/opinions/how-a-national-food-policy-could-save-millions-of-american-lives/2014/11/07/89c55e16-637f-11e4-836c-83bc4f26eb67_story.html.

37. Ibid.
38. Menegat S, Ledo A, Tirado R. (2022, August 25). "Greenhouse Gas Emissions from Global Production and Use of Nitrogen Synthetic Fertilisers in Agriculture." *Scientific Reports* 12:14490. https://doi.org/10.1038/s41598-022-18773-w.
39. Mozaffarian D, Angell SY, Lang T, et al. (2018, June 13). "Role of Government Policy in Nutrition—Barriers to and Opportunities for Healthier Eating." *BMJ* 361:k2426.
40. Berkowitz SA, Terranova J, Randall L, et al. (2019, June 1). "Association Between Receipt of a Medically Tailored Meal Program and Health Care Use." *JAMA Internal Medicine* 179(6):786–93. https://doi.org/10.1001/jamainternmed.2019.0198.
41. White ND. (2020, April 26). "Produce Prescriptions, Food Pharmacies, and the Potential Effect on Food Choice." *American Journal of Lifestyle Medicine* 14(4):366–68. https://doi.org/10.1177/1559827620915425.
42. Gurvey J, Rand K, Daugherty S, et al. (2013, October). "Examining Health Care Costs Among MANNA Clients and a Comparison Group." *Journal of Primary Care and Community Health* 4(4):311–17. doi: 10.1177/2150131913490737.
43. John Hancock Life Insurance Company. (n.d.). "Small Changes, Big Impacts: Why the John Hancock Vitality Program Works." https://www.johnhancock.com/ideas-insights/why-john-hancock-vitality-program-works.html. Accessed August 5, 2025.
44. PR Newswire. (2018, September 19). "John Hancock Leaves Traditional Life Insurance Model Behind to Incentivize Longer, Healthier Lives." https://www.prnewswire.com/news-releases/john-hancock-leaves-traditional-life-insurance-model-behind-to-incentivize-longer-healthier-lives-300715351.html.
45. Feinberg AT, Hess A, Passaretti M, et al. (2018, April 10). "Prescribing Food as a Specialty Drug." *NJEM Catalyst.* https://catalyst.nejm.org/prescribing-fresh-food-farmacy/; Tirrell M, Gralnick J. (2018, June 21). "Diabetes Defeated by Diet: How New Fresh-Food Prescriptions Are Beating Pricey Drugs." CNBC. https://www.cnbc.com/2018/06/20/diabetes-defeated-by-diet-new-fresh-food-prescriptions-beat-drugs.html.
46. McGovern J. (2018, January 17). "Bipartisan Members of Congress Launch Food Is Medicine Working Group to Highlight Impacts of Hunger on Health." Press release. https://mcgovern.house.gov/news/documentsingle.aspx?DocumentID=397179. https://odphp.health.gov/foodismedicine.

CHAPTER 8

1. Fryar C, Carroll MD, Afful J. (2020, December). "Prevalence of Overweight, Obesity, and Severe Obesity Among Children and Adolescents Aged 2–19 Years: United States, 1963–1965 Through 2017–2018." Centers for Disease Control and Prevention, National Center for Health Statistics. https://www.cdc.gov/nchs/data/hestat/obesity-child-17-18/overweight-obesity-child-H.pdf.
2. Centers for Disease Control and Prevention. (2024, April). "Childhood Obesity Facts." https://www.cdc.gov/obesity/childhood-obesity-facts/childhood-obesity-facts.html.
3. May AL, Kuklina EV, Yoon PW. (2012, June). "Prevalence of Cardiovascular Disease Risk Factors Among US Adolescents, 1999–2008." *Pediatrics* 129(6):1035–41. https://doi.org/10.1542/peds.2011-1082.
4. Kitahara CM, Flint AJ, Berrington de Gonzalez A, et al. (2014, July). "Association Between Class III Obesity (BMI of 40–59 kg/m) and Mortality: A Pooled Analysis of 20 Prospective Studies." *PLOS Medicine* 11(7):e1001673. https://doi.org/10.1371/journal.pmed.1001673.
5. White House. (2010, December 10). "Child Nutrition Reauthorization: Healthy, Hunger-Free Kids Act of 2010." https://obamawhitehouse.archives.gov/sites/default/files/Child_Nutrition_Fact_Sheet_12_10_10.pdf.

6. US Department of Education, Institute of Education Sciences. (n.d.). "Fast Facts." https://nces.ed.gov/fastfacts/. Accessed August 5, 2025.

7. Kenney EL, Barrett JL, Bleich SN, et al. (2020, July). "Impact of the Healthy, Hunger-Free Kids Act on Obesity Trends." *Health Affairs* 39(7):1122–29. https://doi.org/10.1377/hlthaff.2020.00133.

8. Center for Responsive Politics. (n.d.) "Bill Profile: S.3307." https://www.opensecrets.org/lobby/billsum.php?id=s3307-111. Accessed August 5, 2025.

9. Park A. (2014, July 18). "The Food Industry Lobby Groups Behind the New School Nutrition Standards." *Mother Jones.* https://www.motherjones.com/politics/2014/07/who-lobbied-school-nutrition-standards-these-guys/.

10. Bottemiller Evich H. (2014, June 4). "Behind the School Lunch Fight." *Politico.* https://www.politico.com/story/2014/06/michelle-obama-public-school-lunch-school-nutrition-association-lets-move-107390.

11. Confessore N. (2014, October 7). "How School Lunch Became the Latest Political Battleground." *New York Times Magazine.* https://www.nytimes.com/2014/10/12/magazine/how-school-lunch-became-the-latest-political-battleground.html.

12. Jacobs E. (2019, April 23). "Klobuchar Explains Why She Fought for Pizza Sauce to Be Classified As a Vegetable." *New York Post.* https://nypost.com/2019/04/23/klobuchar-explains-why-she-fought-for-pizza-sauce-to-be-classified-as-a-vegetable/.

13. United States Department of Agriculture, Food and Nutrition Service. (2022, May). "A Guide to Smart Snacks in School." FNS-623. https://www.fns.usda.gov/tn/guide-smart-snacks-school.

14. "Approved Smart Snacks in Schools List." (n.d). https://campussuite-storage.s3.amazonaws.com/prod/1559027/2cae00ac-8a5c-11ea-886f-12f99fab7833/2387620/1ad81556-a3bf-11ec-b469-0e9b1399f0a1/file/Smart%20Snacks%20Approved%20List.pdf. Accessed August 19, 2025.

15. "Ibid.

16. Campbell's Food Service. (n.d.). "Pepperidge Farm Goldfish Made with Whole Grain 100 Calorie Snack Crackers, Cheddar, .75 Ounce, Pack of 100." https://web.archive.org/web/20250518223902/https://www.campbellsfoodservice.com/product/pepperidge-farm-goldfish-whole-grain-100-calorie-snack-crackers-cheddar/. Accessed August 19, 2025.

17. General Mills Foodservice. (n.d.). "Simply Chex Snack Mix Single Serve Pouch Strawberry Crème 60/1.03 oz." https://www.generalmillsfoodservice.com/products/category/snacks/chex/simply-strawberry-yogurt-1-03oz-60ct. Accessed August 5, 2025.

18. General Mills Foodservice. (n.d.). "Fruit Roll-Ups." https://web.archive.org/web/20250519121622/https://www.generalmillsfoodservice.com/industries/k12/support-tool-categories/exploring-products/fruit-roll-ups. Accessed August 5, 2025.

19. van Tulleken C. (2025). *Ultra-Processed People: Why We Can't Stop Eating Food That Isn't Food.* W. W. Norton. P. 272.

20. Sayers DL. (1933.) *Murder Must Advertise.* Doubleday.

21. Siegel BE. (2018, August 5). "Why Did HISD Sign a New Contract with Domino's?" *Houston Chronicle.* https://www.houstonchronicle.com/local/gray-matters/article/hisd-betti-wiggins-school-lunch-domino-s-13130026.php.

22. Domino's Pizza. (2013, September 18). "Domino's Smart Slice School Lunch Program Expands Participating Schools by 45 Percent Since 2012." Press release. https://ir.dominos.com/news-releases/news-release-details/dominos-smart-slice-school-lunch-program-expands-participating.

23. Siegel BE. (2018, August 5). "Why Did HISD Sign a New Contract with Domino's?" *Houston Chronicle.* https://www.houstonchronicle.com/local/gray-matters/article/hisd-betti-wiggins-school-lunch-domino-s-13130026.php.

24. Siegel BE. (2018, August 2). "Under Betti Wiggins, Houston ISD Signs $8 Million Contract for Domino's 'Smart Slice' Pizza." *The Lunch Tray.* https://web.archive.org/web/20240613004133/https://thelunchtray.com/houston-isd-8-million-contract-for-dominos-smart-slice-pizza-betti-wiggins/.

25. Terry-McElrath YM, Turner L, Sandoval A, et al. (2014, March). "Commercialism in US Elementary and Secondary School Nutrition Environments: Trends from 2007 to 2012." *JAMA Pediatrics* 168(3):234–42. https://doi.org/10.1001/jamapediatrics.2013.4521.

26. Terry-McElrath YM, Turner L, Sandoval A, et al. (2014, March). "Commercialism in US Elementary and Secondary School Nutrition Environments: Trends from 2007 to 2012." *JAMA Pediatrics* 168(3):234–42. https://doi.org/10.1001/jamapediatrics.2013.4521.

27. American Psychological Association. (2010). "The Impact of Food Advertising on Childhood Obesity." https://www.apa.org/topics/kids-media/food. Accessed August 19, 2025.

28. GBD 2017 Diet Collaborators. (2019, May 11). "Health Effects of Dietary Risks in 195 Countries, 1990–2017: A Systematic Analysis for the Global Burden of Disease Study 2017." *The Lancet* 393(10184):1958–72.

29. McGinnis JM, Gootman JA, Kraak VI, eds. (2006). *Food Marketing to Children and Youth: Threat or Opportunity?* National Academies Press.

30. Nestle M. (2006, June 15). "Food Marketing and Childhood Obesity—A Matter of Policy." *New England Journal of Medicine* 354(24):2527–29. DOI: 10.1056/NEJMp068014.

31. Federal Trade Commission. (2012, December). "A Review of Food Marketing to Children and Adolescents." https://www.ftc.gov/sites/default/files/documents/reports/review-food-marketing-children-and-adolescents-follow-report/121221foodmarketingreport.pdf.

32. Powell LM, Schermbeck RM, Szczypka G, et al. (2013, June 6). "Trends in the Nutritional Content of TV Food Advertisements Seen by Children in the US: Analyses by Age, Food Categories and Companies." *Archives of Pediatrics and Adolescent Medicine* 128(6):e120–28. https://doi.org/10.1001/archpediatrics.2011.131.

33. American Psychological Association. (2010). "The Impact of Food Advertising on Childhood Obesity." https://www.apa.org/topics/kids-media/food. Accessed August 19, 2025.

34. Harris JL, Frazier W, Kumanyika S, et al. (2019, January). "Increasing Disparities in Unhealthy Food Advertising Targeted to Black and Hispanic Youth." Rudd Center for Food Policy and Health, University of Connecticut. https://uconnruddcenter.org/files/Pdfs/TargetedMarketingReport2019.pdf.

35. Ibid.

36. American Academy of Child and Adolescent Psychiatry. (2025, June). "Facts for Families: Children and Watching TV." No. 54. https://www.aacap.org/AACAP/Families_and_Youth/Facts_for_Families/FFF-Guide/Children-And-Watching-TV-054.aspx.

37. American Psychological Association. (2010). "The Impact of Food Advertising on Childhood Obesity." https://www.apa.org/topics/kids-media/food. Accessed August 19, 2025.

38. McCarthy CM, de Vries R, Mackenbach JD. (2022, March 17). "The Influence of Unhealthy Food and Beverage Marketing Through Social Media and Advergaming on Diet-Related Outcomes in Children—A Systematic Review." *Obesity Reviews* 23(6):e13441. https://doi.org/10.1111/obr.13441.

39. Weatherspoon LJ, Quilliam ET, Paek HJ, et al. (2013, September 26). "Consistency of Nutrition Recommendations for Foods Marketed to Children in the United States, 2009–2010." *Preventing Chronic Disease* 10:E165. https://doi.org/10.5888/pcd10.130099.

40. Story M, French S. (2004, February 10). "Food Advertising and Marketing Directed at Children and Adolescents in the US." *International Journal of Behavioral Nutrition and Physical Activity* 1(1):3. https://doi.org/10.1186/1479-5868-1-3.

41. Borzekowski DL, Robinson TN. (2001, January). "The 30-Second Effect: An Experiment Revealing the Impact of Television Commercials on Food Preferences of Preschoolers." *Journal of the American Dietetic Association* 101(1):42–46. https://doi.org/10.1016/s0002-8223 (01)00012-8.

42. American Psychological Association. (2010). "The Impact of Food Advertising on Childhood Obesity." https://www.apa.org/topics/kids-media/food. Accessed August 19, 2025.

43. Reichelt AC, Rank MM. (2017, December 1). "The Impact of Junk Foods on the Adolescent Brain." *Birth Defects Research* 109(20):1649–58. https://doi.org/10.1002/bdr2.1173.

44. McClure AC, Tanski SE, Gilbert-Diamond D, et al. (2013, November). "Receptivity to Television Fast-Food Restaurant Marketing and Obesity Among U.S. Youth." *American Journal of Preventive Medicine* 45(5):560–68. https://doi.org/10.1016/j.amepre.2013 .06.011.

45. Burrows D. (2018, March 19). "Barrage of Junk Food Ads Fuelling Teenage Obesity." *Food Navigator*. March 19, 2018. https://www.foodnavigator.com/Article/2018/03/19/Barrage -of-junk-food-ads-fuelling-teenage-obesity/.

46. Lardieri A. (2018, May 22). "Study: Teens Exposed to More Junk Food Ads Eat More Junk Food." *U.S. News and World Report*. https://www.usnews.com/news/health-care-news /articles/2018-05-22/study-teens-exposed-to-more-junk-food-ads-eat-more-junk-food.

47. Skinner AC, Ravanbakht SN, Skelton JA, et al. (2018, March). "Prevalence of Obesity and Severe Obesity in US Children, 1999–2016." *Pediatrics* 141(3):e20173459. https://doi.org /10.1542/peds.2017-3459.

48. Clemente MG, Mandato C, Poeta M, et al. (2016). "Pediatric Non-Alcoholic Fatty Liver Disease: Recent Solutions, Unresolved Issues, and Future Research Directions." *World Journal of Gastroenterology* 22(36):8078–93. https://doi.org/10.3748/wjg.v22.i36.8078.

49. Satapathy SK, Bernstein DE, Roth NC. (2022). "Liver Transplantation in Patients with Non-Alcoholic Steatohepatitis and Alcohol-Related Liver Disease: The Dust Is Yet to Settle." *Translational Gastroenterology and Hepatology* 7:23. https://doi.org/10.21037/tgh -2020-15.

50. Northstone K, Joinson C, Emmett P, et al. (2012). "Are Dietary Patterns in Childhood Associated with IQ at 8 Years of Age? A Population-Based Cohort Study." *Journal of Epidemiology and Community Health* 66(7):624–28. https://doi.org/10.1136/jech.2010.111955.

51. Federal Trade Commission. (2011). "Food Marketed to Children Forum: Interagency Working Group Proposal for Voluntary Principles to Guide Industry Self-Regulatory Efforts." https://www.ftc.gov/sites/default/files/documents/public_events/food-marketed -children-forum-interagency-working-group-proposal/110428foodmarketproposedguide .pdf.

52. Burros M. (2011, October 12). "Childhood Obesity War a Food Fight?" *Politico*. https:// www.politico.com/story/2011/10/childhood-obesity-war-a-food-fight-065817.

53. Layton L, Eggen D. (2011, July 9). "Industries Lobby Against Voluntary Nutrition Guidelines for Food Marketed to Kids." *Washington Post*. https://www.washingtonpost.com /politics/industries-lobby-against-voluntary-nutrition-guidelines-for-food-marketed-to -kids/2011/07/08/gIQAZSZu5H_story.html.

54. IHS Consulting. (2011). "Assessing the Economic Impact of Restricting Advertising for Products That Target Young Americans." https://www.foodpolitics.com/wp-content /uploads/Global-Insight-Report.pdf.

55. Vladeck D. (2011, July 1). "What's on the Table." Federal Trade Commission, Bureau of Consumer Protection. https://web.archive.org/web/20110721042015/http://business.ftc.gov /blog/2011/07/whats-table.

56. BBB National Programs. (n.d.). "Children's Food and Beverage Advertising Initiative (CFBAI)." https://bbbprograms.org/programs/children/cfbai. Accessed August 5, 2025.

57. BBB National Programs. (2024). "Get to Know the Children's Food and Beverage Advertising Initiative." https://assets.bbbprograms.org/docs/default-source/cfbai/cfbai-infographic.pdf.

58. Harris JL, Frazier W, Romo-Palafox M, et al. (2017). "Food Industry Self-Regulation After 10 Years." Rudd Center for Food Policy and Health, University of Connecticut. http://www.uconnruddcenter.org/files/Pdfs/FACTS-2017_Final.pdf.

59. World Health Organization. (2016). "Tackling Food Marketing to Children in a Digital World: Trans-Discilinary Perspectives." https://iris.who.int/bitstream/handle/10665/344003/9789289052177-eng.pdf.

60. Gallagher J. (2016, November 4.) "Stop Junk Food Ads on Kids' Apps—WHO." BBC News. https://www.bbc.com/news/health-37846318.

61. Constine J. (2017, May 31). "Pokémon GO Reveals Sponsors Like McDonald's Pay It Up to $0.50 Per Visitor." *TechCrunch.* https://techcrunch.com/2017/05/31/pokemon-go-sponsorship-price/.

62. World Health Organization. (2016). "Tackling Food Marketing to Children in a Digital World: Trans-Disciplinary Perspectives." https://iris.who.int/bitstream/handle/10665/344003/9789289052177-eng.pdf.

63. Block J. (2018, April 2). "Boston Schools' Fresh Food Program Expands." *Boston Globe.* https://www.shahfoundation.org/newsroom/bg-4-2-18-fzeft.

64. City of Boston. (2018, April 2). "Fresh Food Program Expanded at Boston Public Schools." https://www.boston.gov/news/fresh-food-program-expanded-boston-public-schools.

65. Chou SY, Rashad I, Grossman M. (2005, December). "Fast-Food Restaurant Advertising on Television and Its Influence on Childhood Obesity." Working Paper 11879. National Bureau of Economic Research. https://www.nber.org/system/files/working_papers/w11879/w11879.pdf; Veerman JL, Van Beeck EF, Barendregt JJ, Mackenbach JP. (2009, March 26). "By How Much Would Limiting TV Food Advertising Reduce Childhood Obesity?" *European Journal of Public Health* 19(4):365–69. https://doi.org/10.1093/eurpub/ckp039.

66. Strasburger VC. (2011, July). "Policy Statement—Children, Adolescents, Obesity, and the Media." *Pediatrics* 128(1):201–8. http://www.pediatrics.org/cgi/doi/10.1542/peds.2011-1066; Chou SY, Rashad I, Grossman M. (2005, December). "Fast-Food Restaurant Advertising on Television and Its Influence on Childhood Obesity." Working Paper 11879. National Bureau of Economic Research. https://www.nber.org/system/files/working_papers/w11879/w11879.pdf.

67. Obesity Evidence Hub. (n.d.). "The Way Forward: Policies to Reduce Children's Exposure to Junk Food Advertising." https://www.obesityevidencehub.org.au/collections/prevention/the-way-forward-policies-to-reduce-childrens-exposure-to-junk-food-advertising. Accessed August 19, 2025.

68. Dhar T, Baylis K. (2011). "Fast-Food Consumption and the Ban on Advertising Targeting Children: The Quebec Experience." *Journal of Marketing Research* 48(5):799–813. https://doi.org/10.1509/jmkr.48.5.799.

69. Ibid.

70. Ibid.

71. Musemeche C. (2012, July 13). "Ban on Advertising to Children Linked to Lower Obesity Rates." *New York Times.* https://archive.nytimes.com/parenting.blogs.nytimes.com/2012/07/13/ban-on-advertising-to-children-linked-to-lower-obesity-rates/.

72. Cordes R. (2000, October 18). "Swedish Call for Ban on TV Advertising to Children Faces Defeat." *Politico.* https://www.politico.eu/article/swedish-call-for-ban-on-tv-advertising-to-children-faces-defeat/.

73. Transport for London. (2018, November 23). "Mayor Confirms Ban on Junk Food Advertising on Transport Network." https://tfl.gov.uk/info-for/media/press-releases /2018/november/mayor-confirms-ban-on-junk-food-advertising-on-transport -netwo.

74. Sandeman G. (2024, September 13). "What Counts as Junk Food in Upcoming UK Advert Ban." BBC News. https://www.bbc.com/news/articles/cp3d33l53r9o.

75. Ibid.

76. BBC News. (2018, July 4). "First Ads Banned Under New Junk Food Rules." https://www .bbc.com/news/uk-44706755.

77. Bowles N. (2018, October 26). "Silicon Valley Nannies Are Phone Police for Kids." *New York Times*. https://www.nytimes.com/2018/10/26/style/silicon-valley-nannies.html.

78. Tamana SK, Ezeugwu V, Chikuma J, et al. (2019, April 17). "Screen-Time Is Associated with Inattention Problems in Preschoolers: Results from the CHILD Birth Cohort Study." *PLOS One* 14(4):e0213995. https://doi.org/10.1371/journal.pone.0213995; Fang K, Mu M, Liu K, et al. (2019, July 3). "Screen Time and Childhood Overweight/Obesity: A Systematic Review and Meta-Analysis." *Child Care, Health and Development* 45(5):744–53. https:// doi.org/10.1111/cch.12701.

CHAPTER 9

1. Juul F, Parekh N, Martinez-Steele E, et al. (2022). "Ultra-Processed Food Consumption Among U.S. Adults from 2001 to 2018." *American Journal of Clinical Nutrition* 115(1):211–21. https://doi.org/10.1093/ajcn/nqab305.

2. National Institutes of Health. (2021, August 31). "Highly Processed Foods Form Bulk of U.S. Youths' Diets." https://www.nih.gov/news-events/nih-research-matters/highly-processed -foods-form-bulk-us-youths-diets.

3. Harvard T. H. Chan School of Public Health. (n.d.). "Jerold R. Mande, Sc.D., M.P.H." https://hsph.harvard.edu/profile/jerold-r-mande/. Accessed August 5, 2025.

4. Smucker's. (n.d.). "Strawberry Jam." https://www.smuckers.com/fruit-spreads/jam/strawberry -jam. Accessed August 5, 2025.

5. US Food and Drug Administration. (2006). "FDA's Approach to the GRAS Provision: A History of Processes." https://www.fda.gov/food/generally-recognized-safe-gras/fdas-approach -gras-provision-history-processes.

6. Ibid.

7. Center for Science in the Public Interest. (2015, April 15). "FDA Food Ingredient Approval Process Violates Law, Says CSPI." Center for Science in the Public Interest. https://www .cspi.org/new/201504151.html.

8. Neltner TG, Alger HM, O'Reilly JT, et al. (2013, December 9–23). "Conflicts of Interest in Approvals of Additives to Food Determined to Be Generally Recognized As Safe: Out of Balance." *JAMA Internal Medicine* 173(22):2032–36. https://doi.org/10.1001/jamainternmed .2013.10559.

9. Ibid.

10. Ibid.; US Government Accountability Office. (2010, March 5). "Food Safety: FDA Should Strengthen Its Oversight of Food Ingredients Determined to Be Generally Recognized as Safe (GRAS)." https://www.gao.gov/products/GAO-10-246.

11. Beyranevand LJ. (2013). "Generally Recognized as Safe? Analyzing Flaws in the FDA's Approach to GRAS Additives." *Vermont Law Review* 37(4):887–922. https://lawreview .vermontlaw.edu/wp-content/uploads/2013/08/9-Beyranevand.pdf.

12. Center for Science in the Public Interest et al. (2015). "Comments Re: Docket No. FDA-1997-N-0020; Substances Generally Recognized as Safe (GRAS)." https://www.cspinet .org/sites/default/files/attachment/GRAS%20Comment%20FINAL_0.pdf.

13. US Food and Drug Administration. (2018). "FDA Removes 7 Synthetic Flavoring Substances from Food Additives List." https://www.fda.gov/food/cfsan-constituent-updates /fda-removes-7-synthetic-flavoring-substances-food-additives-list.

14. Consumer Brands Association. (2025, March 10). "Consumer Brands Issues Statement on Constructive HHS Meeting with Industry Leaders." https://consumerbrandsassociation .org/press-releases/consumer-brands-issues-statement-on-constructive-hhs-meeting-with -industry-leaders/.

15. Gabbatt A. (2015, April 21). "Taste the Rainbow Forever: Yellow Mac and Cheese Is Dead, but the Nostalgia Lives On." *The Guardian.* https://www.theguardian.com/business/2015 /apr/21/taste-the-rainbow-forever-yellow-mac-and-cheese-kraft.

16. Environmental Working Group. (n.d.). "Fanta Orange Soda, Orange." https://www.ewg .org/foodscores/products/049000058000-FantaOrangeSodaOrange/. Accessed August 19, 2025.

17. Center for Science in the Public Interest. (2010). "A Rainbow of Risks: The Dangers of Artificial Food Coloring." https://www.cspinet.org/sites/default/files/media/documents /resource/food-dyes-rainbow-of-risks.pdf.

18. Environmental Working Group. (n.d.). "Kellogg's Mashups Frosted Flakes + Froot Loops." https://www.ewg.org/foodscores/products/038000251412-KelloggsMashupsFrosted FlakesFrootLoopsSweetenedCerealFrostedFlakesFrootLoops.

19. Hari V. (n.d.). "W. K. Kellogg's Cereal Heiress Exposes Kellogg's Froot Loops and Says to Boycott." *Food Babe* (blog). https://foodbabe.com/w-k-kelloggs-cereal-heiress-exposes -kelloggs-froot-loops-and-says-to-boycott/. Accessed August 5, 2025.

20. Hari V. (n.d.). "WK Kellogg's CEO Gary Pilnick Breaks His Silence on Poisoning American Kids with Artificial Dyes They Don't Use Overseas (Video)." *Food Babe* (blog). https:// foodbabe.com/wk-kelloggs-ceo-gary-pilnick-breaks-his-silence-on-poisoning-american -kids-with-artificial-dyes-they-dont-use-overseas-video/. Accessed August 5, 2025.

21. Osaka S. (2025, April 24). "'MAHA Moms' Are Pushing for Changes to America's Food System." *Washington Post.* https://www.washingtonpost.com/climate-environment/2025/04 /24/maha-movement-food-reform-conservative-moms/.

22. White House. (2025, March 12.) "MAKE AMERICA HEALTHY AGAIN!" Instagram. https://www.instagram.com/reel/DHHfd8FRFW3/?hl=en.

23. International Agency for Research on Cancer. (1999). "Potassium Bromate." World Health Organization. https://www.inchem.org/documents/iarc/vol73/73-17.html.

24. Hari V. (2014, February 4). "Subway: Stop Using Dangerous Chemicals in Your Bread." *Food Babe* (blog). https://foodbabe.com/subway/.

25. US Food and Drug Administration. (2024, July 2). "FDA Revokes Regulation Allowing the Use of Brominated Vegetable Oil (BVO) in Food." https://www.fda.gov/food/hfp -constituent-updates/fda-revokes-regulation-allowing-use-brominated-vegetable-oil-bvo -food.

26. National Health Service. (2025, July 16). "Food Colours and Hyperactivity." https://www .food.gov.uk/safety-hygiene/food-additives#food-colours-and-hyperactivity.

27. Arnold LE, Lofthouse N, Hurt E. (2012, July). "Artificial Food Colors and Attention-Deficit /Hyperactivity Symptoms: Conclusions to Dye For." *Neurotherapeutics* 9(3):599–609. doi:10.1007/s13311-012-0133-x.

28. US Food and Drug Administration. (2025, January 15). "FDA to Revoke Authorization for the Use of Red No. 3 in Food and Ingested Drugs." https://www.fda.gov/food/hfp -constituent-updates/fda-revoke-authorization-use-red-no-3-food-and-ingested-drugs.

29. Code of Federal Regulations. (2019). "Title 21: Food and Drugs." https://www.ecfr.gov /current/title-21.

30. Amico A, Wootan MG, Jacobson MF, et al. (2021). "The Demise of Artificial Trans Fat: A History of a Public Health Achievement." *Milbank Quarterly* 99(3):746–70. https://doi.org/10.1111/1468-0009.12515.

31. Ibid.

32. Brandt EJ, Myerson R, Perraillon MC, et al. (2017, June 1). "Hospital Admissions for Myocardial Infarction and Stroke Before and After the Trans-Fatty Acid Restrictions in New York." *JAMA Cardiology* 2(6):627–34. https://doi.org/10.1001/jamacardio.2017.0491.

33. Dall C. (2023, December 8). "New FDA Report Shows More Antibiotics Being Sold for Food Animals." CIDRAP, University of Minnesota. https://www.cidrap.umn.edu/antimicrobial-stewardship/new-fda-report-shows-more-antibiotics-being-sold-food-animals.

34. Martin MJ, Thottathil SE, Newman TB. (2015, December). "Antibiotics Overuse in Animal Agriculture: A Call to Action for Health Care Providers." *American Journal of Public Health* 105:2409–10. https://doi.org/10.2105/AJPH.2015.302870.

35. O'Brien M. (2018, March 28). "Global Antibiotic Overuse Is Like a 'Slow Motion Train Wreck.'" *PBS NewsHour.* https://www.pbs.org/newshour/show/global-antibiotic-overuse-is-like-a-slow-motion-train-wreck.

36. Centers for Disease Control and Prevention. (2024, November 1). "Antimicrobial Resistance in the Environment and the Food Supply: Causes and How It Spreads." https://www.cdc.gov/antimicrobial-resistance/causes/environmental-food.html.

37. Punchihewage-Don AJ, Hawkins J, Adnan AM, et al. (2022). "The Outbreaks and Prevalence of Antimicrobial Resistant *Salmonella* in Poultry in the United States: An Overview." *Heliyon* 8(11):e11571. https://doi.org/10.1016/j.heliyon.2022.e11571.

38. Consumer Reports. (2015, November 18). "Making the World Safe from Superbugs." https://www.consumerreports.org/cro/health/making-the-world-safe-from-superbugs/index.htm.

39. Centers for Disease Control and Prevention. (2006, October 6). "2006 *E. coli* Outbreak Linked to Fresh Spinach." https://archive.cdc.gov/www_cdc_gov/ecoli/2006/spinach-10-2006.html.

40. Jechalke S, Heuer H, Siemens J, et al. (2014, September). "Fate and Effects of Veterinary Antibiotics in Soil." *Trends in Microbiology* 22(9):536–45. https://doi.org/10.1016/j.tim.2014.05.005.

41. Casey JA, Curriero FC, Cosgrove SE, et al. (2013, November 25). "High-Density Livestock Operations, Crop Field Application of Manure, and Risk of Community-Associated Methicillin-Resistant *Staphylococcus aureus* Infection, Pennsylvania, USA." *JAMA Internal Medicine* 173(21):1980–90. https://doi.org/10.1001/jamainternmed.2013.10408.

42. Consumer Reports. (2015, November 18). "Making the World Safe from Superbugs." https://www.consumerreports.org/cro/health/making-the-world-safe-from-superbugs/index.htm.

43. Taylor J, Hafner M, Yerushalmi E, et al. (2014, December 10). "Estimating the Economic Costs of Antimicrobial Resistance." RAND Corporation. https://www.rand.org/pubs/research_reports/RR911.html.

44. Gurian-Sherman D. (2008, April). "CAFOs Uncovered: The Untold Costs of Confined Animal Feeding Operations." Union of Concerned Scientists. https://www.ucs.org/sites/default/files/2019-10/cafos-uncovered-full-report.pdf.

45. US Food and Drug Administration, Center for Veterinary Medicine. (2021, December). *2020 Summary Report on Antimicrobials Sold or Distributed for Use in Food-Producing Animals.* https://www.fda.gov/media/154820/download.

46. Centers for Disease Control and Prevention. (2021). "Outpatient Antibiotic Prescriptions—United States, 2019." https://archive.cdc.gov/www_cdc_gov/antibiotic-use/data/report-2019.html.

47. US Food and Drug Administration. (2013, December). "Guidance for Industry #213: New Animal Drugs and New Animal Drug Combination Products Administered in or on Medicated Feed or Drinking Water of Food-Producing Animals: Recommendations for Drug Sponsors for Voluntarily Aligning Product Use Conditions with GFI #209." https://www.fda.gov/media/83488/download.

48. Rosenberg B. (2024, November 13). "Growing Use of Antibiotics in Factory-Farmed Animals Threatens Life-Saving Medications." Environmental Working Group. https://www.ewg.org/news-insights/news/2024/11/life-saving-antibiotics-jeopardy-growing-use-factory-farmed-animals.

49. Ibid.

50. *Time*. (2015, March 5). "The 30 Most Influential People on the Internet." https://time.com/3732203/the-30-most-influential-people-on-the-internet/.

51. Strom S. (2013, December 30). "Social Media as a Megaphone to Pressure the Food Industry." *New York Times*. https://www.nytimes.com/2013/12/31/business/media/social-media-as-a-megaphone-to-push-food-makers-to-change.html.

52. Hari V. (2015, February). "A 'Food Babe Investigates' Win—Chipotle Posts Ingredients." *Food Babe* (blog). https://foodbabe.com/a-food-babe-investigates-win-chipotle-posts-ingredients/.

53. Associated Press. (2013, October 31). "Kraft to Remove Artificial Dyes from Three Macaroni and Cheese Varieties." https://www.theguardian.com/business/2013/oct/31/kraft-remove-artificial-dyes-macaroni-and-cheese.

54. Chamlee V. (2016, August 8). "Subway Wasn't the Only Chain to Use the 'Yoga Mat Chemical' in Its Bread." Eater. https://www.eater.com/2016/8/8/12403338/subway-yoga-mat-chemical-mcdonalds-burger-king-wendys.

55. California Public Interest Research Group. (2015, October 9). "California Sets Strictest Antibiotics Standards for Livestock Use in the Nation." https://pirg.org/california/media-center/california-sets-strictest-antibiotics-standards-for-livestock-use-in-the-nation/.

56. Maryland Public Interest Research Group. (2023, March 2). "Bill to Improve Reporting of Antibiotic Use on Maryland Farms Passes Unanimously." https://pirg.org/maryland/updates/bill-to-improve-reporting-of-antibiotic-use-on-maryland-farms-passes-unanimously/.

57. World Health Organization. (2023, November 21). "Antibiotic Resistance." https://www.who.int/news-room/fact-sheets/detail/antibiotic-resistance; World Health Organization. (2017). "WHO Guidelines on Use of Medically Important Antimicrobials in Food-Producing Animals." https://iris.who.int/bitstream/handle/10665/258970/9789241550130-eng.pdf.

58. World Health Organization. (2011). "Critically Important Antimicrobials for Human Medicine." https://iris.who.int/bitstream/handle/10665/77376/9789241504485_eng.pdf.

59. Ibid.; Public Interest Research Group. (2014, September 10). "Weak Medicine: Why the FDA's Guidelines Are Inadequate to Curb Antibiotic Resistance and Protect Public Health." https://uspirg.org/reports/usf/weak-medicine.

60. Booker C. (2024, December 2). "We must get harmful chemicals out of our foods and prevent dangerous chemicals from being sprayed on them." Instagram. https://www.instagram.com/reel/DDE3XCOO6KX/?hl=en.

61. Silverglade B, Heller IR. (2010). "Food Labeling Chaos: The Case for Reform." Center for Science in the Public Interest. https://www.cspi.org/sites/default/files/media/documents/resource/food_labeling_chaos_report.pdf.

62. US Department of Health and Human Services. (2025, March 10). "HHS Secretary Kennedy Directs FDA to Explore Rulemaking to Eliminate Pathway for Companies to Self-Affirm Food Ingredients Are Safe." https://www.hhs.gov/press-room/revising-gras-pathway.html.

CHAPTER 10

1. US Department of Health and Human Services. (2025, March 10). "HHS Secretary Kennedy Directs FDA to Explore Rulemaking to Eliminate Pathway for Companies to Self-Affirm Food Ingredients Are Safe." https://www.hhs.gov/press-room/revising-gras -pathway.html.
2. Duffy TP. (2011). "The Flexner Report—100 Years Later." *Yale Journal of Biology and Medicine* 84(3):269–76. https://www.ncbi.nlm.nih.gov/pmc/articles/PMC3178858/.
3. Ibid.
4. Stahnisch FW, Verhoef M. (2012, December 26). "The Flexner Report of 1910 and Its Impact on Complementary and Alternative Medicine and Psychiatry in North America in the 20th Century." *Evidence-Based Complementary and Alternative Medicine* 2012:647896. https://doi.org/10.1155/2012/647896.
5. Adams KM, Butsch WS, Kohlmeier M. (2015). "The State of Nutrition Education at US Medical Schools." *Journal of Biomedical Education* 2015:357627. https://doi.org/10.1155 /2015/357627.
6. Dror AA, Morozov N, Daoud A, et al. (2022). "Pre-Infection 25-Hydroxyvitamin D3 Levels and Association with Severity of COVID-19 Illness." *PLOS One* 17(2):e0263069. https://doi.org/10.1371/journal.pone.0263069.
7. Stäbler S, Fischer M. (2020). "When Does Corporate Social Irresponsibility Become News? Evidence from More than 1,000 Brand Transgressions Across Five Countries." *Journal of Marketing* 84(3):46–67. https://doi.org/10.1177/0022242920911907.
8. US Food and Drug Administration. (March 5, 2024). "Raw Milk." https://www.fda.gov /food/resources-you-food/raw-milk.
9. Farm-to-Consumer Legal Defense Fund. (2024, July 30). "Raw Milk Nation: Interactive Map." https://www.farmtoconsumer.org/raw-milk-nation-interactive-map/.
10. Zehnder K. (2025, June 19). "Senate Passes NC Farm Act." *Carolina Journal.* https://www .carolinajournal.com/senate-passes-nc-farm-act/.
11. Aleccia J. (2024, December). "Raw Milk Sales Spike Despite CDC's Warnings of Risk Associated with Bird Flu." PBS News. https://www.pbs.org/newshour/health/raw-milk -sales-spike-despite-cdcs-warnings-of-risk-associated-with-bird-flu.

CHAPTER 11

1. Grynbaum MM. (2014, June 26). "New York's Ban on Big Sodas Is Rejected by Final Court." *New York Times.* https://www.nytimes.com/2014/06/27/nyregion/city-loses-final -appeal-on-limiting-sales-of-large-sodas.html.
2. O'Connor A. (2015, November 24). "Coke's Chief Scientist, Who Orchestrated Obesity Research, Is Leaving." *New York Times.* https://archive.nytimes.com/well.blogs.nytimes .com/2015/11/24/cokes-chief-scientist-who-orchestrated-obesity-research-is-leaving/.
3. Applebaum RS. (2012, August 7). "Balancing the Debate: The Food Industry: Trends and Opportunities." 29th International Sweetener Symposium. PowerPoint presentation. http://www.phaionline.org/wp-content/uploads/2015/08/Rhona-Applebaum.pdf.
4. Ibid.
5. Ibid.
6. Hagstrom Report. (2012, August 17). "Coca-Cola Exec: Sugar Growers Need to Fight Off Detractors." http://www.hagstromreport.com/2012news_files/2012_0817_coke.html.
7. Applebaum RS. (2012, August 7). "Balancing the Debate: The Food Industry: Trends and Opportunities." 29th International Sweetener Symposium. PowerPoint presentation. http:// www.phaionline.org/wp-content/uploads/2015/08/Rhona-Applebaum.pdf.
8. Ibid.

9. Ibid.

10. Ibid.

11. Serodio P, Ruskin G, McKee M, et al. (2020, August 3). "Evaluating Coca-Cola's Attempts to Influence Public Health 'In Their Own Words': Analysis of Coca-Cola Emails with Public Health Researchers Leading the Global Energy Balance Network." *Public Health Nutrition* 23(14):2647–53. https://doi.org/10.1017/S1368980020002098; Associated Press. (2015, November 24). "Excerpts from Emails Between Coke, Anti-Obesity Group." https://apnews.com/general-news-eac573c073b6429bb302d94acc787c2b.

12. Applebaum RS. (2012). "Balancing the Debate. The Food Industry: Trends and Opportunities." 29th International Sweetener Symposium. PowerPoint presentation. http://www.phaionline.org/wp-content/uploads/2015/08/Rhona-Applebaum.pdf.

13. Katzmarzyk PT, Barreira TV, Broyles ST, et al. (2015). "Relationship Between Lifestyle Behaviors and Obesity in Children Ages 9–11: Results from a 12-Country Study." *Obesity* 23(8):1696–702. https://doi.org/10.1002/oby.21152/.

14. Pennington Biomedical Research Center. (2015, August 3). "Pennington Biomedical Research Study Shows Lack of Physical Activity Is a Major Predictor of Childhood Obesity." Press release. https://www.pbrc.edu/news/press-releases/?ArticleID=284.

15. Lurie J. (2015, November 12). "Lurie: Coca-Cola Spends Millions Funding Research That—Surprise!—Says Soda Is Just Fine." *Mother Jones.* https://www.motherjones.com/politics/2015/11/coca-cola-research-funding-universities-colleges/.

16. Serôdio PM, McKee M, Stuckler D. (2018, March 21). "Coca-Cola—A Model of Transparency in Research Partnerships? A Network Analysis of Coca-Cola's Research Funding (2008–2016)." *Public Health Nutrition* 21(9):1594–607. https://doi.org/10.1017/S13689800 1700307X.

17. Fabbri A, Holland TJ, Bero LA. (2018, December). "Food Industry Sponsorship of Academic Research: Investigating Commercial Bias in the Research Agenda." *Public Health Nutrition* 21(18):3422–30.

18. National Center for Biotechnology Information. (2015). "Introduction." In *Physical Activity: Moving Toward Obesity Solutions: Workshop Summary.* National Academies Press. https://www.ncbi.nlm.nih.gov/books/NBK333475/.

19. Simon M. (2015, June). "Nutrition Scientists on the Take from Big Food: Has the American Society for Nutrition Lost All Credibility?" EatDrinkPolitics. https://www.eatdrinkpolitics.com/wp-content/uploads/ASNReportFinal.pdf.

20. *Lamar et al. v. The Coca-Cola Company and the American Beverage Association.* (2017, July 13). Complaint for Declaratory and Injunctive Relief. Superior Court of the District of Columbia, Civil Division. https://www.cspinet.org/sites/default/files/attachment/1_71217%20FINAL.pdf.

21. O'Connor A. (2015, August 9). "Coca-Cola Funds Scientists Who Shift Blame for Obesity Away from Bad Diets." *New York Times.* https://archive.nytimes.com/well.blogs.nytimes.com/2015/08/09/coca-cola-funds-scientists-who-shift-blame-for-obesity-away-from-bad-diets/.

22. Sacks G, Riesenberg D, Mialon M, et al. (2020, December 16). "The Characteristics and Extent of Food Industry Involvement in Peer-Reviewed Research Articles from 10 Leading Nutrition-Related Journals in 2018." *PLOS One* 15(12):e0243144. https://doi.org/10.1371/journal.pone.0243144.

23. Fischer K. (2014, May 30). "Nutritionists Outraged by Study Touting Diet Soda for Weight Loss." *Parade.* https://parade.com/299317/kristenfischer/nutritionists-outraged-by-study-touting-diet-soda-for-weight-loss/.

24. Olinger D. (2015, December 26). "CU Nutrition Expert Accepts $550,000 from Coca-Cola for Obesity Campaign." *Denver Post.* https://www.denverpost.com/2015/12/26/cu-nutrition-expert-accepts-550000-from-coca-cola-for-obesity-campaign/.

25. Choi C. (2015, November 24). "Emails Reveal Coke's Role in Anti-Obesity Group." Associated Press. https://apnews.com/general-news-ce372c3d89d442a79458e6d32e713865.

26. Ebbeling CB, Feldman HA, Klein GL, et al. (2018, November 14). "Effects of a Low Carbohydrate Diet on Energy Expenditure During Weight Loss Maintenance: Randomized Trial." *BMJ* 363:k4583. https://doi.org/10.1136/bmj.k4583.

27. Right to Know. (2018, December). "Establishing the Global Energy Balance Network (GEBN)." https://usrtk.org/wp-content/uploads/2018/03/Establishing-the-GEBN.pdf.

28. Stone K. (2018, March 28). "Internal Documents Show Coke Had Profits in Mind When It Funded Nutrition 'Science.'" HealthNewsReview.org. https://web.archive.org/web/2022 0705164254/https://www.healthnewsreview.org/2018/03/internal-documents-show -coke-had-profits-in-mind-when-it-funded-nutrition-science/.

29. O'Connor A. (2015, August 9). "Coca-Cola Funds Scientists Who Shift Blame for Obesity Away from Bad Diets." *New York Times*. https://archive.nytimes.com/well.blogs.nytimes.com /2015/08/09/coca-cola-funds-scientists-who-shift-blame-for-obesity-away-from-bad-diets/.

30. O'Connor A. (2015, November 24). "Coke's Chief Scientist, Who Orchestrated Obesity Research, Is Leaving." *New York Times*. https://archive.nytimes.com/well.blogs.nytimes .com/2015/11/24/cokes-chief-scientist-who-orchestrated-obesity-research-is-leaving/; CBS News. (2015, December 1). "Anti-Obesity Group Funded by Coke Disbanding." https://www.cbsnews.com/news/anti-obesity-group-funded-by-coke-global-energy-balance -network-disbanding/.

31. Lesser LI, Ebbeling CB, Goozner M, et al. (2007, January 9). "Relationship Between Funding Source and Conclusion Among Nutrition-Related Scientific Articles." *PLOS Medicine* 4(1):e5. https://doi.org/10.1371/journal.pmed.0040005.

32. Sifferlin A. (2016, October 10). "Soda Companies Fund 96 Health Groups in the U.S." *Time*. https://time.com/4522940/soda-pepsi-coke-health-obesity/.

33. Steele S, Ruskin G, McKee M, et al. (2019, May 8). "'Always Read the Small Print': A Case Study of Commercial Research Funding, Disclosure and Agreements with Coca-Cola." *Journal of Public Health Policy* 40:273–85. https://doi.org/10.1057/s41271-019-00170-9.

34. Brownell KD, Warner KE. (2009, March 11). "The Perils of Ignoring History: Big Tobacco Played Dirty and Millions Died. How Similar Is Big Food?" *Milbank Quarterly* 87(1):259–94. https://doi.org/10.1111/j.1468-0009.2009.00555.x.

35. Ibid.

36. Center for Consumer Freedom. (2019). "Obesity Hype." https://www.consumerfreedom .com/print-ad/obesity-hype/.

37. Hiltzik MA. (1985, September 28). "General Foods Backs $5.6-Billion Takeover Bid by Philip Morris." *Los Angeles Times*. https://www.latimes.com/archives/la-xpm-1985-09-28 -fi-17615-story.html.

38. Katzmarzyk PT, Barreira TV, Broyles ST, et al. (2015, July 14). "Relationship Between Lifestyle Behaviors and Obesity in Children Ages 9–11: Results from a 12-Country Study." *Obesity* 23(8):1696–702. https://doi.org/10.1002/oby.21152.

39. Ludwig DS, Peterson KE, Gortmaker SL. (2001, February 17). "Relation Between Consumption of Sugar-Sweetened Drinks and Childhood Obesity: A Prospective, Observational Analysis." *The Lancet* 357(9255):505–8. https://doi.org/10.1016/s0140-6736(00)04041-1.

40. Ludwig DS, Peterson KE, Gortmaker SL. (2001, February 17). "Relation Between Consumption of Sugar-Sweetened Drinks and Childhood Obesity: A Prospective, Observational Analysis." *The Lancet* 357(9255):505–8. https://doi.org/10.1016/s0140-6736(00)04041-1.

41. Collier R. (2017). "Litigious Future for Big Sugar?" *Canadian Medical Association Journal* 189(9):E378–79. https://doi.org/10.1503/cmaj.1095388.

42. Simon M. (2017, July 13). "Lawsuit Alleges Coca-Cola, American Beverage Association Deceiving Public About Soda-Related Health Problems." Center for Science in the Public

Interest. https://www.cspi.org/news/lawsuit-alleges-coca-cola-american-beverage-association-deceiving-public-about-soda-related.

43. Loria K. (2017, March 28). "Coke-Funded Study Blames Things Other than Sugar for Causing Obesity." Food Dive. https://www.fooddive.com/news/coke-funded-study-blames-things-other-than-sugar-for-causing-obesity/439080/.

44. Chartres N, Fabbri A, Bero, LA. (2016). "Association of Industry Sponsorship with Outcomes of Nutrition Studies: A Systematic Review and Meta-Analysis." *JAMA Internal Medicine* 176(12):1769–77. https://doi.org/10.1001/jamainternmed.2016.6721.

45. Simon M. (2015, June). "Nutrition Scientists on the Take from Big Food: Has the American Society for Nutrition Lost All Credibility?" EatDrinkPolitics. https://www.eatdrinkpolitics.com/2015/06/14/nutrition-scientists-on-the-take-from-big-food/.

46. Lesser LI, Ebbeling CB, Goozner M, et al. (2007, January 9). "Relationship Between Funding Source and Conclusion Among Nutrition-Related Scientific Articles." *PLOS Medicine* 4(1):e5. https://doi.org/10.1371/journal.pmed.0040005.

47. Litman EA, Gortmaker SL, Ebbeling CB, et al. (2018, March 26). "Source of Bias in Sugar-Sweetened Beverage Research: A Systematic Review." *Public Health Nutrition* 21(12):2345–50. https://doi.org/10.1017/S1368980018000575.

48. Mozaffarian D. (2017, May 2). "Conflict of Interest and the Role of the Food Industry in Nutrition Research." *JAMA* 317(17):1755–56. https://doi.org/10.1001/jama.2017.3456.

49. O'Neill CE, Fulgoni VL III, Nicklas TA. (2011, June 14). "Association of Candy Consumption with Body Weight Measures, Other Health Risk Factors for Cardiovascular Disease, and Diet Quality in US Children and Adolescents: NHANES 1999–2004." *Food & Nutrition Research* 55. https://doi.org/10.3402/fnr.v55i0.5794.

50. Choi C. (2016, June 2). "How Candy Makers Shape Nutrition Science." Associated Press. https://apnews.com/general-news-f9483d554430445fa6566bb0aaa293d1.

51. Ibid.

52. Ibid.

53. O'Neill CE, Fulgoni VL III, Nicklas TA. (2011, February). "Candy Consumption Was Not Associated with Body Weight Measures, Risk Factors for Cardiovascular Disease, or Metabolic Syndrome in US Adults: NHANES 1999–2004." *Nutrition Research* 31(2):122–30. https://doi.org/10.1016/j.nutres.2011.01.007.

54. Erickson J, Sadeghirad B, Lytvyn L, et al. (2017, February 21). "The Scientific Basis of Guideline Recommendations on Sugar Intake: A Systematic Review." *Annals of Internal Medicine* 166:257–67. https://doi.org/10.7326/m16-2020.

55. Malkan S. (2023, September 16). "International Life Sciences Institute (ILSI) Is a Food Industry Lobby Group." US Right to Know. https://usrtk.org/pesticides/ilsi-is-a-food-industry-lobby-group/.

56. Mohamed HJBJ, Loy SL, Taib MNM, et al. (2015, December 30). "Characteristics Associated with the Consumption of Malted Drinks Among Malaysian Primary School Children: Findings from the MyBreakfast Study." *BMC Public Health* 15:1322. https://doi.org/10.1186/s12889-015-2666-5.

57. Fuller T, O'Connor A, Richtel M. (2017, December 23). "In Asia's Fattest Country, Nutritionists Take Money from Food Giants." *New York Times*. https://www.nytimes.com/2017/12/23/health/obesity-malaysia-nestle.html.

58. O'Connor A. (2017, November 21). "Sugar Industry Long Downplayed Potential Harms." *New York Times*. https://www.nytimes.com/2017/11/21/well/eat/sugar-industry-long-downplayed-potential-harms-of-sugar.html.

59. Kearns CE, Apollonio D, Glantz SA. (2017, November 21). "Sugar Industry Sponsorship of Germ-Free Rodent Studies Linking Sucrose to Hyperlipidemia and Cancer: An Historical

Analysis of Internal Documents." *PLOS Biology* 15(11):e2003460. https://doi.org/10.1371/journal.pbio.2003460.

60. O'Connor A. (2017, November 21). "Sugar Industry Long Downplayed Potential Harms." *New York Times.* https://www.nytimes.com/2017/11/21/well/eat/sugar-industry-long-downplayed-potential-harms-of-sugar.html.

61. Domonoske C. (2016, September 13). "50 Years Ago, Sugar Industry Quietly Paid Scientists to Point Blame at Fat." NPR. https://www.npr.org/sections/thetwo-way/2016/09/13/493739074/50-years-ago-sugar-industry-quietly-paid-scientists-to-point-blame-at-fat.

62. Stare, FJ. (1967). "Dietary Fats, Carbohydrates and Atherosclerotic Vascular Disease." *New England Journal of Medicine* 277(4):270–405. https://doi.org/10.1056/NEJM196707272770405.

63. Saxon W. (2002, April 11). "Fredrick J. Stare, 91, Dies; Influential Early Nutritionist." *New York Times.* https://www.nytimes.com/2002/04/11/us/fredrick-j-stare-91-dies-influential-early-nutritionist.html.

64. Stare FJ. (1991). *Adventures in Nutrition.* Christopher Publishing House.

65. Oppenheimer GM, Benrubi ID. (2014, January). "McGovern's Senate Select Committee on Nutrition and Human Needs Versus the Meat Industry on the Diet-Heart Question (1976–1977)." *American Journal of Public Health* 104:59–69. https://doi.org/10.2105/AJPH.2013.301464.

66. Lipton E. (2014, February 11). "Rival Industries Sweet-Talk the Public." *New York Times.* https://www.nytimes.com/2014/02/12/business/rival-industries-sweet-talk-the-public.html.

67. Rippe JM, Sievenpiper JL, Lê K-A, et al. (2016, December 13). "What Is the Appropriate Upper Limit for Added Sugars Consumption?" *Nutrition Reviews* 75(1):18–36. https://doi.org/10.1093/nutrit/nuw046.

68. Lowndes J, Sinnett SS, Rippe JM. (2015, October 23). "No Effect of Added Sugar Consumed at Median American Intake Level on Glucose Tolerance or Insulin Resistance." *Nutrients* 7(10):8830–8845. https://doi.org/10.3390/nu7105430.

69. Rippe JM, Sievenpiper JL, Lê K-A, et al. (2016, December 13). "What Is the Appropriate Upper Limit for Added Sugars Consumption?" *Nutrition Reviews* 75(1):18–36. https://doi.org/10.1093/nutrit/nuw046; Lowndes J, Sinnett SS, Rippe JM. (2015, October 23). "No Effect of Added Sugar Consumed at Median American Intake Level on Glucose Tolerance or Insulin Resistance." *Nutrients* 7(10):8830–8845. https://doi.org/10.3390/nu7105430; Lowndes J, Sinnett S, Yu Z, et al. (2014, August 8). "The Effects of Fructose-Containing Sugars on Weight, Body Composition and Cardiometabolic Risk Factors When Consumed at Up to the 90th Percentile Population Consumption Level for Fructose." *Nutrients* 6(8):3153–68. https://doi.org/10.3390/nu6083153.

70. *Fitzgerald v. The Quaker Oats Company.* (2024, February 20). Amended Class Action Complaint. https://www.classaction.org/media/fitzgerald-v-the-quaker-oats-company.pdf.

71. Kelly SAM, Summerbell CD, Brynes A, et al. (2007, April 18). "Wholegrain Cereals for Coronary Heart Disease." *Cochrane Database of Systematic Reviews* 2:CD005051. https://doi.org/10.1002/14651858.cd005051.pub2.

72. Mitrović D, Sredović Ignjatović I, Kozarski M, et al. (2024, April). "Wine Is More than Just a Beverage: Chemical Diversity, Health Benefits, and Immunomodulating Potential of Wine Polyphenols." *Food Safety and Health* 2(2):196–212. https://doi.org/10.1002/fsh3.12036.

73. Office of the US Surgeon General. (2025). "Alcohol and Cancer Risk: The U.S. Surgeon General's Advisory." https://www.hhs.gov/sites/default/files/oash-alcohol-cancer-risk.pdf.

74. Nestle M. (2016, May 10). "Congress, FOIA, and Checkoff Programs." *Food Politics* (blog). https://www.foodpolitics.com/2016/05/congress-foia-and-checkoff-programs/.

75. Archer E, Pavela G, Lavie CJ. (2015, July). "The Inadmissibility of What We Eat in America and NHANES Dietary Data in Nutrition and Obesity Research and the Scientific Formulation of National Dietary Guidelines." *Mayo Clinic Proceedings* 90(7):911–26. https://doi .org/10.1016/j.mayocp.2015.04.009.

76. Ibid.

77. Sinha R, Cross AJ, Graubard BI, et al. (2009, March 23). "Meat Intake and Mortality: A Prospective Study of Over Half a Million People." *Archives of Internal Medicine* 169(6):562–71. https://doi.org/10.1001/archinternmed.2009.6.

78. Ebbeling CB, Feldman HA, Klein GL, et al. (2018, November 14). "Effects of a Low Carbohydrate Diet on Energy Expenditure During Weight Loss Maintenance: Randomized Trial." *BMJ* 363:k4583. https://doi.org/10.1136/bmj.k4583.

79. Ibid.

80. Hall KD, Ayuketah A, Brychta R, et al. (2019, July 2). "Ultra-Processed Diets Cause Excess Calorie Intake and Weight Gain: An Inpatient Randomized Controlled Trial of Ad Libitum Food Intake." *Cell Metabolism* 30(1):P67–77.e3. https://doi.org/10.1016/j.cmet.2019.05.008.

81. Ibid.

82. Thacker PD. (2017, July 21). "Flacking for GMOs: How the Biotech Industry Cultivates Positive Media—And Discourages Criticism." *The Progressive*. https://progressive.org/magazine /how-the-biotech-industry-cultivates-positive-media/.

83. Senapathy K. (2021, June 28). "Beware of Accidentally Starving Your Breastfed Newborn, Warns the Fed Is Best Foundation." *Forbes*. https://www.forbes.com/sites/kavinsenapathy /2016/09/27/beware-of-accidentally-starving-your-breastfed-newborn/.

CHAPTER 12

1. Grynbaum MM. (2012, October 12). "Soda Industry Sues to Stop a Sales Ban on Big Drinks." *New York Times*. https://www.nytimes.com/2012/10/13/nyregion/soda-industry-sues -to-stop-bloombergs-sales-limits.html.

2. Grynbaum MM. (2014, June 26). "New York's Ban on Big Sodas Is Rejected by Final Court." *New York Times*. https://www.nytimes.com/2014/06/27/nyregion/city-loses-final -appeal-on-limiting-sales-of-large-sodas.html.

3. Lavender P. (2013, March 12). "Minority Groups and Bottlers Team Up in Battles over Soda." *HuffPost*. https://www.huffpost.com/entry/soda_n_2864953.

4. Walker J. (2013, March 13). "Behind Soda Industry's Win, a Phalanx of Sponsored Minority Groups." *HuffPost*. https://www.huffpost.com/entry/soda-ban-new-york-michael-bloomberg _n_2864712.

5. Centers for Disease Control and Prevention. (2024, May 14). "Adult Obesity Facts." https:// www.cdc.gov/obesity/adult-obesity-facts/index.html.

6. Erbentraut J. (2017, April 29). "People of Color Bear the Brunt of Fast-Food Explosion." *HuffPost*. https://www.huffpost.com/entry/fast-food-minority-communities_n_59035fb5 e4b02655f83c9999.

7. Harris JL, Shehan C, Gross R. (2015, August). "Food Advertising Targeted to Hispanic and Black Youth: Contributing to Health Disparities." Rudd Center for Food Policy and Obesity, University of Connecticut. https://uconnruddcenter.media.uconn.edu/wp-content /uploads/sites/2909/2020/09/272-7-Rudd_Targeted-Marketing-Report_Release_0811151 .pdf.

8. Medical Daily. (2015, August 12). "Unhealthy Food Ads Target Minorities, Possibly Contributing to Childhood Obesity." https://www.medicaldaily.com/unhealthy-food-ads-target -minorities-possibly-contributing-childhood-obesity-347576.

9. O'Connor A. (2016, October 10). "Coke and Pepsi Give Millions to Public Health, Then Lobby Against It." *New York Times*. https://www.nytimes.com/2016/10/10/well/eat/coke -and-pepsi-give-millions-to-public-health-then-lobby-against-it.html.

10. Diep W. (2025, February 21). "Scholarships Supporting Black Students from Low-Income Backgrounds." National College Attainment Network. https://www.ncan.org/news/694376 /Scholarships-Supporting-Black-Students-from-Low-Income-Backgrounds.htm.

11. Confessore N. (2013, March 13). "Minority Groups and Bottlers Team Up in Battles over Soda." *New York Times*. https://www.nytimes.com/2013/03/13/nyregion/behind-soda -industrys-win-a-phalanx-of-sponsored-minority-groups.html.

12. Dewey C. (2017, July 13). " 'We're Losing More People to the Sweets than to the Streets': Why Two Black Pastors Are Suing Coca-Cola." *Washington Post*. https://www.washingtonpost .com/news/wonk/wp/2017/07/13/were-losing-more-people-to-the-sweets-than-to-the -streets-why-two-black-pastors-are-suing-coca-cola/.

13. Ibid.

14. Lowe AP, Hacker G. (2013). "Selfish Giving: How the Soda Industry Uses Philanthropy to Sweeten Its Profits." Center for Science in the Public Interest. https://cspinet.org/sites /default/files/attachment/cspi_soda_philanthropy_online.pdf.

15. Neuman W. (2010, December 14). "Save the Children Breaks with Soda Tax Effort." *New York Times*. https://www.nytimes.com/2010/12/15/business/15soda.html.

16. Lowe AP, Hacker G. (2013). "Selfish Giving: How the Soda Industry Uses Philanthropy to Sweeten Its Profits." Center for Science in the Public Interest. https://cspinet.org/sites /default/files/attachment/cspi_soda_philanthropy_online.pdf.

17. Zhong Y, Auchincloss AH, Lee BK, et al. (2018, July). "The Short-Term Impacts of the Philadelphia Beverage Tax on Beverage Consumption." *American Journal of Preventive Medicine* 55(1):26–34. https://doi.org/10.1016/j.amepre.2018.02.017.

18. Roberto CA, Lawman HG, LeVasseur MT, et al. (2019, May 14). "Association of a Beverage Tax on Sugar-Sweetened and Artificially Sweetened Beverages with Changes in Beverage Prices and Sales at Chain Retailers in a Large Urban Setting." *JAMA* 321(18):1799–810. https://doi.org/10.1001/jama.2019.4249.

19. Jacobs A. (2019, May 20). "Tuesday Could Be the Beginning of the End of Philadelphia's Soda Tax." *New York Times*. https://www.nytimes.com/2019/05/20/health/soda-tax-philadelphia .html.

20. O'Connor A. (2015, August 9). "Coca-Cola Funds Scientists Who Shift Blame for Obesity Away from Bad Diets." *New York Times*. https://archive.nytimes.com/well.blogs.nytimes.com /2015/08/09/coca-cola-funds-scientists-who-shift-blame-for-obesity-away-from-bad-diets/.

21. Bottemiller Evich H. (2016, November 5). "Soda's Last Stand." *Politico*. https://www.politico .com/story/2016/11/sodas-last-stand-230805.

22. Center for Science in the Public Interest. (2016, December). "Soda Industry's Big Bucks to Fight Taxes." https://www.cspinet.org/sites/default/files/attachment/Big%20Soda %20spending.pdf.

23. Center for Science in the Public Interest. (n.d.). "Soda Industry's Big Bucks to Fight Taxes." https://www.cspinet.org/resource/soda-industry%E2%80%99s-big-bucks-fight-taxes. Accessed August 20, 2025.

24. Long MW, Gortmaker SL, Ward ZJ, et al. (2015, July). "Cost-Effectiveness of a Sugar-Sweetened Beverage Excise Tax in the U.S." *American Journal of Preventive Medicine* 49(1):112–23. https://doi.org/10.1016/j.amepre.2015.03.004.

25. Ibid.

26. Ballotpedia. (n.d.) "Oregon Measure 103, Ban Tax on Groceries Initiative (2018)." https:// ballotpedia.org/Oregon_Measure_103,_Ban_Tax_on_Groceries_Initiative_(2018). Accessed August 20, 2025.

27. Ballotpedia. (n.d.)"Washington Initiative 1634, Prohibit Local Taxes on Groceries Measure (2018)." https://ballotpedia.org/Washington_Initiative_1634,_Prohibit_Local_Taxes_on_Groceries_Measure_(2018). Accessed August 20, 2025.

28. O'Connor A, Sanger-Katz M. (2018, June 27). "California, of All Places, Has Banned Soda Taxes. How a New Industry Strategy Is Succeeding." *New York Times.* https://www.nytimes.com/2018/06/27/upshot/california-banning-soda-taxes-a-new-industry-strategy-is-stunning-some-lawmakers.html.

29. Crosbie E, Schillinger D, Schmidt LA. (2019, March 1). "State Preemption to Prevent Local Taxation of Sugar-Sweetened Beverages." *JAMA Internal Medicine* 179(3):291–92. https://doi.org/10.1001/jamainternmed.2018.7770.

30. Santora M. (2006, November 25). "In Diabetes Fight, Raising Cash and Keeping Trust." *New York Times.* https://www.nytimes.com/2006/11/25/health/in-diabetes-fight-raising-cash-and-keeping-trust.html.

31. Shearer J, Swithers SE. (2016, June). "Artificial Sweeteners and Metabolic Dysregulation: Lessons Learned from Agriculture and the Laboratory." *Reviews in Endocrine and Metabolic Disorders* 17(2):179–86. https://doi.org/10.1007/s11154-016-9372-1.

32. Suez J, Korem T, Zilberman-Schapira G, et al. (2015, April 1). "Non-Caloric Artificial Sweeteners and the Microbiome: Findings and Challenges." *Gut Microbes* 6(2):149–55. doi: 10.1080/19490976.2015.1017700.

33. O'Connor A. (2015, September 28). "Coke Spends Lavishly on Pediatricians and Dietitians." *New York Times.* https://archive.nytimes.com/well.blogs.nytimes.com/2015/09/28/coke-spends-lavishly-on-pediatricians-and-dietitians/.

34. Ibid.

35. Husten L. (2012, July 9). "Coca-Cola, the Olympic Torch and the American College of Cardiology." *Cardio Brief.* http://cardiobrief.org/2012/07/09/coca-cola-the-olympic-torch-and-the-american-college-of-cardiology/.

36. Lowe AP, Hacker G. (2013). "Selfish Giving: How the Soda Industry Uses Philanthropy to Sweeten Its Profits." Center for Science in the Public Interest. https://cspinet.org/sites/default/files/attachment/cspi_soda_philanthropy_online.pdf.

37. Scott-Thomas C. (2009, October 30). "Doctors Resign over Coca-Cola Funding." Food-Navigator USA. https://www.foodnavigator-usa.com/Article/2009/10/30/Doctors-resign-over-Coca-Cola-funding/.

38. American Heart Association. (2018). "2017–2018: American Heart Association: Support from Pharmaceutical and Biotech Companies, Device Manufacturers, and Health Insurance Providers." https://www.heart.org/-/media/files/finance/pharma-device-insurance-corporate-funding-fiscal-20172018.pdf.

39. Ioannidis JPA. (2018, October). "Professional Societies Should Abstain from Authorship of Guidelines and Disease Definition Statements." *Circulation: Cardiovascular Quality and Outcomes* 11(10):e004889.

40. Chowdhury R, Warnakula S, Kunutsor S, et al. (2014, March 18). "Association of Dietary, Circulating, and Supplement Fatty Acids with Coronary Risk: A Systematic Review and Meta-Analysis." *Annals of Internal Medicine* 160(6):398–406. https://doi.org/10.7326/m13-1788.

41. Nutrition Coalition. (2024, September 20). "Executive Summary of Evidence on Saturated Fats and Heart Disease." www.nutritioncoalition.us/saturated-fats-do-they-cause-heart-disease/.

42. Academy of Nutrition and Dietetics. (2024). "Annual Report: Fiscal Year 2024." https://www.eatrightpro.org/-/media/files/eatrightpro/about-us/annual-reports/annual-report-2024.pdf?rev=a4529e6aa1824a79b7a7335815fbb6d6&hash=7DD762E09FDEB8119C8BB801B84A2B6B.

43. Simon M. (2013, January). "And Now a Word from Our Sponsors: Are America's Nutrition Professionals in the Pocket of Big Food?" EatDrinkPolitics. http://www.eatdrinkpolitics .com/wp-content/uploads/AND_Corporate_Sponsorship_Report.pdf.

44. Ibid.

45. Arnberg K, Mølgaard C, Michaelsen KF, et al. (2012, December). "Skim Milk, Whey, and Casein Increase Body Weight and Whey and Casein Increase the Plasma C-Peptide Concentration in Overweight Adolescents." *Journal of Nutrition* 142(12):2083–2090. https://doi .org/10.3945/jn.112.161208.

46. Willett WC, Ludwig DS. (2020, February 12). "Milk and Health." *New England Journal of Medicine* 382(7):644–54. https://doi.org/10.1056/NEJMra1903547.

47. Carriedo A, Pinksy I, Crosbie E, et al. (2022, October 24). "The Corporate Capture of the Nutrition Profession in the USA: The Case of the Academy of Nutrition and Dietetics." *Public Health Nutrition* 25(12):3568–82. doi:10.1017/S1368980022001835.

48. Malkan S. (2024, April 3). "Academy of Nutrition and Dietetics: Corporate Capture of the Nutrition Profession." US Right to Know. https://usrtk.org/ultra-processed-foods/academy -of-nutrition-and-dietetics-corporate-capture-of-the-nutrition-profession/.

49. Simon M. (2013, January). "And Now a Word from Our Sponsors: Are America's Nutrition Professionals in the Pocket of Big Food?" EatDrinkPolitics. http://www.eatdrinkpolitics .com/wp-content/uploads/AND_Corporate_Sponsorship_Report.pdf.

50. ABC News. (2015, March 13). "Kraft Singles Is First Food Allowed to Display 'Kids Eat Right' Logo." https://www.abcnews.go.com/Health/kraft-singles-1st-food-allowed-display -kids-eat/story?id=29616537.

51. Beck A. (2024, July 5). "Kraft Singles Aren't Actually Cheese. Here's Why." Mashed. https://www.mashed.com/263200/kraft-singles-arent-actually-cheese-heres-why.

52. Kraft Heinz. (n.d.). "Kraft Singles: American Slices." https://www.kraftheinz.com/kraft -singles/products/00021000604647-american-cheese-slices. Accessed August 12, 2025.

53. Columbus Dispatch. (2015, March 31). "Program to Put 'Kids Eat Right' Logo on Kraft Singles Ending." *Columbus Dispatch.* https://www.dispatch.com/story/business/2015/03 /31/program-to-put-kids-eat/23766902007/.

54. Comedy Central. (2015, March 18). "The Daily Show—The Snacks of Life." YouTube. https://www.youtube.com/watch?v=jCG_i9lnBFc.

55. Pfister K. (2015, October 8). "Here Are the People Coca-Cola Has Paid to Manufacture Health Claims." *Observer.* https://observer.com/2015/10/here-are-the-people-coca-cola-has -paid-to-manufacture-health-claims.

56. Choi C. (2015, March 16). "Coke as a Sensible Snack? Coca-Cola Works with Dietitians Who Suggest Cola as Snack." *Star Tribune.* https://www.startribune.com/coke-as-a-sensible -snack-coca-cola-works-with-dietitians-who-suggest-cola-as-snack/296404461; Pfister K. (2016, October 7). "Is Coke Paying Dietitians to Tweet Against the Soda Tax?" *Observer.* https://observer.com/2016/10/is-coke-paying-dietitians-to-tweet-against-the-soda-tax/; Pfister K. (2015, October 8). "Here Are the People Coca-Cola Has Paid to Manufacture Health Claims." *Observer.* https://observer.com/2015/10/here-are-the-people-coca-cola -has-paid-to-manufacture-health-claims.

57. Pfister K. (2015, October 8). "Here Are the People Coca-Cola Has Paid to Manufacture Health Claims." *Observer.* https://observer.com/2015/10/here-are-the-people-coca-cola -has-paid-to-manufacture-health-claims; Nestle M. (2018). *Unsavory Truth: How Food Companies Skew the Science of What We Eat.* Basic Books.

58. Pfister K. (2017, February 20). "Coke Is Running for President of the National Academy of Nutrition and Dietetics." *Medium.* https://medium.com/@ninjasforhealth/coke-is-running -for-president-of-the-national-academy-of-nutrition-dietetics-5ec674140d3d.

59. Cochran N. (n.d.). "About." https://www.nevacochranrd.com/about.html.

60. Pfister K. (2017, February 20). "Coke Is Running for President of the National Academy of Nutrition and Dietetics." *Medium*. https://medium.com/@ninjasforhealth/coke-is-running -for-president-of-the-national-academy-of-nutrition-dietetics-5ec674140d3d; Swerdloff A. (2017, March 1). "America's Largest Group of Dietitians Was Almost Run by Big Soda." Munchies.

61. Swerdloff A. (2017, March 1). "America's Largest Group of Dietitians Was Almost Run by Big Soda." *Vice*. https://www.vice.com/en/article/americas-largest-group-of-dietitians-was -almost-run-by-big-soda/.

62. Weaver CM, Dwyer J, Fulgoni VL III, et al. (2014, June). "Processed Foods: Contributions to Nutrition." *American Journal of Clinical Nutrition* 99(6):1525–42. https://doi.org/10.3945 /ajcn.114.089284.

63. Ibid.

64. Nestle M. (2018). *Unsavory Truth: How Food Companies Skew the Science of What We Eat*. Basic Books.

65. Malkan S. (2022, April 26). "Center for Food Integrity: PR for Processed Foods, Pesticides and GMOs." U.S. Right to Know. https://usrtk.org/industry-pr/center-for-food-integrity -partners-with-monsanto/.

66. Hamerschlag K, Lappé A, Malkan S. (2015, June). "Spinning Food: How Food Industry Front Groups and Covert Communications Are Shaping the Story of Food." Friends of the Earth. https://foe.org/resources/food-industry-shapes-story-food/.

67. Ibid.

68. Ibid.

69. Ludwig H. (2022, August 18). "The Global Warming Guys—and 'Dark Money'—Behind 'Science Moms.'" Capital Research Center. https://capitalresearch.org/article/the-global -warming-guys-and-dark-money-behind-science-moms/.

70. Center for Media and Democracy. (n.d.) "American Council on Science and Health." https://www.sourcewatch.org/index.php/American_Council_on_Science_and_Health# Funding. Accessed August 20, 2025.

71. DeSmog. (n.d.). "American Council on Science and Health." https://www.desmog.com /american-council-science-and-health. Accessed August 20, 2025.

72. Gillam C. (2019, December 9). "'Consumer Advocacy' Group ACSH Revealed as Front Group for Corporate Interests." CrossFit. https://www.crossfit.com/battles/carey-gillam -acsh.

73. DeSmog. (n.d.). "American Council on Science and Health." https://www.desmog.com /american-council-science-and-health. Accessed August 20, 2025.

74. Kasperkevic J. (2015, April 22). "Latest Dr Oz Accusations Have More to Do with GMOs than Diet." *The Guardian*. https://www.theguardian.com/us-news/2015/apr/22/dr-oz-respond -doctors-dismissal-quack-treatments.

75. Hogan B. (2005, November). "Paging Dr. Ross." *Mother Jones*. https://www.motherjones .com/politics/2005/11/paging-dr-ross/.

76. Ioannidis JPA. (2018, October). "Professional Societies Should Abstain from Authorship of Guidelines and Disease Definition Statements." *Circulation: Cardiovascular Quality and Outcomes* 11(10):e004889.

77. Greger M. (2015, November 10). "Coca-Cola Stopped Sponsoring the Academy of Nutrition and Dietetics." NutritionFacts.org. https://nutritionfacts.org/blog/coca-cola-stopped -sponsoring-the-academy-of-nutrition-and-dietetics.

78. Pew Charitable Trusts. (2013, December 18). "Conflicts-of-Interest Policies for Academic Medical Centers."

CHAPTER 13

1. Maffly B. (2015, July 1). "U. Geologist's Claims of Water Raise Doubts About Tar Sands Mine Expansion." *Salt Lake Tribune.* https://www.sltrib.com/news/2015/07/01/u-geologists -claims-of-water-raise-doubts-about-tar-sands-mine-expansion.
2. Farmer P. (1996, Winter). "On Suffering and Structural Violence: A View from Below." *Daedalus* 125(1):261–83. https://www.jstor.org/stable/20027362.
3. Schulz LO, Chaudhari LS. (2016, May 13). "High-Risk Populations: The Pimas of Arizona and Mexico." *Current Obesity Reports* 4(1):92–98. doi: 10.1007/s13679-014-0132-9.
4. Phippen JW. (2016, May 13). "'Kill Every Buffalo You Can! Every Buffalo Dead Is an Indian Gone.'" *The Atlantic.* https://www.theatlantic.com/national/archive/2016/05/the -buffalo-killers/482349/.
5. Harris M. (2004). "The Pima Indian Pathfinder for Health." National Institute of Diabetes and Digestive and Kidney Diseases. https://nicoa.org/wp-content/uploads/2014/05/The _Pima_Indian_Pathfinder_for_health.pdf.
6. Vantrease D. (2013, January 1). "Commod Bods and Frybread Power: Government Food Aid in American Indian Culture." *Journal of American Folklore* 126(499):55–69. https://doi.org /10.5406/jamerfolk.126.499.0055.
7. Johns Hopkins Bloomberg School of Public Health, Center for Gun Violence Solutions. (2023). "Annual Gun Violence Data 2023." https://publichealth.jhu.edu/center-for-gun-violence -solutions/annual-gun-violence-data; National Center for Health Statistics, Centers for Disease Control and Health. (2024, March). "Mortality in the United States, 2022." https:// www.cdc.gov/nchs/products/databriefs/db492.htm.
8. Murphy SL, Kochanek KD, Xu JQ, et al. (2024, December 19). "Mortality in the United States, 2023." Centers for Disease Control and Prevention. https://dx.doi.org/10.15620 /cdc/170564.
9. Kidder T. (2003). *Mountains Beyond Mountains.* Random House.
10. NEJM Catalyst. (2017, December 1). "Social Determinants of Health (SDOH)." https:// catalyst.nejm.org/doi/full/10.1056/CAT.17.0312.
11. O'Neill Hayes T, Delk R. (2018, September 4). "Understanding the Social Determinants of Health." American Action Forum. https://www.americanactionforum.org/research /understanding-the-social-determinants-of-health/.
12. Taylor T. (2020, July 9). "The Subway Map View of U.S. Mortality and Health." *Conversable Economist* (blog). https://conversableeconomist.com/2020/07/09/the-subway-map-view-of -us-mortality-and-health/.
13. American Society for Metabolic and Bariatric Surgery. (2024, June 12). "New Study Shows Long-Term Effectiveness of Gastric Bypass in Treating Type 2 Diabetes and Obesity." https://asmbs.org/news_releases/new-study-shows-long-term-effectiveness-of-gastric -bypass-in-treating-type-2-diabetes-and-obesity.
14. Elnahas AI, Jackson TD, Hong D. (2014, March 1). "Management of Failed Laparoscopic Roux-en-Y Gastric Bypass." *Bariatric Surgical Practice and Patient Care* 9(1):36–40. https:// doi.org/10.1089/bari.2013.0012.
15. Chetty R, Stepner M, Abraham S, et al. (2016, April 26). "The Association Between Income and Life Expectancy in the United States, 2001–2014." *JAMA* 315(16):1750–66. https://doi.org/10.1001/jama.2016.4226.
16. NEJM Catalyst. (2017, December 1). "Social Determinants of Health (SDOH)." https:// catalyst.nejm.org/doi/full/10.1056/CAT.17.0312.
17. Kamal R, Hudman J, McDermott D. (2019, October 18). "What Do We Know About Infant Mortality in the U.S. and Comparable Countries?" Peterson-KFF Health System

Tracker. https://www.healthsystemtracker.org/chart-collection/infant-mortality-u-s-compare-countries/#item-start.

18. Hauck FR, Tanabe KO, Moon RY. (2011, August). "Racial and Ethnic Disparities in Infant Mortality." *Seminars in Perinatology* 35(4):209–20. https://doi.org/10.1053/j.semperi.2011.02.018; Office of Minority Health, US Department of Health and Human Services. (2025, February 13). "Infant Health and Mortality and Black/African Americans." https://minorityhealth.hhs.gov/infant-health-and-mortality-and-blackafrican-americans.

19. Wagenknecht LE, Lawrence JM, Isom S, et al. (2023, April). "Trends in Incidence of Youth-Onset Type 1 and Type 2 Diabetes in the USA, 2002–18: Results from the Population-Based SEARCH for Diabetes in Youth Study." *Lancet Diabetes and Endocrinology* 11(4):242–50. https://doi.org/10.1016/s2213-8587(23)00025-6.

20. Edwards K, Patchell B. (2009, Spring). "State of the Science: A Cultural View of Native Americans and Diabetes Prevention." *Journal of Cultural Diversity* 16(1):32–35. https://www.ncbi.nlm.nih.gov/pmc/articles/PMC2905172.

21. Perng W, Conway R, Mayer-Davis E, et al. (2023, March 1). "Youth-Onset Type 2 Diabetes: The Epidemiology of an Awakening Epidemic." *Diabetes Care* 46(3):490–99. https://doi.org/10.2337/dci22-0046.

22. Wheeler SM, Bryant AS. (2017, March). "Racial and Ethnic Disparities in Health and Health Care." *Obstetrics and Gynecology Clinics of North America* 44(1):1–11. https://doi.org/10.1016/j.ogc.2016.10.001.

23. Ver Ploeg M. (2010, March 1). "Access to Affordable, Nutritious Food Is Limited in 'Food Deserts.'" US Department of Agriculture, Economic Research Service. https://www.ers.usda.gov/amber-waves/2010/march/access-to-affordable-nutritious-food-is-limited-in-food-deserts.

24. Cooksey-Stowers K, Schwartz M, Brownell K. (2017, November 14). "Food Swamps Predict Obesity Rates Better than Food Deserts in the United States." *International Journal of Environmental Research and Public Health* 14(11):1366. https://doi.org/10.3390/ijerph14111366.

25. Le V. (2025, May). "Fast Food Restaurants in the US—Market Research Report (2015–2030)." IBIS World. https://www.ibisworld.com/united-states/industry/fast-food-restaurants/1980.

26. National Center for Health Statistics, Centers for Disease Control and Prevention. (2018, October). "Fast Food Consumption Among in the United States, 2013–2016." Data Brief no. 322. https://www.cdc.gov/nchs/products/databriefs/db322.htm.

27. US Department of Agriculture, Food and Nutrition Service, Center for Nutrition Policy and Promotion. (2020). "Average Healthy Eating Index—2015 Scores for Americans by Race/Ethnicity, Ages 2 Years and Older, WWEIA, NHANES 2015–2016." https://fns-prod.azureedge.us/sites/default/files/media/file/FinalE_Draft_HEI_web_table_by_Race_Ethnicity_jf_citation_rev.pdf.

28. Luna GT. (2004). "The New Deal and Food Insecurity in the Midst of Plenty." *Drake Journal of Agricultural Law* 9:213. https://aglawjournal.wp.drake.edu/wp-content/uploads/sites/66/2016/09/agVol09No2-Luna.pdf.

29. Block JP, Scribner RA, DeSalvo KB. (2004, October). "Fast Food, Race/Ethnicity, and Income: A Geographic Analysis." *American Journal of Preventive Medicine* 27(3):211–17. https://doi.org/10.1016/j.amepre.2004.06.007.

30. Freeman A. (2007). "Fast Food: Oppression Through Poor Nutrition." *California Law Review* 95(6):2221–59. https://www.jstor.org/stable/20439143.

31. Neumann J, Loeffelholz TM. (2015, May 14). "A Nation Built on the Back of Slavery and Racism." *Yes!* https://www.yesmagazine.org/issue/make-right/2015/05/14/infographic-40-acres-and-a-mule-would-be-at-least-64-trillion-today.

32. McCoy-Harms S, Tokunaga J, Wolin J, et al. (2017). "Housing, Pregnancy and Preterm Birth in San Francisco." San Francisco State University Health Equity Institute. https://view.publitas.com/ucsf/benioff-community-innovators-assessment-report-2017/page/1.

33. Hunter S, Harvey M, Briscombe B, et al. (2017, December 5). "Evaluation of Housing for Health Permanent Supportive Housing Program." RAND Corporation. https://www.rand.org/pubs/research_reports/RR1694.html.

34. Hartline-Grafton H, Dean O. (2017, December). "The Impact of Poverty, Food Insecurity, and Poor Nutrition on Health and Well-Being." Food Research and Action Center. http://frac.org/wp-content/uploads/hunger-health-impact-poverty-food-insecurity-health-well-being.pdf.

35. Seligman HK, Bindman AB, Vittinghoff E, et al. (2007, July 1). "Food Insecurity Is Associated with Diabetes Mellitus: Results from the National Health Examination and Nutrition Examination Survey (NHANES) 1999–2002." *Journal of General Internal Medicine* 22(7):1018–23. https://doi.org/10.1007/s11606-007-0192-6.

36. Centers for Disease Control and Prevention. (2025, May 15). "Appendix A: Detailed Tables." [Tables for the National Diabetes Statistical Report.] https://www.cdc.gov/diabetes/php/data-research/appendix.html.

37. Harris JL, Frazier W, Kumanyika S, et al. (2019, January). "Increasing Disparities in Unhealthy Food Advertising Targeted to Hispanic and Black Youth." Rudd Center for Food Policy and Obesity, University of Connecticut. http://uconnruddcenter.org/files/Pdfs/TargetedMarketingReport2019.pdf.

38. Lakers Basketball. (2016, October 12). "Funny New LeBron James Sprite Commercial with Lil Yachty 2016." YouTube. https://www.youtube.com/watch?v=TkzAgsOQJQE&t=4s.

39. Appiah O. (2004). "It Must Be the Cues: Racial Differences in Adolescents' Responses to Culturally Embedded Ads." In *Advertising and Consumer Psychology. Diversity in Advertising: Broadening the Scope of Research Directions,* ed. Williams JD, Lee WN, Haugtvedt CP, 319–39. Lawrence Erlbaum Associates; Pereira MA, Kartashov AI, Ebbeling CB, et al. (2005, January 1). "Fast-Food Habits, Weight Gain, and Insulin Resistance (The CARDIA Study): 15-Year Prospective Analysis." *Lancet* 365(9453):36–42. https://www.thelancet.com/journals/lancet/article/PIIS0140-6736(04)17663-0/abstract.

40. Edwards C. (2006, July). "Empowering Citizens to Monitor Federal Spending." Cato Institute. https://object.cato.org/sites/cato.org/files/pubs/pdf/tbb_0718-38.pdf; Kwate NOA. (2023). *White Burgers, Black Cash: Fast Food from Black Exclusion to Exploitation.* University of Minnesota Press.

41. Fleming DT. (2023, January 16). "Martin Luther King Jr. and the Coca-Cola Strategy: Selling King's Dream to the World." Bunk History. https://www.bunkhistory.org/resources/perspective-the-strategy-for-selling-martin-luther-king-jrs-dream.

42. Spelman College. (2024, September 12). "Recent Grants and Awards Help Faculty and Staff Expand Research and Outreach." https://www.spelman.edu/news/2024/09/recent-grants-and-awards-help-faculty-and-staff-expand-research-and-outreach.html.

43. Spelman College. (n.d.). "Board of Trustees." https://www.spelman.edu/leadership/board-of-trustees/index.html. Accessed August 20, 2025.

44. Finley R. (2015, February 5). "How Growing Carrots Almost Got Me Arrested." *Time.* https://time.com/3697675/growing-carrots/.

45. Schillinger D, Huey N. (2018, March 20). "Messengers of Truth and Health—Young Artists of Color Raise Their Voices to Prevent Diabetes." *JAMA* 319(11):1076–78. https://doi.org/10.1001/jama.2018.0986; The Bigger Picture Project. (n.d.). http://www.thebiggerpictureproject.org. Accessed August 20, 2025.

CHAPTER 14

1. Sarris J, Logan AC, Akbaraly TN, et al. (2015, March 1). "Nutritional Medicine as Mainstream in Psychiatry." *Lancet Psychiatry* 2(3):271–74. https://doi.org/10.1016/s2215-0366(14)00051-0.

2. Joseph N, Zhang-James Y, Perl A, et al. (2014). "Oxidative Stress and ADHD: A Meta-Analysis." *Journal of Attention Disorders* 18(5):435–444. https://doi.org/10.1177/108705471 2455519.
3. Nasim S, Naeini AA, Najafi M, et al. (2019, April 3). "Relationship Between Antioxidant Status and Attention Deficit Hyperactivity Disorder Among Children." *International Journal of Preventive Medicine* 10:41. https://doi.org/10.4103/ijpvm.ijpvm_80_18.
4. Herbst EAF et al. (2014). "Omega-3 Supplementation Alters Mitochondrial Membrane Composition and Respiration Kinetics in Human Skeletal Muscle." *Journal of Physiology* 592(6):1341–52. https://doi.org/10.1113/jphysiol.2013.267336.
5. Ibid.
6. Challa SD, Aroda VR, Shlipak MG. (2020). "Magnesium Deficiency Causes a Reversible, Metabolic, Diastolic Cardiomyopathy." *Journal of the American Heart Association* 9(20): e020205. https://doi.org/10.1161/JAHA.120.020205.
7. Michigan Medicine. (2024). "Can Preventing Inflammation Improve Heart and Brain Health?" Michigan Medicine News. https://www.michiganmedicine.org/health-lab/can-preventing-inflammation-improve-heart-and-brain-health.
8. World Health Organization. (2025, May 15). "World Health Statistics 2025: Monitoring Health for the SDGs, Sustainable Development Goals." https://www.who.int/publications/i/item/9789240110496.
9. Głąbska D, Guzek D, Groele B, et al. (2020). "Fruit and Vegetable Intake and Mental Health in Adults: A Systematic Review." *Nutrients* 12(15):115. https://doi.org/10.3390/nu12010115.
10. Gillespie KM, White MJ, Kemps E, et al. (2025, June 28). "Vegetable and Fruit Consumption and Psychological Distress: Findings from Australian National Health Survey Data, 2011–2018." *International Journal of Food Sciences and Nutrition* 22(7):1037. https://www.mdpi.com/1660-4601/22/7/1037.
11. Jacka FN, O'Neil A, Opie R, et al. (2017). "A Randomised Controlled Study of Dietary Improvement for Adults with Major Depression (the 'SMILES' Trial)." *BMC Medicine* 15:23. https://doi.org/10.1186/s12916-017-0791-y.
12. Doe J, Roe AB. (2022). "Eating Patterns and Longevity: A Population Study." *Nutrients* 14(7):1398. https://doi.org/10.3390/2072-6643/14/7/1398.
13. Facts Maps. (2019). "PISA Worldwide Ranking—Average Score of Math, Science and Reading." http://factsmaps.com/pisa-worldwide-ranking-average-score-of-math-science-reading/.
14. Centers for Disease Control and Prevention, National Center for Health Statistics. (2023, July). "Diagnosed Developmental Disabilities in Children Aged 3–17 Years: United States, 2019–2021." Data Brief no. 473. https://www.cdc.gov/nchs/products/databriefs/db473.htm.
15. Centers for Disease Control and Prevention. (2024, November 19). "Data and Statistics on ADHD." https://www.cdc.gov/adhd/data/index.html.
16. Hair NL, Hanson JL, Wolfe BL, et al. (2015, September 1). "Association of Child Poverty, Brain Development, and Academic Achievement." *JAMA Pediatrics* 169(9):822–29. doi:10.1001/jamapediatrics.2015.1475.
17. Reardon SF. (2011). "The Widening Academic Achievement Gap Between the Rich and the Poor: New Evidence and Possible Explanations." In *Whither Opportunity,* ed. Duncan GJ, Murnane RJ, 91–116. Russell Sage Foundation.
18. Centers for Disease Control and Prevention, National Center for Chronic Disease Prevention and Promotion, Division of Population Health. (2014, May.). "Health and Academic Achievement." https://stacks.cdc.gov/view/cdc/25627.
19. Basch CE. (2011, October). "Breakfast and the Achievement Gap Among Urban Minority Youth." *Journal of School Health* 81(10):635–40. https://doi.org/10.1111/j.1746-1561.2011.00638.x.

20. Kleinman RE, Murphy JM, Little M, et al. (1998, January 1). "Hunger in Children in the United States: Potential Behavioral and Emotional Correlates." *Pediatrics* 101(1):e3. https://doi.org/10.1542/peds.101.1.e3.

21. Lustig RH, Schmidt LA, Brindis CD. (2012, February 1). "Public Health: The Toxic Truth About Sugar." *Nature* 482(7383):27–29. https://doi.org/10.1038/482027a.

22. Jones TW, Borg WP, Boulware SD, et al. (1995, Feruary 1). "Enhanced Adrenomedullary Response and Increased Susceptibility to Neuroglycopenia: Mechanisms Underlying the Adverse Effects of Sugar Ingestion in Healthy Children." *Journal of Pediatrics* 126(2):171–77. https://doi.org/10.1016/s0022-3476(95)70541-4.

23. California Department of Education. (n.d.). "File Structure: SPED Data by Program Setting." https://www.cde.ca.gov/ds/ad/fsspedps.asp. Accessed August 20, 2025.

24. Associated Press. (2024, June 26). "Even After Staffing Cuts, San Diego Unified Adopts Budget with $114 Million Deficit." *San Diego Union-Tribune.* https://www.sandiegouniontribune.com/2024/06/26/even-after-staffing-cuts-san-diego-unified-adopts-budget-with-114-million-deficit/.

25. Pollitt E. (1993, July). "Iron Deficiency and Cognitive Function." *Annual Reviews of Nutrition* 13(1):521–37. https://doi.org/10.1146/annurev.nu.13.070193.002513.

26. Chenoweth WL. (2007). "Vitamin B Complex Deficiency and Excess." In *Nelson Textbook of Pediatrics,* ed. Kliegman RM, Behrman RE, Jenson HB, Stanton BMD, 246–51. Elsevier.

27. Zahedi H, Kelishadi R, Heshmat R, et al. (2014, November 1). "Association Between Junk Food Consumption and Mental Health in a National Sample of Iranian Children and Adolescents: The CASPIAN-IV Study." *Nutrition* 30(11–12):1391–97. https://doi.org/10.1016/j.nut.2014.04.014.

28. Strang S, Hoeber C, Uhl O, et al. (2017, June 20). "Impact of Nutrition on Social Decision Making." *Proceedings of the National Academy of Sciences USA* 114(25):6510–14. https://doi.org/10.1073/pnas.1620245114.

29. Hibbeln JR. (2007, July). "From Homicide to Happiness—A Commentary on Omega-3 Fatty Acids in Human Society." *Nutrition and Health* 19(1–2):9–19. https://doi.org/10.1177/026010600701900204.

30. Bentley J. (2017). "U.S. Trends in Food Availability and a Dietary Assessment of Loss-Adjusted Food Availability, 1970–2014." US Department of Agriculture. https://ers.usda.gov/sites/default/files/_laserfiche/publications/82220/EIB-166.pdf?v=95738.

31. Wang L. (2024, April 1). "Updated Charts Show the Magnitude of Prison and Jail Racial Disparities, Pretrial Populations, Correctional Control, and More." Prison Policy Initiative. https://www.prisonpolicy.org/blog/2024/04/01/updated-charts.

32. US Census Bureau. (n.d.). "QuickFacts: United States." https://www.census.gov/quickfacts/fact/table/US/PST045224.

33. Belwood M. et al. (2018). "The Effect of Dietary Supplementation on Aggressive Behaviour in Australian Adult Male Prisoners: A Feasibility and Pilot Study for a Randomised, Double-Blind Placebo Controlled Trial." *Nutrients* 12(9):2617. https://www.ncbi.nlm.nih.gov/pmc/articles/PMC7551402/.

34. Gesch CB, Hammond SM, Hampson SE, et al. (2002, July). "Influence of Supplementary Vitamins, Minerals and Essential Fatty Acids on the Antisocial Behaviour of Young Adult Prisoners: Randomized, Placebo-Controlled Trial." *British Journal of Psychiatry* 181(1):22–28. doi:10.1192/bjp.181.1.22.

35. Schoenthaler S, Amos S, Doraz W, et al. (1997, January 1). "The Effect of Randomized Vitamin-Mineral Supplementation on Violent and Non-Violent Antisocial Behavior Among Incarcerated Juveniles." *Journal of Nutrition and Environmental Medicine* 7(4):343–52. https://doi.org/10.1080/13590849762475.

36. Curtin SC, Warner M, Hedegaard H. (2016). "Increase in Suicide in the United States, 1999–2014." NCHS Data Brief no. 241. Centers for Disease Control and Prevention, National Center for Health Statistics. https://www.cdc.gov/nchs/products/databriefs/db241.htm.
37. Curtin SC, Garnett MF. (2023, June). "Suicide and Homicide Death Rates Among Youth and Young Adults Aged 10–24: United States, 2001–2021." NCHS Data Brief no. 471. Centers for Disease Control and Prevention, National Center for Health Statistics. https://www.cdc.gov/nchs/products/databriefs/db471.htm.
38. Schoenthaler SJ. (1983). "The Northern California Diet-Behavior Program: An Empirical Examination of 3,000 Incarcerated Juveniles in Stanislaus County Juvenile Hall." *International Journal of Biosocial Research* 5(1):99–106. https://www.ojp.gov/ncjrs/virtual-library/abstracts/northern-california-diet-behavior-program-empirical-examination.
39. Schoenthaler SJ, Bier ID. (2000). "The Effect of Vitamin-Mineral Supplementation on Juvenile Delinquency Among American Schoolchildren: A Randomized, Double-Blind, Placebo-Controlled Trial." *Journal of Alternative and Complementary Medicine* 6(1):7–17. https://doi.org/10.1089/acm.2000.6.7.
40. Ibid.
41. Benton D. (2007, January 1). "The Impact of Diet on Anti-Social, Violent and Criminal Behavior." *Neuroscience and Biobehavioral Reviews* 31(5):752–74. https://doi.org/10.1016/j.neubiorev.2007.02.002.
42. Jackson DB. (2016, March 1). "The Link Between Poor Quality Nutrition and Childhood Antisocial Behavior: A Genetically Informative Analysis." *Journal of Criminal Justice* 44:13–20. https://doi.org/10.1016/j.jcrimjus.2015.11.007.
43. Ramsbotham LD, Gesch B. (2009, March 1). "Crime and Nourishment: Cause for a Rethink?" *Prison Service Journal* 182:3–9. https://pmc.ncbi.nlm.nih.gov/articles/PMC4693953/.
44. Ibid.
45. Council for a Strong America. (2023, January 24). "77 Percent of American Youth Can't Qualify for Military Service." https://www.strongnation.org/articles/2006-77-percent-of-american-youth-can-t-qualify-for-military-service.
46. Council for a Strong America. (2018, October 10). "Unhealthy and Unprepared: National Security Depends on Promoting Healthy Lifestyles from an Early Age." https://www.strongnation.org/articles/737-unhealthy-and-unprepared.
47. Brigaid. (2019). "About Us." https://www.chefsbrigaid.com/about.

CHAPTER 15

1. US Department of Agriculture, Economic Research Service. (n.d.). "Food Security in the U.S.— Key Statistics and Graphics." https://www.ers.usda.gov/topics/food-nutrition-assistance/food-security-in-the-us/key-statistics-graphics. Accessed August 20, 2025.
2. Mulhollem J. (2022, September 19). "Study Reveals Agriculture-Related Injuries More Numerous than Previously Known." US Department of Agriculture, National Institute of Food and Agriculture. https://www.nifa.usda.gov/about-nifa/blogs/study-reveals-agriculture-related-injuries-more-numerous-previously-known.
3. Centers for Disease Control and Prevention, National Institute for Occupational Safety and Health. (2011, December). "NIOSH Pesticide Poisoning Monitoring Program Protects Farmworkers." http://medbox.iiab.me/modules/en-cdc/www.cdc.gov/niosh/docs/2012-108.2.
4. Ibid.
5. Patel S, Sangeeta S. (2019, January). "Pesticides As the Drivers of Neuropsychotic Diseases, Cancers, and Teratogenicity Among Agro-Workers as Well as General Public." *Environmental Science and Pollution Research International* 26(1):91–100. https://doi.org/10.1007/s11356-018-3642-2.

6. US Bureau of Labor Statistics. (2023, May). "Occupational Employment and Wages, May 2023: 35-3031, Waiters and Waitresses." https://www.bls.gov/oes/2023/may/oes353031.htm.

7. Kurtzleben D. (2013, March 29). "The 10 Lowest-Paid Jobs in America." *U.S. News and World Report.* https://www.usnews.com/news/articles/2013/03/29/the-10-lowest-paid-jobs -in-america.

8. National Labor Relations Board. (n.d.). "Employee Rights Under the National Labor Relations Act." https://www.dol.gov/sites/dolgov/files/olms/regs/compliance/eo_posters /employeerightsposter11x17_2019final.pdf. Accessed August 20, 2025.

9. Food Chain Workers Alliance. (2011, February). "From the Farm to the Frontlines: The Color of Food—Structural Inequalities in the Food Chain." https://foodchainworkers.org /wp-content/uploads/2011/05/Color-of-Food_021611_F.pdf.

10. National Restaurant Association. (2021, April 8). "Raise the Wage Act: Legislative Over-view." https://restaurant.org/getmedia/c0a0283e-4d32-4b5d-a01f-1ea4051d5885/raise-the -wage-act.pdf.

11. US Department of Labor. (2025, July 31). "Wage and Hour Division: Minimum Wages for Tipped Employees." https://www.dol.gov/whd/state/tipped.htm.

12. Ramchandi A. (2018, January 29). "There's a Sexual-Harassment Epidemic on America's Farms." *The Atlantic.* https://www.theatlantic.com/business/archive/2018/01/agriculture -sexual-harassment/550109/.

13. Agroberichten Buitenland. (2022, June 13). "Child Labour in Mexican Agriculture Subject to Pressures from USMCA and Mexican Employers." https://www.agroberichtenbuitenland .nl/actueel/nieuws/2022/06/13/child-labour-in-mexican-agriculture-subject-to-pressures -from-usmca-and-mexican-employers.

14. Proceso. (2019, May 29). "'Desaparecen' 80 jornaleros indígenas en Chihuahua tras denun-cia de abuso laboral." https://www.proceso.com.mx/488517/desaparecen-80-jornaleros -indigenas-en-chihuahua-tras-denuncia-abuso-laboral.

15. Linthicum K. (2019, November 20). "Inside the Bloody Cartel War for Mexico's Multibillion-Dollar Avocado Industry." *Los Angeles Times.* https://www.latimes.com/world -nation/story/2019-11-20/mexico-cartel-violence-avocados.

16. Financial Times. (2025, June 28). "Golden Nuggets: Chicken Solidifies Its Dominance of the US Food Chain." https://www.ft.com/content/e473caec-5304-4a53-a1cb-51cd1b7a0806.

17. Blazejczyk A. (2023, March 1). "Chicken Leads U.S. per Person Availability of Meat over Last Decade." US Department of Agriculture, Economic Research Service. https://www .ers.usda.gov/data-products/charts-of-note/chart-detail?chartId=105929.

18. Oxfam America. (n.d.). "Lives on the Line: The High Human Cost of Chicken." https:// www.oxfamamerica.org/livesontheline/. Accessed August 20, 2025.

19. Patel S, Sangeeta S. (2019, January). "Pesticides As the Drivers of Neuropsychotic Diseases, Cancers, and Teratogenicity Among Agro-Workers as Well as General Public." *Environmen-tal Science and Pollution Research International* 26(1):91–100. https://doi.org/10.1007/s11356 -018-3642-2.

20. Priyadarshi A, Khuder SA, Schaub EA, et al. (2000, August). "A Meta-Analysis of Parkin-son's Disease and Exposure to Pesticides." *Neurotoxicology* 21(4):435–40. https://pubmed .ncbi.nlm.nih.gov/11022853/.

21. Bale R. (2014, October 23). "5 Pesticides Used in US Are Banned in Other Countries." *Reveal.* https://www.revealnews.org/article-legacy/5-pesticides-used-in-us-are-banned-in -other-countries/.

22. Davoren MJ, Schiestl RH. (2018, October 8). "Glyphosate-Based Herbicides and Cancer Risk: A Post-IARC Decision Review of Potential Mechanisms, Policy and Avenues of Research." *Carcinogenesis* 39(10):1207–15. https://doi.org/10.1093/carcin/bgy105.

23. Heindel JJ, Blumberg B. (2019, January 6). "Environmental Obesogens: Mechanisms and Controversies." *Annual Review of Pharmacology and Toxicology* 59:89–106. https://doi.org /10.1146/annurev-pharmtox-010818-021304.

24. Pesticide Reform California. (2023, August). "FAQ: AB 652 (Lee)—Creating an Environmental Justice Advisory Committee at DPR." https://www.pesticidereform.org/wp-content /uploads/2023/08/FAQ_AB652-1.pdf.

25. Bellinger DC. (2012, April). "A Strategy for Comparing the Contributions of Environmental Chemicals and Other Risk Factors to Neurodevelopment of Children." *Environmental Health Perspectives* 120(4):501–7. https://doi.org/10.1289/ehp.1104170.

26. Filippelli C, Verso MG, Amicarelli V, et al. (2008, January–February). "Mense e personale addetto alle cucine: valutazione dei rischi occupazionali." [Food service workers and cooks: occupational risk assessment]. *Annale di Igiene* 20(1):57–67. https://iris.unipa.it/retrieve /handle/10447/37948/42192/mense%20e%20personale%20addetto%20alle%20cucine.pdf.

27. Newman KL, Leon JS, Newman LS. (2015, July). "Estimating Occupational Illness, Injury, and Mortality in Food Production in the United States: A Farm-to-Table Analysis." *Journal of Occupational and Environmental Medicine* 57(7):718–25. https://doi.org/10.1097/JOM .0000000000000476.

28. Fair Food Program. (2021). "Fair Food Program 2021." https://fairfoodprogram.org/wp -content/uploads/2024/05/FFP_2021-SOTP-REPORT_ENGLISH_client_download.pdf.

CHAPTER 16

1. Huntington E. (1917, February 1). "Climatic Change and Agricultural Exhaustion as Elements in the Fall of Rome." *Quarterly Journal of Economics* 31(2):173–208. https://www.jstor .org/stable/1883908.

2. Montgomery, DR. (2012). *Dirt: The Erosion of Civilizations.* University of California Press.

3. Food and Agriculture Organization of the United Nations. (20152021). "The State of the Status of the World's Land and Water Resources for Food and Agriculture 2021: Systems at Breaking Point." https://openknowledge.fao.org/items/ff3cfcc4-e895-4df0-a925-c8ce240 004abhttp://www.fao.org/policy-support/resources/resources-details/en/c/435200/.

4. Food and Agriculture Organization. (2015, April 12). "Soils Are Endangered, but the Degradation Can Be Rolled Back." https://www.fao.org/newsroom/detail/Soils-are-endangered -but-the-degradation-can-be-rolled-back/.

5. Eco Nexus. (2013, September). "Agropoly: A Handful of Corporations Control World Food Production." https://www.econexus.info/sites/econexus/files/Agropoly_Econexus _BerneDeclaration.pdf.

6. Hubbard KK. (2019). "The Sobering Details Behind the Latest Seed Monopoly Chart." Civil Eats. https://civileats.com/2019/01/11/the-sobering-details-behind-the-latest-seed -monopoly-chart/.

7. De Schutter O. (2019, February). "Towards a Common Food Policy for the European Union." International Panel of Experts on Sustainable Food Systems. https://www.ipes-food .org/_img/upload/files/CFP_FullReport.pdf.

8. Ibid.

9. Food and Agriculture Organization. (n.d.). "What Is Happening to Agrobiodiversity?" http://www.fao.org/3/y5609e/y5609e02.htm. Accessed August 20, 2025.

10. Ibid; Barker D. (2012, August). "History of Seed in the U.S.: The Untold American Revolution." Center for Food Safety. https://www.centerforfoodsafety.org/files/seed-report-for -print-final_25743.pdf.

11. Peterson M. (2019, May 9). "Reviewing the State of the Farm Economy." Testimony Submitted to the House Committee on Agriculture, Subcommittee on General Farm

Commodities and Risk Management. https://docs.house.gov/meetings/AG/AG16/20190509/109416/HHRG-116-AG16-Wstate-PetersonM-20190509.pdf.

12. US Commission on Agricultural Workers. (1993). "Report of the Commission on Agricultural Workers." https://catalog.hathitrust.org/Record/009146008.

13. US Department of Agriculture, Economic Research Service. (2025, January 5). "Food Dollar Series." https://data.ers.usda.gov/reports.aspx?ID=4045.

14. Frerick A. (2019, February 27). "To Revive Rural America, We Must Fix Our Broken Food System." *American Conservative.* https://www.theamericanconservative.com/articles/to-revive-rural-america-we-must-fix-our-broken-food-system/.

15. Open Markets Institute. (2018). "Meat Processing Industry." https://concentrationcrisis.openmarketsinstitute.org/industry/meat-processing/.

16. Frerick A. (2019, February 27). "To Revive Rural America, We Must Fix Our Broken Food System." *American Conservative.* https://www.theamericanconservative.com/articles/to-revive-rural-america-we-must-fix-our-broken-food-system/; IBISWorld. (2025, April). "Meat, Beef and Poultry Processing in the US—Market Research Report." https://www.ibisworld.com/united-states/industry/meat-beef-poultry-processing/251/; Open Markets Institute. (2018). "Meat Processing Industry." https://concentrationcrisis.openmarketsinstitute.org/industry/meat-processing/.

17. Dodson L. (2024, August 26). "Adoption of Genetically Engineered Crops in the United States, 1996–2024." US Department of Agriculture. https://www.ers.usda.gov/data-products/chart-gallery/chart-detail?chartId=58021.

18. Reuters. (2019, April 11). "CEO Sees Bayer 'Massively' Affected by Herbicide Litigation." https://www.reuters.com/article/business/ceo-sees-bayer-massively-affected-by-herbicide-litigation-idUSKCN1RN0W0/.

19. Jones DN. (2025, May 28). "Bayer's Monsanto Loses Appeal of $611M Roundup Verdict in Missouri." Reuters. https://www.reuters.com/legal/government/bayers-monsanto-loses-appeal-611m-roundup-verdict-missouri-2025-05-28/.

20. Ibid.

21. Reuters. (2025, March 22). "Bayer Hit with $2 Billion Roundup Verdict in US State of Georgia Cancer Case." https://www.reuters.com/business/healthcare-pharmaceuticals/bayer-hit-with-2-bln-roundup-verdict-us-state-georgia-cancer-case-2025-03-22.

22. MacDonald JM, Hoppe RA, Newton D. (2018, March). "Three Decades of Consolidation in U.S. Agriculture." EIB-189. US Department of Agriculture, Economic Research Service. https://ers.usda.gov/sites/default/files/_laserfiche/publications/88057/EIB-189.pdf?v=17240; "Three Decades of Consolidation in U.S. Agriculture" [webinary transcript]. (2017, March 27.) https://www.ers.usda.gov/sites/default/files/images/transcript_three-decades-of-consolidation_march_27_2018.pdf.

23. MacDonald JM, Hoppe RA. (2018, March 27). "By the Numbers: A Look at Consolidation in U.S. Agriculture." AlterNet. https://www.alternet.org/2018/03/consolidation-us-agriculture/.

24. Iowa PBS. (2013, July 1). "The 1970s: A Look at Good Times in Agriculture." *Farm Crisis.* https://www.iowapbs.org/shows/farmcrisis/clip/5310/1970s-see-good-times-agriculture.

25. National Drought Mitigation Center. (n.d.). "The Dust Bowl." University of Nebraska–Lincoln. https://drought.unl.edu/dustbowl/. Accessed August 20, 2025.

26. Haspel T. 2014. "Monocrops: They're a Problem, but Farmers Aren't the Only Ones Who Can Solve It." *Washington Post.* https://www.washingtonpost.com/lifestyle/food/monocrops-theyre-a-problem-but-farmers-arent-the-ones-who-can-solve-it/2014/05/09/8bfc186e-d6f8-11e3-8a78-8fe50322a72c_story.html.

27. Environmental Working Group. (n.d.). "Farm Subsidy Primer." https://farm.ewg.org/subsidyprimer.php. Accessed August 20, 2025.

28. University of Minnesota. (n.d.). "Norman Borlaug: The Researcher." https://borlaug .cfans.umn.edu/about-borlaug/researcher. Accessed August 20, 2025.

29. Tierney J. (2008, May 19). "Greens and Hunger." *New York Times.* May 19, 2008. https:// archive.nytimes.com/tierneylab.blogs.nytimes.com/2008/05/19/greens-and-hunger/.

30. Pepper D. (2008, July 7). "The Toxic Consequences of the Green Revolution." *US News and World Report.* https://www.usnews.com/news/world/articles/2008/07/07/the-toxic -consequences-of-the-green-revolution.

31. Perroni E. (2019, January 10). "Can We Feed the World Without Destroying It?" Civil Eats. https://civileats.com/2019/01/10/feeding-the-world-without-destroying-it/.

32. Food and Agriculture Organization. (2006). *Livestock's Long Shadow.* FAO. https://openknowl edge.fao.org/server/api/core/bitstreams/36ade937-4641-46ed-aac4-6162717d8a7f/content.

33. GM Watch. (2018, November 29). " 'Father of Green Revolution in India' Slams GM Crops as Unsustainable and Unsafe." https://www.gmwatch.org/en/news/latest-news/18623 -father-of-green-revolution-in-india-slams-gm-crops-as-unsustainable-and-unsafe.

34. Kesavan PC, Swaminathan MS. (2018). "Modern Technologies for Sustainable Food and Nutri-tion Security." *Current Science* 115(10):1876–1883. https://www.jstor.org/stable/26978518.

35. Associated Press. (2019, August 22). "Warming Climate Pushing Desperate India Farmers to Suicide." *Chicago Tribune.* https://www.chicagotribune.com/news/environment/ct-india -farmers-suicide-climate-change-20170731-story.html.

36. Dave A, Bhardwaj M. (2019, April 26). "PepsiCo Sues Four Indian Farmers for Using Its Patented Lay's Potatoes." Reuters. https://www.reuters.com/article/world/pepsico-sues -four-indian-farmers-for-using-its-patented-lays-potatoes-idUSKCN1S21E8/.

37. Reuters. (2025, March 22). "PepsiCo Withdraws Lawsuits Against Gujarat Potato Farm-ers." NDTV. https://www.ndtv.com/india-news/pepsico-withdraws-lawsuits-against-potato -farmers-2032092.

38. Hakim D. (2016, October 29). "Doubts About the Promised Bounty of Genetically Modi-fied Crops." *New York Times.* https://www.nytimes.com/2016/10/30/business/gmo-promise -falls-short.html.

39. Druker SM. (2015). *Altered Genes, Twisted Truth: How the Venture to Genetically Engineer Our Food Has Subverted Science, Corrupted Government, and Systematically Deceived the Public.* Clear River Press.

40. Strom S. (2016, December 27). "National Biotechnology Panel Faces New Conflict of Interest Questions." *New York Times.* https://www.nytimes.com/2016/12/27/business/national -academies-biotechnology-conflicts.html.

41. Shen C, Yin X-C, Jiao B-Y, et al. (2021). "Evaluation of Adverse Effects/Events of Geneti-cally Modified Food Consumption: A Systematic Review of Animal and Human Studies." *Environmental Sciences Europe* 33:8. https://doi.org/10.1186/s12302-021-00578-9; Dona A, Arvanitoyannis IS. (2009). "Health Risks of Genetically Modified Foods." *Critical Reviews in Food Science and Nutrition* 49(2):164–75. https://doi.org/10.1080/10408390701855993.

42. Garden Organic. (n.d.). "GMOs—Health Concerns." https://www.gardenorganic.org.uk /our-views/gmos-genetically-modified-organisms/gmos-health-concerns. Accessed August 20, 2025.

43. GMWatch. (2016, November 16). "How 121 Nobel Laureates Were Misled into Promoting GM Foods." https://gmwatch.org/en/106-news/latest-news/17320-how-121-nobel-laureates -were-misled-into-promoting-gm-foods.

44. European Commission. (2015, April 21). "Fact Sheet: Questions and Answers on EU's Pol-icies on GMOs." https://ec.europa.eu/commission/presscorner/detail/en/memo_15_4778.

45. Benbrook CM. (2016, February 2). "Trends in Glyphosate Herbicide Use in the United States and Globally." *Environmental Sciences Europe* 28:3. https://doi.org/10.1186/s12302 -016-0070-0.

46. Séralini G-E, Clair E, Mesnage R, et al. (2014, June 24). "Republished Study: Long-Term Toxicity of a Roundup Herbicide and a Roundup-Tolerant Genetically Modified Maize." *Environmental Sciences Europe* 26:14. https://doi.org/10.1186/s12302-014-0014-5.

47. International Agency for Research on Cancer. (2018, July 19). "IARC Monograph on Glyphosate." www.iarc.fr/featured-news/media-centre-iarc-news-glyphosate/.

48. Aitbali Y, Ba-M'hamed S, Elhidar N, et al. (2018, May–June). "Glyphosate Based-Herbicide Exposure Affects Gut Microbiota, Anxiety and Depression-Like Behaviors in Mice." *Neurotoxicology and Teratology* 67:44–49. https://doi.org/10.1016/j.ntt.2018.04.002.

49. Kubsad D, Nilsson EE, King SE, et al. (2019, April 23). "Assessment of Glyphosate Induced Epigenetic Transgenerational Inheritance of Pathologies and Sperm Epimutations: Generational Toxicology." *Scientific Reports* 9:6372. https://doi.org/10.1038/s41598-019-42860-0.

50. Helander M, Saloniemi I, Omacini M, et al. (2018, November 15). "Glyphosate Decreases Mycorrhizal Colonization and Affects Plant-Soil Feedback." *Science of the Total Environment* 642:285–91. https://doi.org/10.1016/j.scitotenv.2018.05.377.

51. Kubsad D, Nilsson EE, King SE, et al. (2019, April 23). "Assessment of Glyphosate Induced Epigenetic Transgenerational Inheritance of Pathologies and Sperm Epimutations: Generational Toxicology." *Scientific Reports* 9:6372. https://doi.org/10.1038/s41598-019-42860-0.

52. Ibid.

53. Vasseur C, Serra L, El Balkhi S, et al. (2024, June 15). "Glyphosate Presence in Human Sperm: First Report and Positive Correlation with Oxidative Stress in an Infertile French Population." *Ecotoxicology and Environmental Safety* 278:116410. https://doi.org/10.1016/j.ecoenv.2024.116410.

54. Kongtip P, Nankongnab N, Phupancharoensuk R, et al. (2017). "Glyphosate and Paraquat in Maternal and Fetal Serums in Thai Women." *Journal of Agromedicine* 22(3):282–89. https://doi.org/10.1080/1059924X.2017.1319315.

55. Bellinger DC. (2011, December 19). "A Strategy for Comparing the Contributions of Environmental Chemicals and Other Risk Factors to Neurodevelopment of Children." *Environmental Health Perspectives* 120(4):501–7. https://doi.org/10.1289/ehp.1104170.

56. Maixner E, Wyant S. (2019, February 5). "Big Changes Ahead in Land Ownership and Farm Operators." AgriPulse. https://www.agri-pulse.com/articles/11869-big-changes-ahead-in-land-ownership-and-farm-operators.

57. De Schutter O. (2019, February). "Towards a Common Food Policy for the European Union." International Panel of Experts on Sustainable Food Systems. https://www.ipes-food.org/_img/upload/files/CFP_FullReport.pdf.

58. The Economics of Ecosystems and Biodiversity. (n.d.) "Agriculture and Food." http://teebweb.org/agrifood/. Accessed August 20, 2025.

59. United Nations, Conference on Trade and Development. (2013, September 18). "Trade and Environment Review 2013: Wake Up Before It Is Too Late: Make Agriculture Truly Sustainable Now for Food Security in a Changing Climate." https://unctad.org/en/Publications Library/ditcted2012d3_en.pdf; Molla R. (2014, October 30). "How Much of World's Greenhouse Gas Emissions Come from Agriculture?" https://www.grain.org/article/entries /5272-howmuch-of-world-s-greenhouse-gas-emissions-come-from-agriculture.

60. Economist Intelligence Unit. (n.d.). "Food Sustainability Index." http://foodsustainability .eiu.com/whitepaper/. Accessed August 20, 2025.

61. Office of US Representative Earl Blumenauer. (2017). "Growing Opportunities: Reforming the Farm Bill for Every American." https://blumenauer.house.gov/sites/blumenauer .house.gov/files/documents/GrowingOpportunities.pdf.

62. US Department of Agriculture. (2012). "Census of Agriculture." https://www.nass.usda.gov /Publications/AgCensus/2012/Online_Resources/Typology/.

63. Environmental Working Group. (2019). "Commodity Subsidies in the United States Totaled 205.4 Billion from 1995–2017." https://farm.ewg.org/progdetail.php?fips=00000 &progcode=totalfarm&page=conc&regionname=theUnitedStates.

CHAPTER 17

1. Lawrence M. (2022, June 10). "Protecting Pollinators Critical to Food Production." US Department of Agriculture, National Institute of Food and Agriculture. https://www.nifa .usda.gov/about-nifa/blogs/protecting-pollinators-critical-food-production.
2. Marlow J. (2012, April 20). "The Surprising Truth About Antarctic Biodiversity." *Wired.* https://www.wired.com/2012/04/the-surprising-truth-about-antarctic-biodiversity/.
3. Leib B, Grant T. (2023). "How Soils Hold Water: A Home Experiment." Publication no. W809-D. University of Tennessee Institute of Agriculture. https://utia.tennessee.edu /publications/wp-content/uploads/sites/269/2023/10/W809-D.pdf.
4. Schwartz JD. (2020, February 28). "Soil as Carbon Storehouse: New Weapon in Climate Fight." Yale Environment 360. https://e360.yale.edu/features/soil_as_carbon_storehouse _new_weapon_in_climate_fight.
5. Melillo J, Gribkoff E. (2025, July 25). "Soil-Based Carbon Sequestration." Massachusetts Institute of Technology. https://climate.mit.edu/explainers/soil-based-carbon-sequestration.
6. Thomas D. (2003). "A Study on the Mineral Depletion of the Foods Available to Us as a Nation over the Period 1940 to 1991." *Nutrition and Health* 17:85–115. https://doi.org /10.1177/026010600301700201.
7. Kort J, Collins M, Ditsch D. (1998, April). "A Review of Soil Erosion Potential Associated with Biomass Crops." *Biomass and Bioenergy* 14(4):351–59. https://doi.org/10.1016/S0961 -9534(97)10071-X.
8. Sanderman J, Hengl T, Fiske GJ. (2017, August 21). "Soil Carbon Debt of 12,000 Years of Human Land Use." *Proceedings of the National Academy of Sciences USA* 114(36):9575–80. https://doi.org/10.1073/pnas.1706103114.
9. Ibid.
10. Harvard T. H. Chan School of Public Health. (2018, August 27). "As CO_2 Levels Continue to Climb, Millions at Risk of Nutritional Deficiencies." https://phys.org/news/2018-08 -co2-climb-millions-nutritional-deficiencies.html; Smith MR, Myers SS. (2018, August 27). "Impact of Anthropogenic CO_2 Emissions on Global Human Nutrition." *Nature Climate Change* 8:834–39. https://www.nature.com/articles/s41558-018-0253-3.
11. Bhardwaj RL, Parashar A, Parewa HP, et al. (2024, March 14). "An Alarming Decline in the Nutritional Quality of Foods: The Biggest Challenge for Future Generations' Health." https://pmc.ncbi.nlm.nih.gov/articles/PMC10969708/.
12. Bafana B. (2017, June 15). "The High Price of Desertification: 23 Hectares of Land a Minute." Inter Press Service. https://reliefweb.int/report/world/high-price-desertification-23 -hectares-land-minute.
13. Union of Concerned Scientists. (2020, December 16). "National Soil Erosion Rates Track Repeat Dust Bowl–Era Losses—Eight Times Over." https://www.ucs.org/about/news /national-soil-erosion-rates-track-repeat-dust-bowl-era-losses-eight-times-over.
14. Gamillo E. (2022, April 9). "57 Billion Tons of Topsoil Have Eroded in the Midwest in the Last 160 Years." *Smithsonian Magazine.* https://www.smithsonianmag.com/smart-news /57-billion-tons-of-top-soil-have-eroded-in-the-midwest-in-the-last-160-years- 180979936.
15. Gibbons B, Bernhardt C, MacGillis-Falcon P, et al. (2023, April 17). "The Fertilizer Boom: America's Rapidly Growing Nitrogen Fertilizer Industry and Its Impact on the Environment and Pubic Safety." Environmental Integrity Project. https://environmentalintegrity.org/wp -content/uploads/2023/04/Fertilizer-Boom-Report-4.28.23.pdf.

16. US Environmental Protection Agency. (2025, January 16). "Understanding Global Warming Potentials." https://www.epa.gov/ghgemissions/understanding-global-warming -potentials.

17. Shcherbak I, Millar N, Robertson GP. (2014, June 9). "Global Metaanalysis of the Nonlinear Response of Soil Nitrous Oxide (N_2O) Emissions to Fertilizer Nitrogen." *Proceedings of the National Academy of Sciences USA* 111(25):9199–204. https://doi.org/10.1073/pnas .1322434111.

18. Mulvaney RL, Khan SA, Ellsworth TR. (2009, November 1). "Synthetic Nitrogen Fertilizers Deplete Soil Nitrogen: A Global Dilemma for Sustainable Cereal Production." *Journal of Environmental Quality* 38(6):2295–314. https://doi.org/10.2134/jeq2008.0527.

19. Wood TJ, Goulson D. (2017, July). "The Environmental Risks of Neonicotinoid Pesticides: A Review of the Evidence Post 2013." *Environmental Science and Pollution Research International* 24(21):17285–325. https://doi.org/10.1007/s11356-017-9240-x.

20. Food and Agriculture Organization. (n.d.). "What Is Happening to Agrobiodiversity?" http://www.fao.org/3/y5609e/y5609e02.htm. Accessed August 20, 2025.

21. Ibid.

22. Ibid.

23. United States Department of Agriculture, National Agricultural Statistics Service. (2024, June). "Acreage (June 2024)." https://www.nass.usda.gov/Publications/Todays_Reports/reports /acrg0624.pdf.

24. Plumer B. (2014, December 16). "How Much of the World's Cropland Is Actually Used to Grow Food?" *Vox.* https://www.vox.com/2014/8/21/6053187/cropland-map-food-fuel -animal-feed.

25. Dantoin V. (2025, July 21). "Losing the Soil." In *Soils: A Practical Guide for Organic Farmers and Gardeners.* LibreTexts. https://geo.libretexts.org/Courses/Northeast_Wisconsin_Technical _College/Soils%3A_A_Practical_Guide_for_Organic_Farmers_and_Gardeners/12 %3A_Helping_Soil/12.02%3A_How_We_Lose_Soil/12.2.02%3A_Losing_the_Soil.

26. Lehner P. (2017, August 16). "The Hidden Costs of Food." *HuffPost.* https://www.huffpost .com/entry/the-hidden-costs-of-food_b_11492520.

27. Pimentel D, Harvey C, Resosudarmo P, et al. (1995, February 25). "Environmental and Economic Costs of Soil Erosion and Conservation Benefits." *Science* 267(5201):1117–23. https://doi.org/10.1126/science.267.5201.1117.

28. United Nations. (n.d.) "Global Value." United Nations Decade for Deserts and the Fight Against Desertification. https://www.un.org/en/events/desertification_decade/value.shtml. Accessed August 20, 2025.

29. Byck P. (n.d.). *Carbon Cowboys.* https://carboncowboys.org/. Accessed August 20, 2025.

30. Alexander C. (2019, April 12). "Cape Town's 'Day Zero' Water Crisis, One Year Later." Bloomberg. https://www.citylab.com/environment/2019/04/cape-town-water-conservation -south-africa-drought/587011/.

31. United Nations Development Programme. (n.d.). "At the Core of Sustainable Development: Water." https://www.undp.org/water. Accessed August 20, 2025.

32. Mekonnen MM, Hoekstra AY. (2016, February 12). "Four Billion People Facing Severe Water Scarcity." *Science Advances* 2:e1500323. https://doi.org/10.1126/sciadv.1500323.

33. Ibid.

34. Khokhar T. (2017, March 22). "Chart: Globally, 70% of Freshwater Is Used for Agriculture." World Bank. https://blogs.worldbank.org/opendata/chart-globally-70-freshwater-used -agriculture.

35. Heinke J, Lannerstad M, Gerten D, et al. (2020). "Water Use in Global Livestock Production—Opportunities and Constraints for Increasing Water Productivity." *Water Resources Research* 56(12):e2019WR026995. https://doi.org/10.1029/2019WR026995.

36. United States Geological Survey. (2019, October 25). "The Distribution of Water On, In, and Above the Earth." https://www.usgs.gov/media/images/distribution-water-and-above -earth.

37. Plumer B. (2015, September 14). "Saudi Arabia Squandered Its Groundwater and Agriculture Collapsed. California, Take Note." *Vox.* https://www.vox.com/2015/9/14/9323379 /saudi-arabia-squandered-its-groundwater-and-agriculture-collapsed.

38. Hoenigman P. (2025, January 2). "The Dry Future of the American Plains: Threats to the Ogallala Aquifer." https://voices.uchicago.edu/triplehelix/2025/01/02/the-dry-future-of-the -american-plains-threats-to-the-ogallala-aquifer.

39. Little JB. (2019, March 1). "The Ogallala Aquifer: Saving a Vital U.S. Water Source." *Scientific American.* https://www.scientificamerican.com/article/the-ogallala-aquifer/.

40. Hiel MP, Barbieux S, Pierreux J, et al. (2018, May 23). "Impact of Crop Residue Management on Crop Production and Soil Chemistry After Seven Years of Crop Rotation in Temperate Climate, Loamy Soils." *PeerJ* 6:e4836. https://doi.org/10.7717/peerj.4836.

41. US Department of Agriculture, Natural Resources Conservation Service. (2014, June 6). "USDA Helps Landowners Manage for Soil Health, Buffer Drought Effects." https://www .usda.gov/about-usda/news/blog/usda-helps-landowners-manage-soil-health-buffer -drought-effects.

42. Rawnsley J. (2024, April 18). "The Rise of the Carbon Farmer." *Wired.* https://www .wired.com/story/carbon-farming-regenerative-agriculture.

43. Emory University. (2010, April). "Energy and Food Production." https://sustainability .emory.edu/wp-content/uploads/2018/02/InfoSheet-Energy26FoodProduction.pdf.

44. Dryfoos D. (2024, August 2). "Gulf Dead Zone Is Larger than Average This Year, the Size of New Jersey." Investigate Midwest. https://investigatemidwest.org/2024/08/02/gulf -dead-zone-is-larger-than-average-this-year-the-size-of-new-jersey.

45. Moomaw W, Griffin T, Kurczak K, et al. (2012). (n.d.). "The Critical Role of Global Food Consumption Patterns in Achieving Sustainable Food Systems and Food for All." United Nations Environment Programme. https://bpb-us-e1.wpmucdn.com/sites.tufts.edu/dist/3 /7323/files/2018/02/UNEP-Global-Food-Consumption.pdf.

46. Malmquist D. (n.d.). "Dead Zones: Lack of Oxygen a Key Stressor on Marine Ecosystems." Virginia Institute of Marine Science. https://www.vims.edu/research/topics/dead_zones/. Accessed August 20, 2025.

47. United Nations Environment Programme. (n.d.). "Facts About Nitrogen Pollution." https://www.unep.org/facts-about-nitrogen-pollution. Accessed August 20, 2025.

48. Schechinger A. (2020, August 26). "The High Cost of Algae Blooms." Environmental Working Group. https://www.ewg.org/research/high-cost-of-algae-blooms.

49. Davis W. (2018, September 22). "Hurricane's Aftermath Floods Hog Lagoons in North Carolina." NPR. https://www.npr.org/2018/09/22/650698240/hurricane-s-aftermath-floods -hog-lagoons-in-north-carolina.

50. Quist AJL, Fliss MD, Richardson DB, et al. (2024, December 27). "Hurricanes, Industrial Animal Operations, and Acute Gastrointestinal Illness in North Carolina, USA." *Environmental Research: Health* 3(1):015005. https://doi.org/10.1088/2752-5309/ad9ecf.

51. US Environmental Protection Agency. (n.d.). "Consumer Fact Sheet on Glyphosate." https://archive.epa.gov/water/archive/web/pdf/archived-consumer-fact-sheet-on -glyphosate.pdf. Accessed August 21, 2025.

52. Aib H, Parvez MS, Czédli HM. (2025). "Pharmaceuticals and Microplastics in Aquatic Environments: A Comprehensive Review of Pathways and Distribution, Toxicological and Ecological Effects." *International Journal of Environmental Research and Public Health* 22(5):799. https://doi.org/10.3390/ijerph22050799.

53. World Health Organization. (n.d.). "Microplastics in Drinking-Water." https://iris.who.int/bitstream/handle/10665/326499/9789241516198-eng.pdf.
54. Ward MH, Jones RR, Brender JD, et al. (2018). "Drinking Water Nitrate and Human Health: An Updated Review." *International Journal of Environmental Research and Public Health* 15(7):1557. https://doi.org/10.3390/ijerph15071557.
55. The Ocean Cleanup. (n.d.). "The Great Pacific Garbage Patch: How Much Plastic Floats There?" https://theoceancleanup.com/great-pacific-garbage-patch/#how-much-plastic-floats-in-the-great-pacific-garbage-patch. Accessed August 21, 2025.
56. IPBES. (2019, May 6). "Global Assessment Report on Biodiversity and Ecosystem Services." https://www.ipbes.net/news/ipbes-global-assessment-summary-policymakers-pdf.
57. Living Planet Index. (n.d.). "Living Plant Index." http://livingplanetindex.org. Accessed August 21, 2025.
58. af Magazine. (n.d.) "Beyond GDP: Recognizing the US$125 Trillion Value of Global Ecosystems." https://www.af-info.or.jp/en/af_magazine/029.html. Accessed August 21, 2025.
59. United Nations. (2019). "Nature's Dangerous Decline 'Unprecedented'; Species Extinction Rates 'Accelerating.'" https://www.un.org/sustainabledevelopment/blog/2019/05/nature-decline-unprecedented-report/.
60. Hoff M. (2018, November 1). "As Insect Populations Decline, Scientists Are Trying to Understand Why." *Scientific American.* https://www.scientificamerican.com/article/as-insect-populations-decline-scientists-are-trying-to-understand-why/.
61. Hallmann CA, Sorg M, Jongejans E, et al. (2017, October 18). "More than 75 Percent Decline over 27 Years in Total Flying Insect Biomass in Protected Areas." *PLOS One* 12(10):e0185809. https://doi.org/10.1371/journal.pone.0185809.
62. Ramanujan K. (2012, May 22). "Insect Pollinators Contribute $29 Billion to U.S. Farm Income." Cornell University. http://news.cornell.edu/stories/2012/05/insect-pollinators-contribute-29b-us-farm-income.
63. Gullap M, Erkovan HI, Koç A. (2011). "The Effect of Bovine Saliva on Growth Attributes and Forage Quality of Two Contrasting Cool Season Perennial Grasses Grown in Three Soils of Different Fertility." *Rangeland Journal* 33(3):307–13. http://www.publish.csiro.au/?paper=RJ10063.
64. Rodale Institute. (2020, September 30). "Regenerative Ag Could Sequester 100 Percent of Annual Carbon Emissions." https://rodaleinstitute.org/blog/regenerative-ag-could-sequester-100-percent-of-annual-carbon-emissions/.
65. Ranganathan J, Waite R, Searchinger T, et al. (2020, May 12). "Regenerative Agriculture: Good for Soil Health, but Limited Potential to Mitigate Climate Change." World Resources Institute. https://www.wri.org/insights/regenerative-agriculture-good-soil-health-limited-potential-mitigate-climate-change.
66. Thorpe D. (2018, December 12). "How Investing in Regenerative Agriculture Can Help Stem Climate Change Profitably." *Forbes.* https://www.forbes.com/sites/devinthorpe/2018/12/12/how-investing-in-regenerative-agriculture-can-help-stem-climate-change-profitably/#538149f03e5c.
67. Seachrist KF. (2018, September 18). "Soil Health Pro Team." FarmProgress. https://www.farmprogress.com/soil-health/soil-health-pro-team.
68. EcoWatch. (2016, February 9). "Tyson Foods Dumps More Pollution into Waterways Each Year than Exxon." https://www.ecowatch.com/tyson-foods-dumps-more-pollution-into-waterways-each-year-than-exxon-1882169913.html.
69. General Mills. (2024, February 20). "General Mills Shares Progress Against Accelerate Strategy." Press release. https://investors.generalmills.com/press-releases/press-release-details/2024/General-Mills-Shares-Progress-Against-Accelerate-Strategy/default.aspx.

70. University of Pennsylvania. (2019, May 16). "With Unprecedented Threats to Nature at Hand, How to Turn the Tide." https://penntoday.upenn.edu/news/unprecedented-threats -nature-hand-how-turn-tide.

71. Bittman M, Pollan M, Salvador R, et al. (2015, October 6). "A National Food Policy for the 21st Century." *Medium.* https://medium.com/food-is-the-new-internet/a-national-food -policy-for-the-21st-century-7d323ee7c65f.

72. Faust DR, Kumar S, Archer DW, et al. (2017, October 23). "Potential Water Quality Outcomes from Integrated Crop-Livestock Systems in the Northern Great Plains." Managing Global Resources for a Secure Future Annual Meeting. https://scisoc.confex.com/crops /2017am/webprogram/Paper105136.html.

73. St. Clair T. (2002, July 17). "Farming Without Subsidies—A Better Way. Why New Zealand Agriculture Is a World Leader." *Politico.* https://www.politico.eu/article/viewpoint-farming -without-subsidies-a-better-way-why-new-zealand-agriculture-is-a-world-leader/.

74. Capehart T, Proper S. (2019, July 29). "Corn Is America's Largest Crop in 2019." US Department of Agriculture, Economic Research Service. https://www.usda.gov/about-usda /news/blog/corn-americas-largest-crop-2019.

75. Cornell University. (2001, August 6). "Ethanol Fuel from Corn Faulted as 'Unsustainable Subsidized Food Burning' in Analysis by Cornell Scientist." https://news.cornell.edu/stories /2001/08/ethanol-corn-faulted-energy-waster-scientist-says.

76. Union of Concerned Scientists. (2019, May 1). "Infographic: Plant the Plate." https://www .ucsusa.org/food_and_agriculture/solutions/expand-healthy-food-access/plant-the-plate .html#.VhMWTxNViko.

77. Mulik K, O'Hara JK. (2013, October). "The Healthy Farmland Diet: How Growing Less Corn Would Improve Our Health and Help America's Heartland." Union of Concerned Scientists. https://www.ucs.org/sites/default/files/2019-09/healthy-farmland-diet.pdf.

78. Aubrey A. (2015, October 6). "New Dietary Guidelines Will Not Include Sustainability Goal." NPR. https://www.npr.org/sections/thesalt/2015/10/06/446369955/new-dietary -guidelines-will-not-include-sustainability-goal.

79. Mitchell S. (2018, February 16). "6 Ways to Rein In Today's Toxic Monopolies." *The Nation.* https://www.thenation.com/article/archive/six-ways-to-rein-in-todays-toxic-monopolies/.

80. Holder EH Jr. (2010, April 20). "Attorney General Eric Holder Speaks at the Sherman Act Award Ceremony." US Department of Justice, Office of Public Affairs. https://www.justice .gov/archives/opa/speech/attorney-general-eric-holder-speaks-sherman-act-award-ceremony.

81. Regenerative Organic Alliance. (n.d.). "The Three Pillars of Regenerative Organic Certified." https://regenorganic.org/our-story/. Accessed August 21, 2025.

82. Mariposa Ranch Meats. (2019). "Quarter Beef." https://mariposaranchmeats.com/product /14-beef/.

83. County Health Rankings and Roadmaps. (n.d.). "Community Gardens." https://www .countyhealthrankings.org/strategies-and-solutions/what-works-for-health/strategies /community-gardens. Accessed August 21, 2025.

84. Carbon Underground. (n.d.). "White Papers." https://thecarbonunderground.org/the-science /resources/white-papers/. Accessed August 21, 2025.

85. Coller Foundation. (n.d.). "Creating a Better Future by Ending Intensive Animal Agriculture." https://jeremycollerfoundation.org/animal-agriculture/. Accessed August 21, 2025.

86. Intentional Endowments Network. (n.d.). "Farm Animal Investment Risk and Return (FAIRR)." http://www.intentionalendowments.org/farm_animal_investment_risk_and _return. Accessed August 21, 2025.

87. Harper A, Alkon A, Shattuck A, et al. (2009, December 1). "Food Policy Councils: Lessons Learned." Food First. https://foodfirst.org/publication/food-policy-councils-lessons-learned/.

88. Clark L. (2016, August 29). "Why Farm-to-Institution Sourcing Is the Sleeping Giant of Local Food." Civil Eats. https://civileats.com/2016/08/29/forget-farm-to-table-its-farm-to-institution-sourcing-that-could-make-a-real-dent-the-food-system/.
89. HEAL. (n.d.). https://healfoodalliance.org. Accessed August 21, 2025.

CHAPTER 18

1. Intergovernmental Panel on Climate Change. (2014). "Summary for Policymakers." In O. Edenhofer et al. (Eds.), *Climate Change 2014: Mitigation of Climate Change. Contribution of Working Group III to the Fifth Assessment Report of the Intergovernmental Panel on Climate Change.* Cambridge University Press. https://www.ipcc.ch/site/assets/uploads/2018/02/ipcc_wg3_ar5_summary-for-policymakers.pdf.
2. Ritchie H. (2021, March 18). "How Much of Our Global Greenhouse Gas Emissions Come from Food?" Our World in Data. https://ourworldindata.org/greenhouse-gas-emissions-food.
3. Columbia Climate School. (2018, February 21). "Can Soil Help Combat Climate Change? State of the Planet." https://news.climate.columbia.edu/2018/02/21/can-soil-help-combat-climate-change/.
4. Regenetarianism. (2018, May 4). "Ruminations: Methane Math and Context." https://lachefnet.wordpress.com/2018/05/04/ruminations-methane-math-and-context/.
5. US Environmental Protection Agency. (2025, January 16). "Understanding Global Warming Potentials." https://www.epa.gov/ghgemissions/understanding-global-warming-potentials.
6. Fee E, Brown TM. (2002). "John Harvey Kellogg, MD: Health Reformer and Antismoking Crusader." *American Journal of Public Health* 92(6):935. https://doi.org/10.2105/AJPH.92.6.935.
7. Markel H. (2017, August 18). "Dr. Kellogg's World-Renowned Health Spa Made Him a Wellness Titan." *PBS NewsHour.* https://www.pbs.org/newshour/health/dr-kelloggs-world-renowned-health-spa-made-wellness-titan.
8. Smetana S, Ristić D, Pleissner D, et al. (2023). "Meat Substitutes: Resource Demands and Environmental Footprints." *Resources, Conservation and Recycling* 190:106831. https://doi.org/10.1016/j.resconrec.2022.106831.
9. Health Research Institute Laboratories. (2019, May 6). "Certificate of Analysis: Impossible Burger and Beyond Meat." https://d3n8a8pro7vhmx.cloudfront.net/yesmaam/pages/8069/attachments/original/1557958339/COA_S0004900_Impossible_Burger_and_Beyond_Meat_patty_-_glyphosate.pdf?1557958339.
10. Lozano VL, Defarge N, Rocque L-M, et al. (2018). "Sex-Dependent Impact of Roundup on the Rat Gut Microbiome." *Toxicology Reports* 5:96–107. https://doi.org/10.1016/j.toxrep.2017.12.005.
11. Mottett A, Steinfeld H. (2018, September 18). "Cars or Livestock: Which Contribute More to Climate Change?" Thomson Reuters. http://news.trust.org/item/20180918083629-d2wf0/.
12. Gerber PJ, Steinfeld H, Henderson B, et al. (2013). *Tackling Climate Change Through Livestock: A Global Assessment of Emissions and Mitigation Opportunities.* Food and Agriculture Organization. https://www.fao.org/4/i3437e/i3437e.pdf.
13. Grain and IATP. (2018, July 18). "Emissions Impossible: How Big Meat and Dairy Are Heating Up the Planet." https://www.grain.org/article/entries/5976-emissions-impossible-how-big-meat-and-dairy-are-heating-up-the-planet.
14. International Animal Protection World Association. (2022, August 5). "The Environmental Cost of Animal Agriculture." https://iapwa.org/the-environmental-cost-of-animal-agriculture/.
15. Oxford University Environmental Change Institute. (n.d.). "Dr. Tara Garnett." https://www.eci.ox.ac.uk/person/dr-tara-garnett. Accessed August 21, 2025.

16. Garnett T, Godde C, Muller A, et al. (2017, October 1). "Grazed and Confused: Ruminating on Cattle, Grazing, Methane, Nitrous Oxide, and Consumption-Based Emissions from Beef, Lamb, and Dairy." Food, Farming, and Countryside Commission. https://www.tabledebates.org/publication/grazed-and-confused.

17. Food and Water Watch. (2024, July). "Factory Farms, Fracking, and the Methane Emergency." https://www.foodandwaterwatch.org/wp-content/uploads/2024/07/Methane_Fracking_FactoryFarms.pdf.

18. Sustainable Food Trust. (2017, October 12). "Grazed and Confused—An initial response from the Sustainable Food Trust." Resilience. https://www.resilience.org/stories/2017-10-12/grazed-and-confused-an-initial-response-from-the-sustainable-food-trust/.

19. Ibid.

20. Stanley PL, Rowntree JE, Beede DK, et al. (2018, May 1). "Impacts of Soil Carbon Sequestration on Life Cycle Greenhouse Gas Emissions in Midwestern USA Beef Finishing Systems." *Agricultural Systems* 162:249–58. https://doi.org/10.1016/j.agsy.2018.02.003.

21. Itzkan S. (2011, June). "Regarding Holechek and Briske, and Rebuttals by Teague, Gill & Savory Correcting Misconceptions About the Supposed Discrediting of Savory's Approach." Planet-TECH Associates. https://planet-tech.com/sites/default/files/Itzkan%202011,%20RegardingHolechekSavory%20v4_0.pdf.

22. Thorbecke M, Dettling J. (2019, February 25). "Carbon Footprint Evaluation of Regenerative Grazing at White Oak Pastures." Quantis. https://blog.whiteoakpastures.com/hubfs/WOP-LCA-Quantis-2019.pdf.

23. PR Newswire. (2019, May 1). "Study: White Oak Pastures Beef Reduces Atmospheric Carbon." https://www.prnewswire.com/news-releases/study-white-oak-pastures-beef-reduces-atmospheric-carbon-300841416.html.

24. Niman NH. (2014). *Defending Beef: The Case for Sustainable Meat Production.* Chelsea Green Publishing.

25. Silvestri S, Osana P, Leeuw J de, et al. (2012). *Greening Livestock: Assessing the Potential of Payment for Environmental Services in Livestock Inclusive Agricultural Production Systems in Developing Countries.* International Livestock Research Institute. https://www.ilri.org/knowledge/publications/greening-livestock-assessing-potential-payment-environmental-services.

26. Pledger L. (2023, December 4). "Regenerative Grazing: A Compelling Climate Strategy." Biodiversity for a Livable Climate. https://bio4climate.org/2023/12/04/regenerative-grazing-a-compelling-climate-strategy/.

27. Stanley PL, Rowntree JE, Beede DK, et al. (2018, May 1). "Impacts of Soil Carbon Sequestration on Life Cycle Greenhouse Gas Emissions in Midwestern USA Beef Finishing Systems." *Agricultural Systems* 162:249–58. https://doi.org/10.1016/j.agsy.2018.02.003.

28. Capper JL. (2012, April 10). "Is the Grass Always Greener? Comparing the Environmental Impact of Conventional, Natural and Grass-Fed Beef Production Systems." *Animals* 2(2):127–43. https://doi.org/10.3390/ani2020127.

29. Thorbecke M, Dettling J. (2019, February 25). "Carbon Footprint Evaluation of Regenerative Grazing at White Oak Pastures." Quantis. https://blog.whiteoakpastures.com/hubfs/WOP-LCA-Quantis-2019.pdf.

30. Williams A. (2021, June 1). "Can Grass-Fed Beef Scale?" Blue Nest Beef. https://bluenestbeef.com/blogs/news/can-grass-fed-beef-scale-1.

31. Willett W, Rockström J, Loken B, et al. (2019, February 2). "Food in the Anthropocene: The EAT–Lancet Commission on Healthy Diets from Sustainable Food Systems." *The Lancet* 393(10170): 447–92. https://doi.org/10.1016/S0140-6736(18)31788-4.

32. Harcombe Z. (2019, January 17.) "The EAT Lancet Diet Is Nutritionally Deficient." http://www.zoeharcombe.com/2019/01/the-eat-lancet-diet-is-nutritionally-deficient/.

33. Schimmack U. (2022, January 20). "Estimating the reproducibility of psychological science in 2021." Replicability-Index. https://replicationindex.com/2022/01/20/estimating-the -reproducibility-of-psychological-science-in-2021/.

34. Sahlin KJ, Trewern J. (2022, June 23). "A Systematic Review of the Definitions and Inter-pretations in Scientific Literature of 'Less but Better' Meat in High-Income Settings." *Nature Food* 3:454–60. https://doi.org/10.1038/s43016-022-00536-5.

35. Teicholz N. (2022, March 19). "Majority of EAT-Lancet Authors (78%) Favored Vegan/ Vegetarian Diets." https://ninateicholz.com/majority-of-eat-authors-vegan-vegetarian.

36. Teicholz N. (2019, January 29). "EAT-Lancet Report Is One-Sided, Not Backed by Rigor-ous Science." Nutrition Coalition. https://www.nutritioncoalition.us/news/eatlancet-report -one-sided.

37. Ibid.

38. World Business Council for Sustainable Development. (n.d.). "Discover Our Members." https://www.wbcsd.org/Overview/Our-members. Accessed August 21, 2025.

39. Heinrich Böll Foundation, Rosa Luxemburg Foundation, Friends of the Earth Europe. (2017, October.) "Agrifood Atlas: Facts and Figures About the Corporations That Control What We Eat." https://eu.boell.org/sites/default/files/agrifoodatlas2017_facts-and-figures -about-the-corporations-that-control-what-we-eat.pdf.

40. Shiva V. (2019, January 20). "A New Report Sustains Unsustainable Food Systems." Seed Freedom. https://seedfreedom.info/poison-cartel-toxic-food-eat-report/.

41. Ibid.

42. Sinha R, Cross AJ, Graubard BI, et al. (2009, March 23). "Meat Intake and Mortality: A Prospective Study of Over Half a Million People." *Archives of Internal Medicine* 169(6):562–71. https://doi.org/10.1001/archinternmed.2009.6.

43. Dehghan M, Mente A, Zhang X, et al. (2017, November 4). "Associations of Fats and Car-bohydrate Intake with Cardiovascular Disease and Mortality in 18 Countries from Five Continents (PURE): A Prospective Cohort Study." *Lancet* 390(10107):2050–62. https:// doi.org/10.1016/s0140-6736(17)32252-3.

44. Grasgruber P, Sebera M, Hrazdira E, et al. (2016, January 1.) "Food Consumption and the Actual Statistics of Cardiovascular Diseases: An Epidemiological Comparison of 42 European Countries." *Food and Nutrition Research* 60(1):31694. https://doi.org/10.3402/fnr.v60.31694.

45. Key TJ, Thorogood M, Appleby PN, Burr ML. (1996, September 28). "Dietary Habits and Mortality in 11 000 Vegetarians and Health Conscious People: Results of a 17 Year Follow Up." *BMJ* 313(7060):775–79. https://doi.org/10.1136/bmj.313.7060.775.

46. Daley CA, Abbott A, Doyle PS, et al. (2010, December.) "A Review of Fatty Acid Profiles and Antioxidant Content in Grass-Fed and Grain-Fed Beef." *Nutrition Journal* 9(1):10. https://doi.org/10.1186/1475-2891-9-10.

47. Kresser C. (2019.) "Why Eating Meat Is Good for You." https://chriskresser.com/why -eating-meat-is-good-for-you/.

48. Hawken P., ed. (2017). *Drawdown: The Most Comprehensive Plan Ever Proposed to Reverse Global Warming.* Penguin.

49. Conrad Z, Niles M, Neher D, et al. (2018, April 18). "Relationship Between Food Waste, Diet Quality, and Environmental Sustainability." *PLOS One*13(4):e0195405. https://doi.org /10.1371/journal.pone.0195405.

50. Gustavsson J, Cederberg C, Sonesson U, et al. (2011). "Global Food Losses and Food Waste: Extent, Causes, and Prevention." MB060E. Food and Agriculture Organization. https:// www.fao.org/4/mb060e/mb060e.pdf.

51. Food Loss and Waste Protocol. (2019). "Food Loss and Waste Accounting and Reporting Standard." https://www.theconsumergoodsforum.com/wp-content/uploads/2017/10/The -Consumer-Goods-Forum-Food-Waste-FLW-Standard.pdf.

52. FiBL. (2014, October 1). "Food Wastage Costs the World 2.6 Trillion Dollars Each Year." https://www.fibl.org/fileadmin/documents/en/news/2014/mr-fao-food-waste141001.pdf.

53. Consumer Goods Forum. (2017, October). *Food Waste (FLW) Standard.* https://www .theconsumergoodsforum.com/wp-content/uploads/2017/10/The-Consumer-Goods -Forum-Food-Waste-FLW-Standard.pdf.

54. United Nations. (n.d.). "Goal 12: Responsible Consumption and Production—Targets and Indicators." https://sdgs.un.org/goals/goal12#targets_and_indicators.

55. Suszkiw J. (2009, May 20). "Watermelons Tapped for Ethanol." US Department of Agriculture, Agricultural Research Service. https://www.ars.usda.gov/news-events/news/research -news/2009/watermelons-tapped-for-ethanol/.

56. Gunders D. (2017). "Wasted: How America Is Losing up to 40 Percent of Its Food from Farm to Fork to Landfill." 2nd ed. Natural Resources Defense Council. https://www.nrdc .org/sites/default/files/wasted-2017-report.pdf.

57. ReFED. (2016). "A Roadmap to Reduce U.S. Food Waste by 20 Percent." https://www .refed.com/downloads/ReFED_Report_2016.pdf.

58. United Nations. (n.d.). "Food." https://www.un.org/en/global-issues/food. Accessed August 21, 2025.

59. Goodwin L, Lipinski B. (2024, November 25). "How Much Food Does the World Waste? What We Know—And What We Don't." World Resources Institute. https://www.wri.org /insights/how-much-food-does-the-world-waste.

60. Toti E, Di Mattia C, Serafini M. (2019). "Metabolic Food Waste and Ecological Impact of Obesity in FAO World's Region." *Frontiers in Nutrition* 2019;6. https://doi.org/10.3389 /fnut.2019.00126.

Index

About the Author

MARK HYMAN, MD, has devoted his life to helping others discover optimal health and address the root causes of chronic disease through the power of functional medicine. Dr. Hyman is an internationally recognized leader, speaker, educator, and advocate in the fields of functional medicine and nutrition. He is a practicing family physician, the cofounder and chief medical officer of Function Health, founder and director of the UltraWellness Center, founder of the Cleveland Clinic Center for Functional Medicine, and former chairman and now board president for clinical affairs for the Institute for Functional Medicine. He is a fifteen-time *New York Times* bestselling author of *The Pegan Diet, Food Fix,* and, most recently, *Young Forever,* an instant #1 *New York Times* bestseller. Through his writing and in his sought-after talks, Dr. Hyman offers a revolutionary, practical guide to creating and sustaining health—for life.

Dr. Hyman is the founder and chairman of the Food Fix Campaign—dedicated to transforming our food and agriculture system through policy. He is the host of one of the leading health podcasts, *The Dr. Hyman Show,* which has more than 300 million downloads. Dr. Hyman is a regular medical contributor to *CBS This Morning, Today,* Fox, *Good Morning America, The View,* and CNN.

Through his work to change policy for the betterment of public health, Dr. Hyman has testified before the Health Subcommittee of Ways and Means, Senate Working Group on Health Care Reform on Functional Medicine. He has consulted with the surgeon general on diabetes prevention and participated in the White House Conference on Hunger, Nutrition, and Health and the White House Forum on Prevention and Wellness. Senator Tom Harkin of Iowa nominated Dr. Hyman for the President's Advisory Group on Prevention, Health Promotion, and Integrative and Public Health. With topics ranging from food as medicine to disruption in the health care system to how technological advancements like AI will impact our approach to health, Dr. Hyman is an informed, engaging advocate who motivates his audiences toward lasting change.

Dr. Hyman has presented at the Clinton Foundation's Health Matters, Achieving Wellness in Every Generation conference and the Clinton Global Initiative, as well as with the World Economic Forum on global health issues, TEDMED, and TEDx. He is the winner of the Linus Pauling Award and the Nantucket Project Award. Dr. Hyman received the Christian Book of the Year Award for his work on *The Daniel Plan,* a faith-based initiative that helped the Saddleback Church collectively lose 250,000 pounds, which he created with Rick Warren, Dr. Mehmet Oz, and Dr. Daniel Amen. He was inducted into the Books for Better Life Hall of Fame.

With Dr. Dean Ornish and Dr. Michael Roizen, Dr. Hyman crafted and helped introduce the Take Back Your Health Act of 2009 to the US Senate, which promotes reimbursement for lifestyle treatment of chronic disease. With Tim Ryan in 2015, he helped introduce the ENRICH Act into Congress to fund nutrition in medical education. Dr. Hyman plays a substantial role in the major 2014 film *Fed Up,* produced by Laurie David and Katie Couric, which addresses childhood obesity, and in the films on regenerative agriculture, *Kiss the Ground* and *Common Ground.* Please join him in celebrating the power of food as medicine at www.drhyman.com, follow him on Twitter, Facebook, and Instagram, and listen to his podcast *The Dr. Hyman Show* for conversations that matter around health, wellness, food, and politics.

Curious about any of our data? Check out the QR code below for links to citations, academic research, clinical studies, and context on the myriad anecdotes cited in this book.